CELLULAR NEUROBIOLOGY

PROGRESS IN CLINICAL AND BIOLOGICAL RESEARCH

Series Editors

Robert Grover

George J. Brewer   Kurt Hirschhorn   Sidney Udenfriend

Vincent P. Eijsvoogel   Seymour S. Kety   Jonathan W. Uhr

CELLULAR NEUROBIOLOGY

Proceedings of the ICN–UCLA Symposium on Neurobiology
held at Squaw Valley, California
February 1976

Editors:

ZACH HALL
University of California, San Francisco

REGIS KELLY
University of California, San Francisco

C. FRED FOX
University of California, Los Angeles

Alan R. Liss, Inc. • New York • 1977

© 1977 by Alan R. Liss, Inc.

Address all inquiries to the publisher:
   Alan R. Liss, Inc.
   150 Fifth Avenue
   New York, New York 10011

Printed in the United States of America

Library of Congress Cataloging in Publication Data

ICN-UCLA Symposium on Neurobiology, Squaw Valley,
   Calif., 1976.
   Cellular neurobiology.

   (Progress in clinical and biological research;
15)
   Includes bibliographical references and index.
   1. Neurobiology—Congresses. 2. Neurophysiology—Congresses. I. Hall, Zach W.
II. Kelly, Regis. III. Fox, C. Fred, IV. Title
V. Series. [DNLM: 1. Neurophysiology—Congresses. 2. Neurochemistry—Congresses. W1 PR668
v. 15 / WL102 1104n 1976]
QP356.I16 1976   599'.01'88   77-3386
ISBN 0-8451-0015-7

NOTE

Pages 1–60 are reprinted from the Journal of Supramolecular Structure, Volume 5, 1976. The page numbers in the Table of Contents, Author Index, and Subject Index of this volume correspond to the page numbers in parentheses on these pages.

Contents

Preface

In late February 1976, a symposium was held at Squaw Valley, California on the subject of Cellular Neurobiology, a topic which was new to the ICN–UCLA series of symposia. To sustain the spirit of novelty, we chose to avoid reviewing the well-established success stories of neurobiology, and looked instead to some of the newer problems. We tried to assemble a group of people that cut across disciplinary lines and included electro-physiologists, morphologists, biochemists and immunobiologists. The common bond was an interest in how membranes mediate signalling and cellular interactions in the nervous system.

We were rewarded by one of the lowest attendances in the Symposia history, but also having assembled for a week a group of more than a hundred people who shared a similar viewpoint of cellular neurobiology and its future directions. Some of the excitement that most of us felt at that meeting will hopefully be captured by this symposium volume.

We are indebted to ICN Pharmaceuticals for the financial support of this meeting and to the ICN–UCLA staff for their organizational efforts. We are especially grateful to Fran Stusser for her help before, during, and after the meeting.

Regis Kelly
Zach Hall

Journal of Supramolecular Structure 5:397 (1)–407 (11) (1976)

Interactions of Neurotoxins With the Action Potential Na$^+$ Ionophore

William A. Catterall and Radharaman Ray

Laboratory of Biochemical Genetics, National Heart and Lung Institute, National Institutes of Health, Bethesda, Maryland 20014

Four neurotoxins that activate the action potential Na$^+$ ionophore of electrically excitable neuroblastoma cells interact with two distinct classes of sites, one specific for the alkaloids veratridine, batrachotoxin, and aconitine, and the second specific for scorpion toxin. Positive heterotropic cooperativity is observed between toxins bound at these two classes of sites. Tetrodotoxin, a specific inhibitor of the action potential Na$^+$ current, inhibits activation by each of these toxins in a noncompetitive manner (K_I = 4–8 nM). These results suggest the existence of three functionally separable components of the action potential Na$^+$ ionophore: two regulatory components, which bind activating neurotoxins and interact allosterically in controlling the activity of a third ion-transport component, which binds tetrodotoxin. The dissociation constant for scorpion toxin binding is increased 10-fold by depolarization of the cells with K$^+$, suggesting that the scorpion toxin binding site is located on a voltage-sensitive regulatory component of the ionophore.

INTRODUCTION

Several neurotoxins cause repetitive action potentials and persistent depolarization of nerves. This group of toxins includes the alkaloids veratridine (1, 2), batrachotoxin (3), and aconitine (4, 5), grayanotoxin (6), and the polypeptide toxins of scorpion venom (7–11) and coelenterate nematocysts (12). Since the action of these toxins is blocked by tetrodotoxin, a specific inhibitor of the action potential Na$^+$ current (13, 14), their effects have been ascribed to activation of the action potential Na$^+$ ionophore. These toxins, therefore, are potentially important tools in studying the mechanism of action potential generation.

Clonal lines of mouse neuroblastoma cells grown in vitro are electrically excitable (15, 16). The Na$^+$-dependent portion of the action potential is inhibited by tetrodotoxin at low concentration, suggesting that an action potential Na$^+$ ionophore identical with that in nerve axons is present in these cells (17, 18). Variant cell clones have been obtained which specifically lack the depolarizing phase of the action potential (18, 19). In this report we describe the interaction of veratridine, batrachotoxin, aconitine, and scorpion toxin with the action potential Na$^+$ ionophore of cultured neuroblastoma cells using isotopic flux measurements to detect the permeability changes caused by the toxins and ligand binding methods to study the formation of the toxin-ionophore complex.

METHODS

Detailed descriptions of the methods used in these experiments have been published elsewhere. Neuroblastoma cells were grown in vitro and changes in Na^+ permeability were measured by $^{22}Na^+$ uptake experiments as described previously (20–23). In brief, neuroblastoma cells grown to saturation in multiwell plates are incubated with neurotoxins in Na^+-free solution at 36°C to allow activation of the Na^+ ionophore without increasing the intracellular Na^+ concentration. Initial rate of $^{22}Na^+$ uptake is then measured in a medium containing 10 mM Na^+ with choline as an Na^+ replacement to maintain osmolarity (except where indicated) and with 5 mM ouabain added to inhibit active transport of Na^+. The Na^+ concentration is selected so that the dependence of uptake on Na^+ concentration is linear when the ionophore is maximally activated to ensure that the rate of $^{22}Na^+$ influx is not limited by fluxes of counterions (Cl^- moving in and K^+ moving out) required to maintain charge balance.

Scorpion toxin was purified from the venom of Leiurus quinquestriatus by ion exchange chromatography as described previously (23). The purified toxin was iodinated by standard procedures and the labeled toxin separated from unlabeled toxin by ion exchange chromatography. This procedure will be described in detail in a subsequent manuscript.

RESULTS AND DISCUSSION

Treatment of electrically excitable neuroblastoma cells such as clone N18 with veratridine, batrachotoxin, aconitine, scorpion toxin, or combinations of these agents causes an increase in Na^+ permeability that is reflected in an increased initial rate of uptake of $^{22}Na^+$ (Fig. 1, left). Similar treatment of electrically inexcitable cells such as clone N103 (Fig. 1, right) leads to no detectable increase in $^{22}Na^+$ uptake. In studies of over 20 clonal lines derived from mouse neuroblastoma C1300, clonal lines and primary cultures

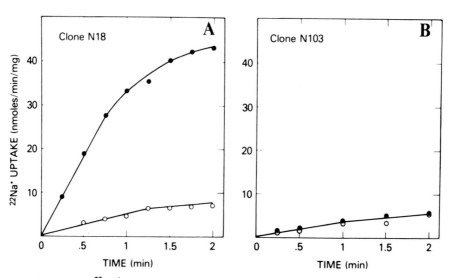

Fig. 1. Stimulation of $^{22}Na^+$ uptake by veratridine and scorpion toxin. Neuroblastoma cells of clone N18 (A) or N103 (B) were incubated for 30 min at 36°C in Na^+-free medium (○) or in Na^+-free medium containing 20 μM veratridine and 128 ng/ml scorpion toxin (●). Initial rate of $^{22}Na^+$ uptake was then determined.

of skeletal muscle cells, primary cultures of cardiac muscle cells, and clonal lines derived from various non-neuronal tissues including glial, fibroblast, liver, and kidney, a complete correlation has been found between electrical excitability and increase of Na$^+$ permeability by neurotoxins (reference 20 and unpublished results).

The increase in ^{22}Na$^+$ uptake caused by treatment with these neurotoxins is completely inhibited by tetrodotoxin (20, 21), a specific inhibitor of action potential Na$^+$ current (13, 14). Half-maximal inhibition is obtained at 4–8 nM tetrodotoxin for all neuroblastoma lines tested and for primary cultures of chick skeletal and cardiac muscle (20, 21, and unpublished experiments). However, rat muscle cells, in which Na$^+$-dependent action potentials are relatively resistant to inhibition by tetrodotoxin (24), require approximately 1 μM tetrodotoxin for half-maximal inhibition (25).

Both these series of experiments provide strong evidence in favor of the conclusion that these neurotoxins act specifically on the Na$^+$ permeability pathway involved in the action potential by activating the action potential Na$^+$ ionophore in the absence of an electrical stimulus.

The action of these toxins does not require the presence of either ion gradients or a membrane potential. Figure 2 illustrates the increase in ^{22}Na$^+$ uptake caused by treatment with veratridine plus scorpion venom in a medium with extracellular cation concentrations ([K$^+$] = 135.5 mM, [Na$^+$] = 15 mM, [Ca^{++}] = 0) which mimic intracellular concentrations. The membrane potential (measured with microelectrodes) is zero under these conditions. These results support the conclusion that these neurotoxins activate the action potential Na$^+$ ionophore by a direct chemical mechanism.

Na$^+$ permeability of cells treated with one of the three alkaloid toxins (aconitine, veratridine, or batrachotoxin) increases with time to an equilibrium level that is concentration dependent (reference 21 and unpublished experiments). Figure 3 illustrates equilibrium concentration-response curves for aconitine, batrachotoxin, and veratridine.

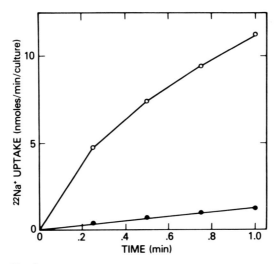

Fig. 2. Stimulation of ^{22}Na$^+$ uptake by veratridine and scorpion toxin in the absence of ion gradients. Neuroblastoma cells of clone N18 were incubated for 30 min at 36°C in medium with 130 mM KCl, 15 mM NaCl, and no CaCl$_2$ in the presence (O) or absence (●) of 20 μM veratridine and 128 ng/ml scorpion toxin. Initial rate of ^{22}Na$^+$ uptake was then determined in medium with the same ion concentrations.

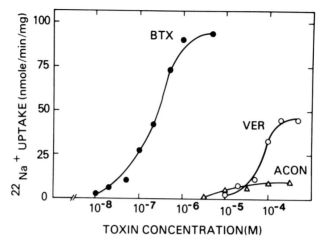

Fig. 3. Concentration dependence of activation by veratridine, batrachotoxin, and aconitine. Neuro-blastoma cells of clone N18 were incubated for 30 min at 36°C in Na^+-free medium containing the indicated concentrations of aconitine (△), veratridine (○), or batrachotoxin (●). Initial rate of $^{22}Na^+$ uptake was then determined in medium containing 50 mM NaCl and Tris-Cl as as osmotic replacement.

Both the maximum rates of uptake of $^{22}Na^+$ (V_∞) and the concentrations required for half-maximal activation ($K_{0.5}$) differ markedly: batrachotoxin, V_∞ = 100 nmol/min/mg, $K_{0.5}$ = 0.3 μM; veratridine, V_∞ = 42 nmol/min/mg, $K_{0.5}$ = 80 μM; aconitine, V_∞ = 10 nmol/min/mg, $K_{0.5}$ = 8 μM. If these three toxins activate the action potential Na^+ ionophore by interaction with an identical class of binding sites, the rate of $^{22}Na^+$ uptake in the presence of saturating concentrations of any two toxins should not be greater than in the presence of batrachotoxin alone. Furthermore, as an excess of a less effective activator (such as aconitine) is added, batrachotoxin should be displaced from the common binding site and the rate of $^{22}Na^+$ uptake should be reduced. Such competitive interactions are ob-served among the three alkaloid neurotoxins (references 21 and 22, and unpublished results).

The measured uptake velocity (v) in the presence of two neurotoxins that interact competitively can be described quantitatively as the sum of the activity due to toxin 1 modified by competition with toxin 2 (v_1), and the activity due to toxin 2 modified by competition with toxin 1 (v_2).

$v = v_1 + v_2 = V_1 s_1/(K_1(1 + s_2/K_2) + s_1) + V_2 s_2/(K_2(1 + s_1/K_1) + s_2)$ where s is the concentration of toxin. If toxin 2 is aconitine, then v_2 is always small ($\leqslant$ 10 nmol/min/mg) and can be calculated from independent measurements of V_2, K_2, and K_1. It is possible, then, to test whether aconitine is a strictly competitive inhibitor of activation by batracho-toxin and veratridine by plotting $1/(v-v_2)$ against $1/s_1$ at different fixed aconitine con-centrations (s_2) in the form of a Michaelis-Menten double reciprocal plot. The results of such experiments (Fig. 4) confirm that aconitine is a competitive inhibitor of activation by veratridine and batrachotoxin.

These results show that aconitine, veratridine, and batrachotoxin bind to a saturable class of binding sites during activation of the action potential Na^+ ionophore. The three toxins are lipophilic and veratridine has been shown to interact with lipid monolayers to cause expansion (26). These observations form the basis of the hypothesis that veratridine acts by perturbing the lipid structure of the membrane (26). Since interaction of the

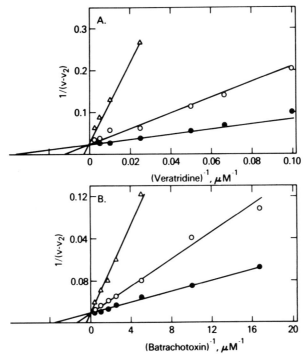

Fig. 4. Competitive inhibition of veratridine-dependent and batrachotoxin-dependent ^{22}Na$^+$ uptake by aconitine. Neuroblastoma cells were incubated for 30 min at 36°C in Na$^+$-free medium in the presence of the indicated concentrations of veratridine (A) or batrachotoxin (B) plus 0 μM (●), 20 μM (○), or 50 μM (△) aconitine, and the rates of ^{22}Na$^+$ uptake were measured in the presence of the same concentrations of toxin. The results are plotted according to the equation given in the text with K_2 = 8 μM, V_2 = 10 nmol/min/mg, and K_1 = 40 μM for veratridine and 0.25 μM for batrachotoxin as determined in companion experiments.

lipophilic toxins with the lipid phase of the membrane should be nonsaturable, the demonstration of competitive interactions among these toxins makes this mechanism unlikely. It is more likely that these three toxins bind to a specific site on the action potential Na$^+$ ionophore that is involved in the regulation of the ion transport activity of the ionophore.

In contrast to the competitive interactions observed among the three alkaloid toxins, scorpion venom interacts cooperatively with each of the alkaloid toxins. Experiments in which cells were treated with varying concentrations of the alkaloid toxins in the presence or absence of scorpion venom and then tested for Na$^+$ permeability are presented in Fig. 5. Scorpion venom causes a reduction in apparent K_D for each of the alkaloid toxins. It also causes an increase in the maximum velocity of ^{22}Na$^+$ uptake at saturating concentrations.

We have purified a toxic polypeptide from scorpion venom using its ability to cause cooperative activation of the action potential Na$^+$ ionophore in the presence of veratridine as an assay (23). The purified protein appears homogeneous in gel electrophoretic and isoelectric focusing studies, has a molecular weight of 6,700 and an isoelectric point of approximately 9.7, and lacks methionine and histidine (23). Treatment of cells with 1–10 nM scorpion toxin and varying concentrations of batrachotoxin or aconitine gives

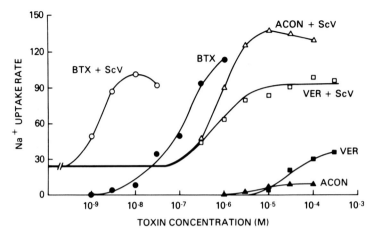

Fig. 5. Effect of scorpion venom on the concentration dependence of activation by veratridine, batrachotoxin, and aconitine. Neuroblastoma cells were incubated for 30 min at 36°C in Na^+-free medium in the presence of the indicated concentrations of veratridine, batrachotoxin, and aconitine plus 10 μg/ml scorpion venom where indicated. Initial rate of $^{22}Na^+$ uptake was measured in the presence of the same toxin concentrations in medium containing 50 mM NaCl and Tris-Cl as an osmotic replacement.

the concentration-response curves illustrated in Fig. 6. The purified protein reduces $K_{0.5}$ for aconitine, batrachotoxin, and veratridine 3-fold, 12-fold, and 4-fold respectively. As with the venom, V_∞ is increased for aconitine and veratridine but not for bactracho-toxin. Thus, batrachotoxin alone can induce the maximum rate of $^{22}Na^+$ uptake under these conditions.

These results demonstrate that the scorpion toxin acts at a site that is different from the binding site for the alkaloid toxins discussed above and that binding of scorpion toxin to that site causes an increase in the affinity of the alkaloid toxins for their binding site. These cooperative interactions between the alkaloid toxins and scorpion toxin imply that these two sites are allosterically coupled and exhibit positive heterotropic cooperativity, i.e. positive cooperativity between nonidentical binding sites.

In contrast to the whole venom, the purified scorpion toxin has little capacity to activate the action potential Na^+ ionophore unless an alkaloid toxin is also present (23). In order to determine whether alkaloid toxins affect apparent K_D for scorpion toxin, cells were treated for 30 min with various concentrations of scorpion toxin in the presence or absence of 20 μM veratridine, then washed and treated with 20 μM veratridine for 2 min, and finally, Na^+ permeability was determined. Since the action of scorpion toxin is only slowly reversible (23), sequential treatment with scorpion toxin and veratridine should give activation equivalent to simultaneous treatment with both toxins if veratridine does not affect apparent K_D for scorpion toxin. Equivalent activation is observed with these two different experimental protocols (Fig. 7), indicating that veratridine does not affect the affinity for scorpion toxin but is required to observe the effect of the toxin on Na^+ permeability. The cooperativity observed between alkaloid toxins and scorpion toxins is therefore not reciprocal. The mechanism of this cooperative interaction remains uncertain.

Studies of activation of the action potential Na^+ ionophore by veratridine and batrachotoxin did not reveal homotropic cooperativity in this process. The scorpion

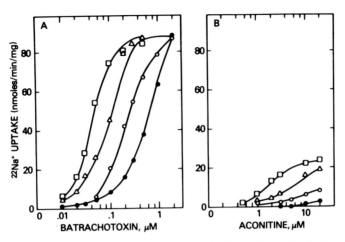

Fig. 6. Effect of purified scorpion toxin on the concentration dependence of activation by batracho-toxin and aconitine. Neuroblastoma cells were incubated for 30 min at 36°C in Na$^+$-free medium containing the indicated concentrations of batrachotoxin (left) or aconitine (right), with 0 ng/ml (●), 6.4 ng/ml (○). 32 ng/ml (△), or 320 ng/ml (□) purified scorpion toxin. Initial rates of ^{22}Na$^+$ uptake were then determined.

toxin titration data of Fig. 7 are also fit by a simple Langmuir isotherm. Thus, these ligands exhibit heterotropic cooperativity but not homotropic cooperativity.

This interpretation of scorpion toxin action implies that reversible, noncovalent interaction of the toxin with the Na$^+$ ionophore is sufficient to cause activation. Experimental evidence not presented in this report supports this conclusion. The toxin acts without a lag time (23), the extent of activation is concentration dependent (23), and the activation by the toxin is completely reversible (23). In addition, assays for proteolytic activity using denatured casein as substrate and for phospholipase activity using egg lecithin as substrate were negative (unpublished experiments).

Tetrodotoxin, a specific inhibitor of the action potential Na$^+$ current (13, 14), inhibits the increase in ^{22}Na$^+$ uptake caused by veratridine and batrachotoxin in a non-competitive manner with $K_I = 8$ nM (21). Incubation of cells with increasing scorpion toxin concentrations in the presence or absence of tetrodotoxin followed by measurements of Na$^+$ permeability gives the concentration response curves illustrated in Fig. 8. These best fit curves are drawn for a common apparent K_D and different V_∞. Thus, tetrodotoxin is also a noncompetitive inhibitor of scorpion toxin action.

Tetrodotoxin and saxitoxin have been shown to compete for a common class of binding sites in nerve axon membranes (27, 28). The characteristics of inhibition of binding by cations has led to the hypothesis that this site represents a coordination site for transported cations (29).

The interactions of neurotoxins with the action potential Na$^+$ ionophore therefore define three functionally separable components of the action potential Na$^+$ ionophore. The alkaloid toxins and scorpion toxin interact with two regulatory components that bind these toxins specifically and interact cooperatively in controlling the ion transport activity of the ionophore. Tetrodotoxin and saxitoxin inhibit the ionophore by interaction with a third component that is directly involved in transport of ions and may contain an ion coordination site for transported cations.

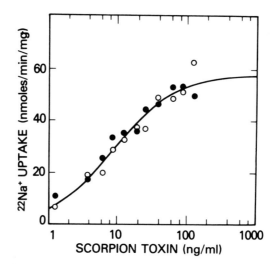

Fig. 7. Effect of veratridine on the concentration dependence of activation by scorpion toxin. Neuro-blastoma cells were incubated for 30 min at 36°C in Na$^+$-free medium containing the indicated concentrations of purified scorpion toxin with (●) or without (○) 20 μM veratridine. Cells were rinsed and incubated for 2 min with 20 μM veratridine in Na$^+$-free medium and initial rates of ^{22}Na$^+$ uptake were determined.

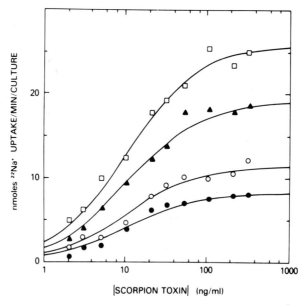

Fig. 8. Inhibition of scorpion toxin-dependent ^{22}Na$^+$ uptake by tetrodotoxin. Neuroblastoma cells were incubated for 30 min at 36°C in Na$^+$-free medium containing the indicated concentrations of purified scorpion toxin and 0 nM (□), 2 nM (▲), 5 nM (○), or 10 nM (●) tetrodotoxin. Initial rates of ^{22}Na$^+$ uptake were then determined in medium containing the same tetrodotoxin concentrations.

If these postulated regulatory components are involved in the normal voltage-dependent regulation of ionophore activity, it might be possible to detect membrane potential-dependent changes in toxin binding. In this experimental system, membrane potential can be controlled by alteration of the extracellular K$^+$ concentration during incubation with toxin in Na$^+$-free medium. In preliminary experiments we have not detected large changes in apparent dissociation constant for alkaloid toxins at different K$^+$ concentrations. Extracellular K$^+$ concentration has a large effect on the apparent K$_D$ for scorpion toxin, however (Fig. 9). The apparent K$_D$ is increased from 2.4 to 28 nM by increasing extracellular K$^+$ from 5.4 mM to 130 mM. Measurements of the rate of reversal of scorpion toxin activation under these conditions demonstrate that the change in K$_D$ reflects at least in part an increase in the unimolecular off rate constant. These results suggest that depolarization of the cells causes a conformation change in the Na$^+$ ionophore that is reflected in a 10-fold increase in apparent K$_D$ for scorpion toxin. The scorpion toxin binding component of the ionophore is therefore implicated in the voltage-dependent regulation of ionophore activity.

In order to show directly that depolarization inhibits the binding of scorpion toxin and not a subsequent step in its action, we have studied the binding of ^{125}I-labeled scorpion toxin. Excitable neuroblastoma cells (clone N18) have a saturable component of ^{125}I-scorpion toxin binding that is displaced by unlabeled toxin (Fig. 10). Clone N103, which is electrically inexcitable and does not respond to veratridine or scorpion toxin (Fig. 1), does not have a similar saturable component of binding (unpublished results). Binding of labeled toxin is inhibited by unlabeled toxin with a dissociation constant approximately

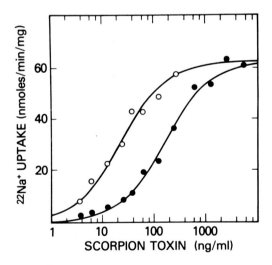

Fig. 9. Effect of extracellular K$^+$ concentration on activation by purified scorpion toxin. Neuroblastoma cells were incubated for 30 min at 36°C in Na$^+$-free medium containing the indicated concentrations of scorption toxin and either 135 mM KCl (●) or 130 mM choline Cl plus 5.4 mM KCl (○). Initial rates of ^{22}Na$^+$ uptake were then determined in medium containing 10 mM NaCl and 120 mM choline Cl to maintain osmolarity.

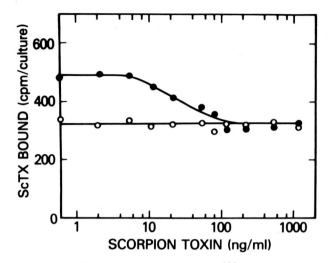

Fig. 10. Effect of extracellular K^+ concentration on binding of ^{125}I-labeled scorpion toxin. Neuro-blastoma cells were incubated for 30 min at 36°C in Na^+-free medium containing ^{125}I-labeled scorpion toxin (0.5 nM ^{125}I), the indicated concentrations of unlabeled scorpion toxin, and either 135 mM KCl (○) or 130 mM choline Cl plus 5.4 mM KCl (●) to maintain osmolarity. Cells were washed to remove free toxin, and bound toxin was measured by gamma counting.

equal to its apparent K_D for activation of the Na^+ ionophore (compare Figs. 7 and 10). These results support the conclusion that the saturable component of binding observed represents binding to the site causing activation of the ionophore.

The saturable component of binding is much reduced in medium containing 135 mM K^+ (Fig. 10). These results confirm that the effect of K^+ is on the binding of toxin and also provide further support for the conclusion that the saturable binding of toxin represents binding to the Na^+ ionophore. Scorpion toxin thus provides a sensitive probe of a change in ionophore structure that is involved in membrane potential-dependent regulation of ionophore activity.

The neurotoxins discussed in this report appear to provide specific probes of three functionally separable components of the Na^+ ionophore. There is little doubt that they will prove useful in understanding the molecular basis of electrical excitability.

ACKNOWLEDGMENTS

We thank Mrs. Cynthia Morrow for excellent technical assistance, Drs. J. Daly and B. Witkop for providing the batrachotoxin, and Mrs. Mary Ellen Miller for typing the manuscript.

Dr. Ray is the recipient of a MARC Faculty Fellowship from the National Institute of General Medical Sciences (Fellowship number 1F32 GM05571-01).

REFERENCES

1. Straub, R., Helv. Physiol. Acta 14:1–28 (1956).
2. Ulbricht, W., Ergeb. Physiol. Biol. Chem. Exp. Pharmakol. 61:18–71 (1969).
3. Albuquerque, E. X., Daly, J. W., and Witkop, B., Science 172:995–1002 (1971).

4. Herzog, W. H., Feibel, R. M., and Bryant, S. H., J. Gen. Physiol. 47:719–733 (1964).
5. Peper, K., and Trautwein, W., Pfluegers Arch. Ges. Physiol. 296:328–336 (1967).
6. Seyama, I., and Narahashi, T., J. Pharm. Exp. Ther. 184:299–307 (1973).
7. Koppenhofer, E., and Schmidt, H., Pflueger's Arch. Ges. Physiol. 303:133–161 (1968).
8. Koppenhofer, E., and Schmidt, H., Experientia 24:41–42 (1967).
9. Narahashi, T., Shapiro, B. I., Deguchi, T., Scuka, M., and Wang, C. M., Am. J. Physiol. 222:850–857 (1972).
10. Cahalan, M. C., J. Physiol. 244:511–534 (1975).
11. Parnas, I., Avgar, D., and Shulov, A., Toxicon 8:67–69 (1970).
12. Narahashi, T., Moore, J. W., and Shapiro, B. I., Science 163:680–681 (1969).
13. Narahashi, T., Moore, J. W., and Scott, W. R., J. Gen. Physiol. 47:965–974 (1964).
14. Evans, M. H., Int. Rev. Neurobiol. 15:83–166 (1972).
15. Nelson, P. G., Ruffner, W., and Nirenberg, M., Proc. Nat. Acad. Sci. U.S.A. 64:1004–1010 (1969).
16. Nelson, P. G., Peacock, J. H., Amano, T., and Minna, J., J. Cell. Physiol. 77:337–352 (1971).
17. Spector, I., Kimhi, Y., and Nelson, P. G., Nature 246:124–126 (1973).
18. Peacock, J., Minna, J., Nelson, P., and Nirenberg, M., Exp. Cell. Res. 73:367–377 (1972).
19. Minna, J., Nelson, P. G., Peacock, J., Glazer, D., and Nirenberg, M., Proc. Nat. Acad. Sci. U.S.A. 68:234–239 (1971).
20. Catterall, W. A., and Nirenberg, M. W., Proc. Nat. Acad. Sci. U.S.A. 70:3759–3763 (1973).
21. Catterall, W. A., J. Biol. Chem. 250:4053–4059 (1975).
22. Catterall, W. A., Proc. Nat. Acad. Sci . U.S.A. 72:1782–1786 (1975).
23. Catterall, W. A., J. Biol. Chem. (1976). In press.
24. Harris, J. B., and Thesleff, S., Acta Physiol. Scan. 83:382–388 (1971).
25. Catterall, W. A., Biochem. Biophys. Res. Commun. 68:136–142 (1976).
26. Shanes, A. M., and Gershfeld, N. L., J. Gen. Physiol. 44:345–363 (1960).
27. Benzer, T. I., and Raftery, M. A., Proc. Nat. Acad. Sci. U.S.A. 69:3634–3637 (1972).
28. Colquhoun, D., Henderson, R., and Ritchie, J. M., J. Physiol. 227:95–126 (1972).
29. Henderson, R., Ritchie, J. M., and Strichartz, G. R., Proc. Nat. Acad. Sci. U.S.A. 71:3936–3940 (1974).

Journal of Supramolecular Structure 5:409 (13)–416 (20) (1976)

Interaction of Charged Lipid Vesicles With Planar Bilayer Lipid Membranes: Detection by Antibiotic Membrane Probes

Joel A. Cohen and Mario M. Moronne

Laboratory of Physiology and Biophysics, University of the Pacific, San Francisco, CA 94115

A technique has been developed for monitoring the interaction of charged phospholipid vesicles with planar bilayer lipid membranes (BLM) by use of the antibiotics Valinomycin, Nonactin, and Monazomycin as surface-charge probes. Anionic phosphatidylserine vesicles, when added to one aqueous compartment of a BLM, are shown to impart negative surface charge to zwitterionic phosphatidylcholine and phosphatidylethanolamine bilayers. The surface charge is distributed asymmetrically, mainly on the vesicular side of the BLM, and is not removed by exchange of the vesicular aqueous solution. Possible mechanisms for the vesicle-BLM interactions are discussed.

Key words: antibiotics, bilayer lipid membranes, surface charge, phospholipid vesicles, fusion

INTRODUCTION

Vesicle-membrane fusion is a common event in cell biology, providing, for example, the pathway for exocytotic discharge of transmitter in the neuromuscular junction during excitation. Although the mechanisms for biological control of the fusion process, including the roles of membrane proteins and filamentous structures, are not yet understood, it has recently become apparent that phospholipid "model" membranes, under appropriate conditions, can fuse spontaneously. Thus, at least in such "artificial" situations, the fusion process is known to be mediated by the phospholipids themselves. It is of interest to ascertain whether such phospholipid interactions can provide the underlying mechanism for biological fusion, with ancillary protein-mediated interactions perhaps exerting control via modulation of factors which affect the lipids (1). Such a hypothesis requires, as a first step, thorough elucidation of the nature of "bare" phospholipid membrane fusion. In this regard, the phenomena of lipid vesicle-vesicle fusion (2–7) and spherical bilayer fusion (8–10) have been investigated by several authors.

We have chosen to examine the possibility of phospholipid vesicle fusion with planar bilayer lipid membranes (BLM). The reasons are threefold: a) The planar BLM provides a geometry more akin to that of the cell membrane (large radius of curvature), as seen by a vesicle, than does another vesicle. The structural instability of small (~ 300 Å diameter) vesicles should render the fusion of vesicles with BLM less favorable energetically than fusion of vesicles with one another. b) Planar BLMs provide a unique geometry for investigation of membrane transport, in that convenient electrical and chemical accessibility to both sides of the BLM are possible. Thus, functional properties of the fused membrane system can be studied; for example, the voltage dependence and specificity of the conductance, or the asymmetry of the transport characteristics. c) An understanding of vesicle-BLM fusion could lead the way toward successful incorporation of biologically functional microsomes into BLM, thus permitting thorough electro-chemical characterization of these membrane preparations.

The interaction of phospholipid vesicles and biological microsomes with planar lipid bilayers has now been reported several times (11–16), always with some speculation regarding the occurrence of fusion. The major purpose of this paper is to report a new technique for monitoring the interaction of charged phospholipid vesicles (or microsomes) with planar BLMs and for determining whether or not such interactions are likely to involve fusion. We shall illustrate the technique by demonstrating the interaction of phosphatidylserine (PS) vesicles with phosphatidylethanolamine (PE), phosphatidyl-choline (PC), and PS BLMs.

Our technique is based on the fact that if interaction of charged vesicles with a BLM injects charged phospholipids into the BLM, then the BLM surface-charge density must be altered. For example, incorporation of anionic PS lipids into a zwitterionic PE BLM must impart negative surface charge to the BLM. A BLM surface-charge monitor could then detect such an interaction. It is well known that membrane surface-charge detectors indeed exist in the form of antibiotics such as Valinomycin, Nonactin, and Monazomycin. In the presesnce of these antibiotics the BLM conductance, which is easily monitored, is a function of the BLM surface-charge density [see McLaughlin and Eisenberg (17) for an excellent review]. Our technique, then, involves the use of standard methods for monitoring the BLM surface-charge density as charged vesicles are added to the aqueous phase.

In addition to sensing an "average" surface-charge density on the BLM, this technique can also detect asymmetries of surface-charge distributions on the two sides of the BLM. Such asymmetries are reflected in the current-voltage characteristic of the anti-biotic-treated BLM. Monazomycin is particularly sensitive to these effects (18). Thus, if charged vesicles are added to one side of a BLM only, it is possible to detect the charge densities appearing on each of the two surfaces of the BLM separately. Appearance of surface charge on the side opposite to which charged vesicles are added is a likely indica-tion of fusion (9, 19–21).

METHODS

Lipid bilayers were formed on a 1 mm diameter hole in a Teflon partition separating 5 and 10 ml aqueous compartments. Electrical measurements were made with a pair of Ag/AgCl electrodes connected to the aqueous solutions through KCl-agar bridges. A standard op-amp circuit was used to clamp the membrane voltage and monitor the mem-brane current. Each membrane was formed in an aqueous solution initially consisting of 10 mM KCl buffered at pH 7.0 with 5 mM Mops/Tris buffer at 22°C. In some cases, 0.2 mM EDTA was also present.

Membranes were made from bacterial phosphatidylethanolamine (Supelco), egg phosphatidylcholine (Sigma, Type VI), and bovine phosphatidylserine (PL Biochemicals).

Each lipid was dissolved in n-decane (Sigma) to give a 1% (w/v) solution. For the Valino-mycin measurements the Val was added directly to the lipid-decane solutions in a concentration range of 0.05–0.3 mg/ml. The Valinomycin-treated membranes typically achieved conductances of 2×10^{-6} to 2×10^{-5} ohms^{-1} cm^{-2}. These values were sufficiently high to provide a convenient baseline above the unmodified bilayer conductance but sufficiently low to avoid the undesirable effects of diffusion polarization or interface-limited kinetics (28). All Valinomycin results were confirmed with Nonactin. Monazomycin, when used for asymmetric surface-charge determinations, was added to the aqueous phase of one side of the BLM at a concentration of 3.1 μg/ml. The Monazomycin was a generous gift from Dr. E. L. Patterson, Lederle Laboratories, and Nonactin from Drs. H. Bickel and F. Jenny, Ciba-Geigy Ltd.

Phosphatidylcholine vesicles were prepared by sonicating an 8.3 mg/ml lipid suspension, buffered to pH 7.0, until a clear bluish solution was obtained. Sonication usually took about 25 min at 40–50°C. Phosphatidylserine vesicles were similarly prepared but required only 5–10 min of sonication at 25°C to give a clear opalescent solution. Sonication was carried out under nitrogen using a Kontes probe-type sonicator. Unless otherwise indicated, all vesicle additions to the aqueous BLM compartments gave 13 μg/ml final concentration.

Aqueous solutions were exchanged in the presence of a bilayer with a peristaltic pump (Cole-Parmer) that provided gentle enough action to avoid excessive disturbance of the bilayer. Exchange rates of $\sim$ 5 ml/min were typically used.

RESULTS

In these measurements Valinomycin was used as the BLM surface-charge detector. The action of this antibiotic has been well characterized (22–24), and its utility in sensing BLM surface-charge density is well known (17). Briefly, Valinomycin (Val) imparts K$^+$ specificity to the BLM conductance, which is then proportional to the K$^+$ concentration (or activity) at the BLM-water interface. If the BLM has surface charge, then [K$^+$] at the interface is altered relative to [K$^+$] in the bulk aqueous phase by electrostatic attraction or repulsion. Thus, the observed Val-mediated BLM conductance (G$^+$) is enhanced by negative, and suppressed by positive, surface charge. Quantitatively, G$^+$ $\propto$ [K$^+$]$_{interface}$ = [K$^+$]$_{bulk}$ exp $(-F \Psi_0/RT)$, where Ψ_0 is the BLM surface potential. Ψ_0 is in turn determined by the surface-charge density and the bulk electrolyte concentrations by the Gouy equation (for simple electrolytes) or Grahame equation (for more complex electrolytes) (25). Changes in surface-charge density can thus be calculated from observed changes in G$^+$ *if* it can be established that the G$^+$ changes are indeed electrostatic in origin.

Figure 1 shows the conductance of a Val-treated PE BLM as a function of time upon addition of 13 μg/ml PS vesicles (A) or PC vesicles (B) to both aqueous compartments. The conductance increases markedly upon addition of the PS vesicles, indicative of anionic surface charge appearing on the BLM. The possibility of this conductance increase arising from PS-induced BLM leakage was investigated by adding PS vesicles to a *non*-Val-treated PE BLM under otherwise identical conditions. The dashed line segment in the lower right corner of Fig. 1A indicates the maximum conductance increase that can be attributed to leakage. The electrostatic origin of the G$^+$ increase in Fig. 1A was further confirmed by the addition of 0.1 M LiCl (final concentration) to both 10 mM KCl

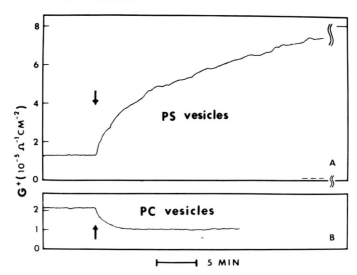

Fig. 1. Conductance of Val-treated PE BLM vs time. Arrows indicate the addition of 13 μg/ml PS vesicles (A) or PC vesicles (B) to both aqueous compartments of the BLM. Voltage clamp = +50 mV. Solutions are 10 mM KCl and 0.2 mM EDTA buffered at pH 7.0 with 5 mM Mops/Tris at 22°C. Dashed line segment in (A) indicates the conductance observed after addition of PS vesicles to a non-Val-treated PE BLM as discussed in the text.

aqueous compartments of the Val-PE BLM. The Li^+ cannot contribute significantly to G^+ due to Val's pronounced K^+ selectivity (24); hence its presence serves merely to increase the ionic strength of the aqueous medium. From the Gouy equation, this should screen the negative surface charge, decrease the magnitude of the surface potential, and hence cause G^+ to drop. In fact, G^+ in Fig. 1A decreases markedly (by ∼ 67%) when the LiCl is added, in approximate concordance with the Gouy theory.

In Fig. 1B the PC vesicles are seen to cause a G^+ decrease of ∼ 50%. Ideally, zwitterionic PC vesicles should not change G^+ at all, since they cannot add surface charge to the BLM. We attribute this G^+ decrease to loss of Val from the BLM. (This idea is confirmed later in Fig. 3.) Conceivably aqueous vesicles deplete the aqueous Val concentration, which then causes Val to diffuse out of the BLM faster than it can be replenished from the torus. This nonelectrostatic effect is undoubtedly superimposed upon the surface-charge-related G^+ increase for PS vesicles in Fig. 1A and must be accounted for in quantitative determinations. Estimates from the steady-state conductances in Fig.1 indicate a negative PS surface-charge density of ∼ 1 charge/700 $Å^2$ appearing on both sides of the PE BLM. The current-voltage relation is slightly superlinear and symmetric.

When PS vesicles are added to one side only of a Val-PE BLM, a conductance increase similar to that of Fig. 1A, but of smaller magnitude, is observed. Now the current-voltage relation is asymmetric, as seen in Fig. 2. (This asymmetry is further evidence against leakage.) The properties of Valinomycin-like carrier transport under asymmetric membrane conditions have been discussed by Stark (23) and by Hall and Latorre (26). The asymmetry seen in Fig. 2 is consistent with the majority of negative surface charge appearing on the side of the BLM to which the vesicles are added. This conclusion is

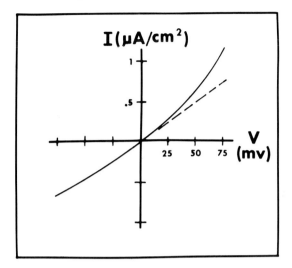

Fig. 2. Current-voltage relation for Val-treated PE BLM after addition of 13 μg/ml PS vesicles to one aqueous compartment. Conditions are the same as for Fig. 1. Dashed line is the tangent at zero voltage. Sign convention: V as indicated = V (vesicle side) $-$V (non-vesicle side).

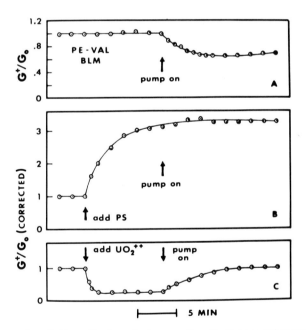

Fig. 3. Perfusion experiment. Normalized conductance vs time for Val-treated PE BLMs. Voltage clamp = +50 mV (sign convention as in Fig. 2). "Pump on" indicates start of exchange of solution in one aqueous compartment with buffered 10 mM KCl. Curve (A) shows decrease in steady-state conductance resulting from loss of Val during exchange. Curves (B) and (C) are corrected for this loss of Val during exchange. (B) shows increase in BLM conductance following addition of PS vesicles (13 μg/ml) to one side of the BLM. Conductance remains unaffected by exchange of vesicle solution. (C) shows membrane conductance drop following addition of 3 μM UO_2^{++} to one compartment. BLM conductance returns to initial value when UO_2^{++} solution is exchanged.

substantiated by screening the highly-charged side of the BLM with 0.1 M impermeant LiCl, which causes the current-voltage curve to become symmetric and the conductance to return to near its original value.

A more quantitative measurement of the asymmetric charge distribution was made with the voltage-sensitive pore-former Monazomycin. The advantage of Monazomycin arises from its extreme sensitivity to asymmetric changes in membrane surface potentials (18). In particular, if Monazomycin is added to one side of a bilayer (which we call the *cis* side), it can readily detect changes of several millivolts in surface potential on the opposite (*trans*) side of the membrane, while remaining relatively insensitive to changes on the cis side. Using this approach, we added PS vesicles to the cis side of a Monazomycin-treated PE bilayer. If surface charge were to appear on the trans side, a significant increase in the Monazomycin conductance would be expected. We found the conductance to increase by a factor of approximately 3 after addition of the vesicles. If all of this conductance increase were attributed to charge appearing on the trans side, the trans charge density would be ~ 1 charge/10,000 Å^2. However, as mentioned above, the Valinomycin data indicate that most of the charge appears on the vesicle side of the BLM. Thus, the charge density on the trans side must in fact be much smaller than the above maximal value. A reasonable estimate is $\leqslant 1$ charge/50,000 Å^2 on the trans side of the membrane or $\leqslant 1$ charge/1,000 phospholipids. This value is $\leqslant 2\%$ of the charge estimated to be on the vesicle side of the BLM.

We find that Val-treated egg-PC BLMs act similarly to Val-PE BLMs with respect to acquisition of surface charge from aqueous PS vesicles. However, Val-PS BLMs do not acquire additional surface-charge density in the presence of PS vesicles. This result is not unexpected and reflects either a) a lack of PS vesicle — PS BLM interaction, conceivably due to charge repulsion, or b) a "saturated" BLM charge density (~ 1 charge/phospholipid) that cannot be exceeded by further PS incorporation.

It is interesting to consider whether the BLM surface charge acquired from PS vesicles is actually incorporated irreversibly into the bilayer structure or, alternatively, is loosely bound on the surface. We attempted to answer this question by perfusing the vesicle-containing aqueous compartment with fresh vesicle-free electrolyte while monitoring the BLM conductance; that is, we attempted to "flush off" the surface charge. The results are given in Fig. 3. Fig. 3A shows the effect of perfusion on a plain Val-PE BLM having no surface charge. The G^+ decrease indicates that about one-third of the Val is lost from the BLM. (This result is similar to that observed in Fig. 1B and supports the mechanism described there; i.e., depletion of aqueous Val indeed causes a G^+ decrease.) Figs. 3B and 3C compare the effects due to addition of PS liposomes and UO$_2^{++}$ to one side of Val-PE BLM, with subsequent perfusion. These curves are corrected for the loss of Val shown in Fig. 3A. Uranyl ion is known to bind strongly to lipid membranes ($K_D \sim 10^{-5}$ M for PE) and therefore to impart positive surface charge to BLMs (25). This effect is evident in Fig. 3C from the sharp G^+ decrease upon addition of 3 μM uranyl acetate to one aqueous compartment. However, perfusion removes the positive surface charge completely, implying the existence of a reversible equilibrium between aqueous and membrane-bound UO$_2^{++}$. Thus the uranyl, although bound strongly, is not bound irreversibly. On the other hand, the negative surface charge from the PS liposomes is *not* removed by perfusion (Fig. 3B). The PS surface charge seems to be irreversibly incorporated into the PE BLM structure.

DISCUSSION

Our results have shown that addition of PS vesicles to the aqueous phase of Valino-mycin-treated PE or PC BLMs causes negative surface charge to appear on the BLMs. This charge is irreversibly bound to the BLM and appears mainly on the side of the BLM to which the vesicles are added.

There are several a priori mechanisms that could explain these effects: a) lipid monomer transfer from vesicles to BLM via the aqueous phase; b) lipid transfer from vesicles to BLM via direct contact, either transitory or long-lived; c) irreversible adhesion of vesicles to BLM; d) semi-fusion, in which apposing vesicle and BLM monolayers fuse, but the back monolayers do not; e) full fusion; f) assorted combinations of the above.

In order to test for possibility a), we added one-tenth the normal concentration of PS dispersion to the aqueous phase of Val-PE BLM, the rationale being that since our PS solution ($\sim$ 16 μM) is far above the PS critical micelle concentration, a tenfold reduction in lipid concentration should reduce the vesicle population but not affect the aqueous monomer population. Thus, a decreased effect would indicate the interaction to be vesicle-mediated (or micelle-mediated), and an unchanged effect would indicate the inter-action to be monomer-mediated. We found that the effect virtually disappeared for the reduced PS situation, implying vesicle or micelle mediation. We do not, however, feel that this simple test entirely rules out the possibility of aqueous monomer transfer.

Mechanism b) is fully consistent with our observations. The possibility of exchange of hydrophobic molecules from one membrane to another upon close contact was considered by Pohl et al. (11). Exchange of amphiphilic lipids should be equally possible.

It is difficult to envision how mechanism c) could affect the BLM conductance significantly, unless it also involved lipid transfer, that is, mechanism b). A vesicle adhered to the BLM would simply remove the vesicle-BLM adhesion area from contact with the electrolyte, thus reducing the conductive area of the BLM. Possibly that part of the vesicular surface charge lying outside the contact area, but within a Debye length of the BLM surface, could affect local ionic concentrations at the BLM-water interface over small regions, giving rise to small conductance effects.

In mechanism d) PS lipids could spread over the "front" side of the BLM by lateral diffusion, producing the types of effects we have seen. Under the assumption that ad-hered or semi-fused vesicles might fuse fully with BLM if suitably perturbed, we tried adding decane "chasers" (16), lysolecithin, and heating to 50°C. These manipulations produced no discernible change in the Val-BLM charge distributions.

Full fusion, mechanism e), should deposit some surface charge on the "back" side of the BLM, that is, the side opposite to which the vesicles are added. Monitoring charge density on the back BLM surface is thus the most reliable indicator of fusion provided by our technique. Other mechanisms listed above cannot deposit surface charge on the back of the BLM unless they also manage to enhance lipid flip-flop rates significantly. Our semiquantitative determination of back-side surface-charge density for PS vesicles and PE BLM ($\leqslant$ 1 charge/50,000 Å^2 and $\leqslant$ 2% of the front charge density) indicates that most of the observed interaction is not fusion.

In conclusion, we have shown that surface-charge-sensitive antibiotic probes can be used to detect and monitor the interaction of charged vesicles with planar BLMs. For the case of PS liposomes with PE or PC BLMs, a definite interaction occurs and implants anionic surface charge irreversibly on the BLM. The charge appears mainly, if not completely, on the side of the BLM to which the vesicles are added. Thus this interaction is *not* likely to be fusion.

ACKNOWLEDGMENTS

This work was supported by the National Institutes of Health (HL-16607) and the National Science Foundation (PCM 76-11950).

REFERENCES

1. Ahkong, Q. F., Fisher, D., Tampion, W., and Lucy, J. A., Nature 253:194 (1975).
2. Papahadjopoulos, D., Poste, G., Schaeffer, B. E., and Vail, W. J., Biochim. Biophys. Acta 352:10 (1974).
3. van der Bosch, J., and McConnell, H. M., Proc. Nat. Acad. Sci. USA 72:4409 (1975).
4. Taupin, C., and McConnell, H. M., FEBS Symposium 28:219 (1972).
5. Kantor, H. L., and Prestegard, J. H., Biochem. 14:1790 (1975).
6. Prestegard, J. H., and Fellmeth, B., Biochem. 13:1122 (1974).
7. Miller, C., and Racker, E., J. Memb. Biol. 26:319 (1976).
8. Breisblatt, W., and Ohki, S., J. Memb. Biol. 23:385 (1975).
9. Neher, E., Biochim. Biophys. Acta 373:327 (1974).
10. Liberman, E. A., and Nenashev, V. A., Biofizika 17:1017 (1972).
11. Pohl, G. W., Stark, G., and Trissl, H. W., Biochim. Biophys. Acta 318:478 (1973).
12. Drachev, L. A., Jasaitis, A. A., Kaulen, A. D., Kondrashin, A. A., Liberman, E. A., Nemecek, I. B., Ostroumov, S. A., Semenov, A. Yu., and Skulachev, V. P., Nature 249:321 (1974).
13. Sergeeva, N. S., Poglazov, A. F., and Vladimirov, Yu. A., Biofizika 20:1029 (1975).
14. Cohen, J. A., and Moronne, M. M., Biophys. J. 16:113a (1976).
15. Düzgünes, N., and Ohki, S., Biophys. J. 16:140a (1976).
16. Moore, M. R., Biochim. Biophys. Acta 426:765 (1976).
17. McLaughlin, S., and Eisenberg, M., Ann. Rev. Biophys. Bioeng. 4:335 (1975).
18. Muller, R. U., and Finkelstein, A., J. Gen. Physiol. 60:263 and 285 (1972).
19. Lucy, J. A., Nature 227:815 (1970).
20. Poste, G., and Allison, A. C., Biochim. Biophys. Acta 300:421 (1973).
21. Satir, B., Sci. Am. 233:28 (1975).
22. Stark, G., and Benz, R., J. Memb. Biol. 5:133 (1971).
23. Stark, G., Biochim. Biophys. Acta 298:323 (1973).
24. Läuger, P., Science 178:24 (1972).
25. McLaughlin, S. G. A., Szabo, G., and Eisenman, G., J. Gen. Physiol. 58:667 (1971).
26. Hall, J. E., and Latorre, R., Biophys. J. 16:99 (1976).

Journal of Supramolecular Structure 5:417 (21)–429 (33) (1976)

Central Nervous System Antigen (NS-5) and Its Presence During Murine Ontogenesis

Astrid Zimmermann,* Melitta Schachner,‡ and Joan L. Press§

*Departments of Neurobiology and §Medicine (Immunology), Stanford University
Medical Center, Stanford, California 94305, and
Harvard Medical School, Boston, Massachusetts 02215

An antiserum raised by immunization of C3H.SW/Sn mice with cerebellum from 4-day-old C57BL/6J mice recognizes a cell surface component(s) [NS-5] present in different degrees on various parts of the mouse central nervous system. When analyzed by an antiserum- and complement-mediated cell cytotoxicity test and by the ability of various tissues to absorb anti-NS-5 antiserum activity, the antigen(s) was detectable on cerebellum, retina, olfactory bulb, cortex, basal ganglia, and medulla, but not on nonneural tissues with the exception of mature spermatozoa and 4-day-old kidney. The antigen(s) detected by the anti-NS-5 antiserum was found in similar quantities on young and adult rat and mouse cerebellum; however, it was not detectable on any of 16 clonal cell lines derived from the rat central nervous system. During preimplantation stages of murine development, the antigen could be detected on all cells of (2–4)-cell and (8–16)-cell stages and on the trophoblastic cells of blastocysts by indirect immunofluorescence. Embryos on day 9 of gestation, the earliest stage tested after implantation, expressed the antigen(s), but expression was restricted to the nervous system.

Key words: nervous system — cell surface antigen(s); rat CNS clonal cell lines; preimplantation embryos; indirect immunofluorescence staining

INTRODUCTION

Immunological methodology has proven to be very useful in providing sensitive probes for defining differences between organs or cell types in the adult and developing organism (1–3). In attempts to use this approach to help define different cell populations in the nervous system via their cell surface antigens, several investigators have used antisera raised against nervous tissue and especially against tumors and cloned cell lines derived from the nervous system (4–12). The use of tumors or cloned cell lines as antigenic material may provide a more homogeneous cell population for analysis, but it has disadvantages in that transformed cells may differ in several respects from their normal counterparts [13,14]. Furthermore, some cloned cell lines have been shown to lose or alter the expression of certain cell surface antigens when kept in culture, as opposed to passage in vivo [15]. When normal central or peripheral nervous system tissue is used for immunization, the antigenic material will consist of a wide variety of different cell types and antigens. However, antigens reflecting possible functional and positional properties of the different cells may be preserved and could potentially be recognized. Unfortunately, viable single cell suspensions are difficult, if not impossible, to obtain, depending on the stage of brain development analyzed.

In the studies reported here, the cerebellum of postnatal day 4 mice was used as the tissue source for immunization. The cerebellum is a component of the central nervous system whose anatomy, development, and physiology have been well characterized (16–18). It is easily removed from the brain, and viable single-cell suspensions can readily be prepared from early postnatal stages and kept in culture (19). At postnatal day 4, the mouse cerebellum is not fully matured; instead it is in the midst of its developmental program, the main aspect of which is the proliferation of cells in the external granular layer and their inward migration and formation of the internal granular cell layer (20).

This communication demonstrates that when C3H.SW/Sn mice are immunized with postnatal day 4 C57BL/6J cerebellum, the anti-NS-5 antiserum (21) elicited reacts with a cell surface antigen(s) differentially expressed by tissues of the mouse and rat central nervous system (CNS). Anti-NS-5 antiserum also reacts with a cell surface antigen(s) on sperm, 4-day-old kidney, and cleavage stage embryos (two-cell stage to blastocyst).

MATERIALS AND METHODS

Mice. All inbred strains were obtained from the breeding colonies of the Departments of Neurobiology and Medicine, Stanford University School of Medicine, Stanford, California; from the Department of Neuroscience, Children's Hospital Medical Center, Boston, Massachussetts; and from the Jackson Laboratory, Bar Harbor, Maine.

Antisera. Anti-NS-5 antiserum was raised in C3H.SW/Sn mice against the particulate fractions of homogenates prepared from cerebella of 4-day-old C57BL/6J mice. The preparations of the antigenic material from whole cerebellum and the immunization schedule have been described in detail (9,21).

Preparation of brain cell suspensions. Two to three cerebella from 4-day-old mice were incubated for 10 min at room temperature in 3 ml of EBSS (Earle's Balanced Salt Solution) (International Scientific Industries) containing 0.025% trypsin and 0.0025% DNase I (Worthington Biochemical Co., codes TRL and DP, respectively). After one wash in EBSS, single cells were released from the cerebellum by pipetting up and down in 9 ml containing 0.0075% trypsin and 0.00075% DNase I, using first a wide- then a small-bore fire-polished Pasteur pipette. To inhibit the trypsin 0.4 mg of soybean trypsin inhibitor (Worthington Biochemical Co.) and 1 ml of fetal calf serum (GIBCO) were added. The average yield of cells using this trypsinization procedure is 3×10^6 cells per 4-day-old cerebellum. (For an evaluation of this procedure, see Ref. 9.)

Embryonic brain cells were prepared with the same enzymes, but a one-step procedure was used. The brains were teased into small pieces and incubated for 15 min at room temperature in 5 ml of EBSS containing 0.0125% and 0.00125% DNase I. Single cells were released by carefully pipetting up and down with a 5 ml pipette.

Serological tests. In the complement-mediated cell cytotoxicity test, 0.025 ml of cells (5×10^6 per ml) in Medium 199 (GIBCO) with 10% gamma-globulin-free, heat-inactivated fetal calf serum (FCS), 0.025 ml of antiserum dilution, and 0.025 ml of rabbit complement diluted 1:12 were incubated for 30 min at 37°C in a one-step procedure. Cell death was determined by uptake of Trypan Blue dye; the cytotoxic activity of the antiserum was calculated by determining the percentage of dead cells over background (complement alone). For absorptions, antiserum was used at a concentration of 3–5 serial dilutions below the cytotoxic endpoint (antiserum dilution at which 50% of maximal kill occurs). The diluted antiserum was incubated with washed particulate fractions of tissue homogenates for 30 min at 0°C, using a ratio of 1:1 serum volume to pellet volume of tissue homogenate.

Cell lines. BDIX rats and clonal cell lines derived from the CNS of BDIX rats (22) were a generous gift from Dr. David Schubert, Salk Institute, La Jolla, California. The lines were cultured in Dulbecco's Modified Eagle Medium (GIBCO) containing 5% FCS (GIBCO), in 6 cm Falcon tissue culture dishes in humidified 5% CO_2, 95% air. Cells near confluency were used for cytotoxic tests and absorptions, and were removed from the tissue culture dish either mechanically or with trypsin.

Embryos. Fertilized eggs were obtained from superovulated (BALB/c × 129)F_1 (c129) female mice 5–8 weeks old. Female mice received 5 units of pregnant mare serum (Sigma Laboratories) intraperitoneally (i.p.), followed 48 hr later by an i.p. injection of 2.5 units of human chorionic gonadotropin (Ayerest Laboratory, New York). The mice were mated to male c129 mice immediately after the second injection, then checked for the presence of vaginal plugs the following morning. At 24, 48, and 72 hr following detection of the plug, the female mice were sacrificed and the oviducts (plus uterus for blastocysts) were flushed with Brinster's medium (23) containing 3% bovine serum albumin, and 5% gamma-globulin-free, heat-inactivated fetal calf serum, to obtain (2–4)-cell, (8–16)-cell, and morula-blastocyst stage embryos, respectively. The zona pellucida was removed by digestion with 0.5% pronase (24). The eggs were washed extensively in medium prior to analysis.

Indirect immunofluorescence. The immunoglobulin fraction of a polyvalent rabbit anti-mouse-immunoglobulin antiserum (RAMIg, 20 mg/ml) was provided by Dr. L. Herzenberg, Department of Genetics, Stanford University. Rabbit immunoglobulin, fractionated by DEAE cellulose chromatography and analyzed for purity by immunoelectrophoresis, electrophoretic mobility, and precipitin bands in Ouchterlony gel diffusion (25), was used to immunize a goat to produce goat anti-rabbit-immunoglobulin serum, (GARIg). The immunoglobulin fraction of GARIg was obtained by ion-exchange chromatography, and was fluorescein-conjugated using fluorescein isothiocyanate (26). The fluoresceinated GARIg was fractionated by gradient elution from DEAE-cellulose to obtain fractions with a fluorescein/protein (F/P) ratio between 2 and 4. The final fluoresceinated GARIg (GARIg^F) stock solution (20 mg/ml) had an F/P ratio of 3.4. It was clarified by centrifugation at 100,000 × g and filtered through a sterile millipore membrane. For staining both cells and embryos, RAMIg was used at a 1/120 dilution and GARIg^F at a 1/400 dilution, in medium containing 5% gamma-globulin-free, heat-inactivated FCS and 0.02% sodium azide. A fluoresceinated rabbit anti-mouse gamma globulin (5.8 mg/ml; F/P ratio 1:7) was provided by Dr. M. Iverson, Department of Genetics, Stanford University, and was used undiluted.

A two- or three-step indirect immunofluorescent staining procedure was used. $(1-5) × 10^7$ cells were incubated with 0.05 ml of anti-NS-5 antiserum or preimmune (normal) mouse serum at a 1:3 or 1:6 dilution in Medium 199 (GIBCO) containing 5% gamma-globulin-free, heat-inactivated FCS, and 0.02% sodium azide. The cells were incubated for 15 min at room temperature, underlayered with 1 ml of gamma-globulin-free, heat-inactivated FCS, and centrifuged at 220 × g for 10 min. The cells were resuspended in 0.05 ml of fluoresceinated rabbit anti-mouse gamma globulin (two-step procedure) or

RAMIg (three-step procedure) and incubated for 15 min at room temperature. The cells were underlayered again with FCS, pelleted by centrifugation, and washed. In the two-step procedure, the cells were resuspended in phosphate-buffered saline (PBS) and scored for fluorescence using a Zeiss Universal microscope, or analyzed on the fluorescence-activated cell sorter (FACS) (27). In the three-step procedure, the cells were resuspended on 0.050 ml of GARIgF and incubated for 15 min, following which they were centrifuged through FCS, washed, and analyzed for fluorescence.

Mouse cleavage stage embryos were analyzed by indirect immunofluorescence using a three-step procedure and the reagents described above. The preimplantation stages were incubated either in anti-NS-5 antiserum or normal mouse serum diluted 1:3 in Brinster's medium containing 5% gamma-globulin-free, heat-inactivated FCS and 0.02% sodium azide for 20 min at 37°C in a closed hood aerated with 5% CO_2–95% air. The eggs were washed by successive transfers through 3 droplets of medium, then incubated in RAMIg for 20 min; after washing, the eggs were incubated in GARIgF for 20 min, washed extensively, and transferred under oil to microwell plates. Fluorescence was determined using a Zeiss Universal fluorescence microscope at × 200. Photographs were taken with a Leica Camera, Ektachrome high-speed color slide film (exposure time 2 min).

RESULTS

Antisera (anti-NS-5) raised in C3H.SW/Sn mice against cerebellum of postnatal day 4 (P4) C57BL/6J mice are cytotoxic in the presence of complement for postnatal day 4 cerebellar cells from all mouse strains tested so far: C57BL/6J, C3H.SW/Sn, C3H/HeDiSn, A/J, AKR/J, BALB/c, DBA/2, and 129/J. No quantitative differences in the amount of antigen per volume of packed cerebellar cells were found in absorption experiments using 4-day-old donors from the above strains. When P4 cerebellar cells prepared by trypsinization were analyzed by cytotoxicity tests using anti-NS-5 antiserum and complement, 80–95% of the cells were killed. These variations in maximal kill were not dependent on the number of immunizations of the recipient mice, but were observed for any batch of antiserum from the first to the last bleeding. Therefore, these differences in maximal kill probably reflect differences in the composition of the cerebellar cell suspensions prepared by trypsinization. The antiserum titer at which 50% of maximal kill was observed was 1:100 to 1:300, depending on the number of previous immunizations.

The presence or absence of the antigen(s) recognized by the anti-NS-5 antiserum on cells of various tissues from 4-day-old and adult (2 months or older) C57BL/6J mice, and on tumors of the mouse nervous system, had been determined by antiserum absorptions and/or cytotoxicity tests (21). Table I shows that the antigen(s) recognized by the anti-NS-5 antiserum are not restricted to the cerebellum of postnatal day 4 mice, but are also present on the adult cerebellum, although in lower amounts per volume of packed cells (21); on postnatal day 4 and adult brain minus cerebellum; on neural retina; and on a medulloepithelioma (a tumor of possibly subventricular origin (28). Of nonneural tissues, only mature spermatozoa and postnatal day 4 kidney carried detectable antigen. The anti-NS-5 antiserum was not cytotoxic for the following target cells derived from the peripheral nervous system:Pl superior cervical ganglia cells, the hybrid (strain) cell line NX-31 (29), and the Cl300 neuroblastoma; nor did Cl300 and NX-31 absorb NS-5 antibody activity.

TABLE I. Capacity of Different Mouse Tissues and Tumors to Absorb Cytotoxic Activity From Anti-NS-5 Antiserum

Tissue used for absorptions	Target cells in cytotoxicity test		
	P4 cerebellar cells	P4 retina cells	C3H/Bif B/Ki medulloepithelioma cells
P4/Adult liver	−	−	−
P4/Adult spleen	−	−	−
P4/Kidney	+	+	+
Adult kidney	−	−	−
P4/Adult thymocytes and lymphocytes	−	−	−
P4/Adult epidermis	−	−	−
Adult muscle	−	−	−
Adult testis	−	−	−
Sperm from epididymis and vas deferens	−	−	+
P4/Adult cerebellum	+	+	+
P4/Adult brain minus cerebellum	+	+	+
P4/Adult retina	+	+	+
C3H/Bif B/Ki medulloepithelioma	+	+	+
A/J Neuroblastoma	−	−	−
C57BL/6J Glioblastoma	−	−	−
C57BL/6J Glioblastoma G261	−	n.d.	n.d.
C57BL/6J Glioma G26	−	n.d.	n.d.
C57GL/6J Ependymoblastoma	−	n.d.	n.d.
C57BL/6J Ependymoblastoma EPA	−	n.d.	n.d.

P4 cerebellar, P4 retina, and C3H/Bif B/Ki medulloepithelioma cells were used as target cells in a subsequent cytotoxicity test (21).
+ signifies that absorption tissue absorbs all cytotoxic activity; −, absorbs none; n.d., not determined.

Since cerebellum was used as the immunogen, the antiserum was examined to see if it contained any activity exclusively directed against cerebellar cells. The anti-NS-5 antiserum was repeatedly absorbed with 4-day-old brain from which the cerebellum had been removed, then tested for residual cytotoxic activity on P4 cerebellar target cells. As shown in Fig. 1, extensive absorption with brain minus cerebellum removed all activity for the target cells, whereas the same number of absorptions with liver did not significantly reduce the cytotoxic activity. One absorption with P4 cerebellar cells was sufficient to eliminate all cytotoxic activity.

In order to determine whether there were other "hot spots" (that is, regions with high amounts of antigen) in the brain besides cerebellum, cytotoxic tests and absorptions were done with other parts of the brain of postnatal 1-day-old (P1) C57BL/6J mice. Single-cell suspensions were prepared as described for embryonic brain. Figure 2 shows the results of cytotoxicity tests on cell suspensions from neural retina, cerebellum,

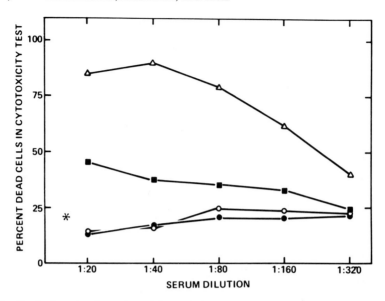

Fig. 1. Result of exhaustive absorption of the anti-NS-5 antiserum with cerebellum and brain minus cerebellum. Absorptions were carried out each time with 0.050 ml of packed tissue and 0.050 ml of anti-NS-5 antiserum dilution. △——△ 3 × liver; ○——○ 3 × brain minus cerebellum; ■——■ 1 × brain minus cerebellum, 2 × liver; ●——● 1 × cerebellum, 2 × liver; * = complement control.

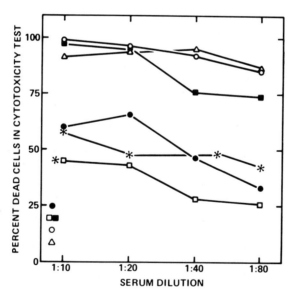

Fig. 2. Expression of NS-5 antigen(s) on various parts of the brain of 1-day-old C57BL/6J mice as measured by direct cytotoxicity. Single-cell suspensions for the cytotoxicity test were prepared from each brain part as described for embryonic brain in Materials and Methods. ○——○, retina; △——△, cerebellum; ■——■, olfactory bulb; ●——●, basal ganglia; □——□, cortex; *——*, medulla.

olfactory bulb, basal ganglia, cortex, and medulla. In the presence of anti-NS-5 antiserum and complement, a high percentage of cells from the retina, cerebellum, and olfactory bulb were killed. More than 50% of the cells in the basal ganglia cell suspension and less than 50% of cells in the cortex cell suspension were killed. There was almost no specific kill on the medulla cells; however, these data are hard to evaluate due to the high values obtained in the complement controls, which reflect the difficulties encountered in preparing viable cell suspensions from this part of the brain at P1. The results of the cytotoxicity tests shown in Fig. 2 are in concordance with the results of absorption analyses, in that cells from parts of the brain that gave the greatest cytotoxicity when used as target cells in the cytotoxicity test also have the highest absorptive capacity. From these results neural retina, cerebellum, and olfactory bulb were judged to have the highest level of antigen expression; cortex and basal ganglia, intermediate; and medulla, low levels. Hippocampus, thalamus, and isocortex have also been shown to express the NS-5 antigen(s), whereas the meninges, a tissue of mesodermal origin on the surface of the brain, was found to be negative (21).

In order to determine which cell type carries the NS-5 antigen(s), 5 tumors of putatively glial cell origin (Table I) derived from the mouse central nervous system had been examined and shown not to express detectable amounts of NS-5 (21). Since the anti-NS-5 antiserum crossreacts with antigens on brain cells from several mammalian species, including rat, rabbit, cat, and human (A. Zimmermann and M. Schachner, unpublished observations), these studies were extended to a number of cell lines derived from the rat central nervous system. Figure 3 shows the results of cytotoxicity tests on mouse P4 cerebellar target cells after absorption of the anti-NS-5 antiserum with adult C57BL/6J

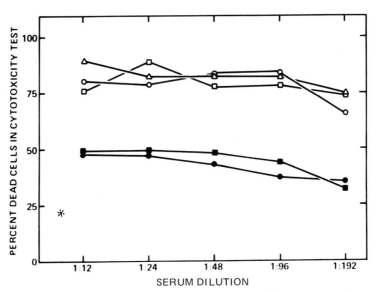

Fig. 3. Expression of NS-5 antigen(s) on cerebellum of adult C57BL/6J mice and BDIX rats as determined by absorption of cytotoxic antibodies, using 0.05 ml of packed tissue and 0.05 ml of antiserum dilution. O——O, BDIX rat liver; ■——■, BDIX rat cerebellum; △——△, C57BL/6J mouse liver; ●——●, C57BL/6J mouse cerebellum; □----□, unabsorbed antiserum; * = complement control.

mouse or BDIX rat cerebellum. The absorptive capacity of adult cerebellum from both species is quite similar; this was also seen with the cerebellum of postnatal day 4 mouse and rat. Previous experiments had shown that the adult mouse neural retina, a part of the central nervous system with neurons comprising more than 90% of its total cell population (M. M. LaVail, personal communication), expressed high levels of NS-5 antigen(s), whereas 5 putative glial tumors of the mouse did not carry detectable antigen(s) (21). It was therefore of special interest to test the rat clonal cell lines classified as neuronal, that is, B103, B104, B35, B50, and B65 (22). Eleven other lines not classified as neuronal, B108, B82, B49, B111, B92, B6, B11, B12, B9, B19, and B23, were also tested. The absorptions were performed using cells that had been cultured to near confluency. Figure 4 presents the results of absorption experiments using the lines B103, B35, B92, and B6. Surprisingly, not one of the 16 clonal cell lines was found to express detectable levels of NS-5 antigen(s). In order to test the possibility that the NS-5 antigen(s) might be expressed when the cell lines were grown in vivo, the lines B82, B108, B103, B35, B65, B50, B92, B11, and B104 were passaged in BDIX rats. After subcutaneous passage for 2–3 weeks, solid tumors derived from these cell lines still did not express detectable NS-5 antigen(s) as judged by absorption tests.

In a previous report, it was shown that NS-5 antigen(s) were present on the brain and spinal cord, but not on gut, liver, or skin during embryonic development (21). These results were obtained by absorbing the anti-NS-5 antiserum with the different parts of the mouse embryo, followed by cytotoxicity tests on P4 cerebellar cells. This type of analysis, however, permits only the demonstration of the presence or absence of cytotoxic antibodies, whereas antibodies that bind to the cell but do not fix complement would remain undetected. In view of the possibility of using for further analysis a fluorescence-activated cell sorter (FACS) (27) to sort NS-5 antigen(s) bearing cells from the developing mouse embryo, it was necessary to determine whether the binding of anti-NS-5 antibodies measured by indirect immunofluorescence followed the same specificity patterns observed in absorption and cytotoxicity tests. Consequently, cells from different parts of the

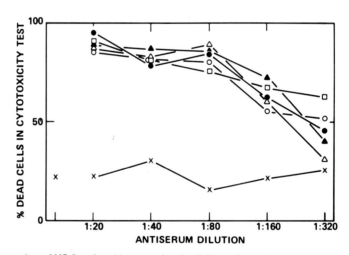

Fig. 4. Representation of NS-5 antigen(s) on rat clonal cell lines of central nervous system origin as judged by absorption of cytotoxic antibodies, using 0.05 ml of packed cells and 0.05 ml of antiserum dilution. X——X, P4 cerebellum; □——□, B103; △——△, B35; ○——○, B92; ▲——▲, B6; ●——●, P4 liver; X = complement control.

mouse embryo were stained with anti-NS-5 antiserum, and the stained cells were then analyzed by fluorescence microscopy or by the cell sorter. Figure 5 shows the result of such an analysis on liver and brain cells from embryonic day 13 (E13) mouse embryos and on thymocytes from adult mice. A three-step staining procedure was employed for liver and thymocytes, tissues that had been shown to be negative by cytotoxicity and absorption assays. This staining procedure would magnify and enable detection of very small amounts of fluorescence over the control staining with normal mouse serum. No specific staining with the NS-5 antiserum was detected by fluorescence microscopy on thymocytes or liver cells. When these cells were analyzed by the FACS, there was only a slight increase in the staining of liver cells and thymocytes with anti-NS-5 antiserum over the preimmunization control serum. In contrast, there is a clear difference between the staining profiles of control serum and anti-NS-5 antiserum on E13 brain cells, using a two-step staining procedure.

Studies were conducted to investigate the presence of the NS-5 antigen(s) on pre-implantation stages of development, using a three-step staining procedure and fluorescence microscopy. The (2–4)-cell stage (Fig. 6); the (8–16)-cell stage; morulae; and the trophoblastic cells of the blastocyst could all be shown to specifically stain with anti-NS-5 antiserum, in comparison to normal mouse serum.

DISCUSSION

The anti-NS-5 antiserum raised in C3H.SW/Sn mice against cerebellum cells of postnatal day 4 C57BL/6J mice detects a cell surface antigen or set of antigens on cells of the central nervous system. Cells of peripheral nervous system origin — C1300, a neuronal tumor of sympathetic origin, superior cervical ganglion cells, and the hybrid cell line NX-31 — do not express detectable NS-5 antigen(s). However, only these three have been tested so far, and only one of them is nontransformed. Therefore it remains to be determined whether other parts of the peripheral nervous system also do not carry the NS-5 antigen(s). Mature spermatozoa and postnatal day 4 (P4), but not adult, kidney cells also express antigen(s) recognized by the anti-NS-5 antiserum (21). Absorptive capacity of sperm could not be demonstrated when either neural retina or cerebellar cells were used as target cells in the cytotoxicity test. However, absorption with sperm, neural retina, or P4 cerebellum completely removes anti-NS-5 antibody activity when medulloepithelioma cells are used as target cells (21). The reaction of anti-NS-5 antiserum with sperm and P4 kidney is interesting, expecially since it is a feature that has been observed with several other, heterologous antisera raised against nervous tissue (4,8,9,11), and with serum from nonimmune C3H mice (10). The potential crossreactivity between brain and sperm antigens may be more than coincidental. For example, a number of neurological mutations in mice, like *quaking (qk)* (30) and *purkinje cell degeneration (pcd)* (31), as well as several mutations in the T locus that affect neuroectodermal development (32), also affect spermatogenesis [for further discussion, see (9,21)].

The NS-5 antigen(s) operationally defined by absorption, cytotoxicity, and indirect immunofluorescence could be detected not only on cerebellar cells, but also on cells from other regions of the brain; for example, neural retina, olfactory bulb, basal ganglia, cortex, and so forth. The anti-NS-5 antiserum does not contain antibody activity directed exclusively against cerebellum, in contrast to another antiserum, anti-Cb1 (8), raised in rabbits against mouse cerebellar cell aggregates. There is a high absorptive capacity of some neuron-rich parts of the central nervous system, like neural retina, early postnatal cerebellum, and olfactory bulb in comparison to a low absorptive capacity of white matter (medulla) regions. These findings, in conjunction with the apparent absence of NS-5 antigen(s) on 5 putative glial cell tumors, may indicate that the NS-5 antigen(s) is associated with neurons rather than glial cells. In view of the abundance of cells in the brain that express NS-5 antigen(s), it was indeed surprising that none of the 16-cell lines from the rat central nervous system expressed detectable NS-5 antigen(s). It is possible

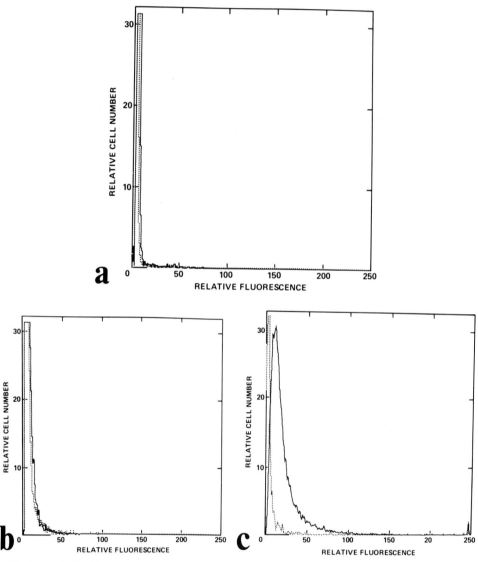

Fig. 5. Analysis of indirect immunofluorescence staining on adult thymocytes, E13 liver cells and E13 brain cells. Laser wavelength: 488 nm, gain: 10; number of cells analyzed: 10,000. a) Thymocytes stained with normal mouse serum (. . . . .) or anti-NS-5 antiserum (——), and rabbit anti-mouse gamma globulin and fluoresceinated goat anti-rabbit gamma globulin; b) E13 liver cells stained as a); c) E13 brain cells stained with normal mouse serum (. . . .) or anti-NS-5 antiserum (——) and fluoresceinated rabbit anti-mouse gamma globulin.

Fig. 6. Indirect immunofluorescence staining on 2-cell-stage embryos as described in Materials and Methods with a) normal mouse serum; b) anti-NS-5 antiserum.

that the cell types from which the different rat cell lines were derived do not normally express NS-5 antigen(s). Alternatively, expression of the antigen(s) might have been lost as a result of transformation, cloning, or in vitro culture. Loss of NS-5 antigen(s) expression due to in vitro culture conditions seems unlikely, however, since the antigen(s) was still not detectable after the rat cell lines were passaged in vivo.

The apparent paradox that the anti-NS-5 antiserum reaction with spermatozoa is detected only when medulloepithelioma cells are used as target cells following anti-NS-5 antiserum absorption with sperm, but not when cerebellar target cells are used, may also pertain to the findings with the rat cell lines. So far, only cerebellar cells have been used as target cells after absorption of anti-NS-5 antisera with the different rat CNS cell lines. It is possible that shared specificities would be detected, if medulloepithelioma cells were used as target cells following antiserum absorption. Given these unknowns, the studies conducted with the mouse tumors and rat clonal cell lines cannot be used to argue for or against the neuronal nature of the cells expressing NS-5 antigen(s).

The delineation of which cell type expresses the NS-5 antigen(s) is important not only for studies on cell interactions in the early postnatal and adult brain, but also for studies on the development of the nervous system, particularly neural cell differentiation. This characterization awaits future studies using horseradish peroxidase staining on brain sections, or using a fluorescence-activated cell sorter to obtain viable NS-5 antigen(s) bearing cells for analysis in cell culture.

We had shown previously that cells of the brain and spinal cord from the developing mouse embryo express the NS-5 antigen(s) as determined by absorptions and cytotoxicity assays, but cells from gut, liver, and skin were found to be negative in these assays (21). The same result has now been obtained by indirect immunofluorescent staining. No specific staining could be detected on liver cells and thymocytes, either by fluorescence microscopy or by the more sensitive analysis on the FACS, whereas brain cells were stained strongly by the NS-5 antiserum in comparison to preimmunization serum. Surprisingly, preimplantation stages of development from two-cell stage to blastocyst are also stained specifically by the NS-5 antiserum. It appeared that all blastomeres at each stage were labeled. No information is as yet available about the inner cell mass of the blastocyst, and further experiments are necessary to ascertain the identity of the antigen(s) recognized on central nervous system cells and on preimplantation embryos. Preliminary experiments have shown, however, that two-cell stages are no longer stained when the antiserum has been preabsorbed with brain.

ACKNOWLEDGMENTS

The authors are grateful to Dr. M. Iverson for running the cell sorter analysis, Dr. D. Schubert for supplying the rat clonal cell lines, and to Ms. Mary Vadeboncoeur, Brenda Job, and Kathy Wortham for their skillful technical assistance. We are especially indebted to Dr. Eric M. Shooter for providing support and facilities for this project and for many helpful discussions. A. Z. would like to thank the DAAD for their support. J. L. P. is a recipient of an Arthritis Foundation Postdoctoral Fellowship.

REFERENCES

1. Cantor, H., and Boyse, E. A.: J. Reticuloendoth. Soc. 17:115 (1975).
2. Goldschneider, I., and Moscona, A. A.: J. Cell Biol. 53:435 (1972).

3. Raff, M. C., Nase, S., and Mitchison, N. A.: Nature 230:50 (1971).
4. Martin, S. E.: Nature 249:71 (1974).
5. Akeson, R., and Herschman, H.: Nature 249:620 (1974).
6. Schachner, M.: Proc. Nat. Acad. Sci. USA 71:1795 (1974).
7. Schachner, M., and Carnow, T. B.: Brain Res. 88:394 (1975).
8. Seeds, N. K.: Proc. Nat. Acad. Sci. USA 72:4110 (1975).
9. Schachner, M., Wortham, K. A., Carter, L. D., and Chaffee, J. K.: Develop. Biol. 44:313 (1975).
10. Martin, S. E., and Martin, W. J.: Proc. Nat. Acad. Sci. USA 72:1036 (1975).
11. Fields, K. L., Gosling, C., Megson, M., and Stein, P. L.: Proc. Nat. Acad. Sci. USA 72:1296 (1975).
12. Stallcup, W. B., and Cohn, M.: Exptl. Cell Res. 98:285 (1976).
13. Pollack, R. E., and Hough, P. V. C.: Ann. Rev. Medicine 25:431 (1974).
14. Hogg, N. M.: Proc. Nat. Acad. Sci. USA 71:489 (1974).
15. Sundaraj, N., Schachner, M., and Pfeiffer, S. E.: Proc. Nat. Acad. Sci. USA 72:1927 (1975).
16. Eccles, J. H., Ho, M., and Szentagothi, J.: "The Cerebellum as a Neuronal Machine." Berlin: Springer-Verlag, 1967.
17. Palay, S., and Chan-Palay, V.: "Cerebellar Cytology and Organization." Berlin-Heidelberg—New York: Springer-Verlag, 1973.
18. Eccles, J. C.: J. Physiol. (London) 229:1 (1973).
19. Nelson, P. G., and Peacock, J. H.: Brain Res. 61:163 (1973).
20. Rakic, P.: J. Comp. Neurol. 141:283 (1971).
21. Zimmermann, A., and Schachner, M.: Brain Res. 115:297 (1976).
22. Schubert, D., Heinemann, S., Carlisle, W., Tarikas, H., Hines, B., Patrick, J., Steinbach, J. H., Culp, W., and Brandt, B. L.: Nature 249:224 (1974).
23. Brinster, R. L.: J. Reprod. Fertility 10:227 (1965).
24. Mintz, B.: Science 138:594 (1962).
25. Ouchterlony, O.: Progr. Allergy 6:30 (1962).
26. Cebra, J. J., and Goldstein, G.: J. Immunol. 95:230 (1965).
27. Hulett, H. R., Bonner, W. A., Sweet, R. G., and Herzenberg, L. A.: Clin. Chem. 19:813 (1973).
28. Chaffee, J. K., and Schachner, M.: Manuscript in preparation.
29. Chalazonitis, A., Greene, L. A., and Shain, W.: Exptl. Cell Res. 96:225 (1975).
30. Bennett, W. I., Gale, A. M., Southard, J. L., and Sidman, R. L.: Biol. of Reprod. 5:30 (1971).
31. Mullen, R. J., Eicher, E. M., and Sidman, R. L.: Proc. Nat. Acad. Sci. USA 73:208 (1976).
32. Bennett, D. Cell 6:441 (1975).

Journal of Supramolecular Structure 5:431 (35)–451 (55) (1976)

The Structure of the Gramicidin A Transmembrane Channel

William Veatch

Department of Molecular Biophysics and Biochemistry, Yale University, New Haven, Connecticut 06520

Gramicidin A is a linear polypeptide antibiotic that facilitates the diffusion of monovalent cations across lipid bilayer membranes by forming channels. It has been proposed that the conducting channel is a dimer which is in equilibrium with nonconducting monomers in the membrane. To directly test this model in several independent ways, we have prepared and purified a series of gramicidin C derivatives. All of these derivatives are fully active analogs of gramicidin A, and each derivative has a useful chromophore esterified to the phenolic hydroxyl of tyrosine #11.

Simultaneous conductance and fluorescence measurements on planar lipid bilayer membranes containing dansyl gramicidin C yielded four conclusions: 1) A plot of the logarithm of the membrane conductance versus the logarithm of the membrane fluorescence had a slope of 2.0 ± 0.3, over a concentration range for which nearly all the gramicidin was monomeric. Hence, the active channel is a dimer of the nonconducting species. 2) In a membrane in which nearly all of the gramicidin was dimeric, the number of channels was approximately equal to the number of dimers. Thus, most dimers are active channels and so it should be feasible to carry out spectroscopic studies of the conformation of the transmembrane channel. 3) The association constant for dimerization is more than 1,000-fold larger in a glycerolester membrane with 26 Å-hydrocarbon thickness than in a 47 Å-glycerolester membrane. The dimerization constant in a 48 Å-phosphatidyl choline membrane was 200 times larger than in a 47 Å-glycerolester membrane, showing that it depends on the type of lipid as well as on the thickness of the hydrocarbon core. 4) We were readily able to detect 10^{-14} mole cm^{-2} of dansyl gramicidin C in a bilayer membrane, which corresponds to 60 fluorescent molecules per square μm. The fluorescent techniques described here should be sufficiently sensitive for fluorescence studies of reconstituted gates and receptors in planar bilayer membranes.

An alternative method of determining the number of molecules of gramicidin in the channel is to measure the fraction of hybrid channels present in a mixture of 2 chemically different gramicidins. The single-channel conductance of p-phenylazo-benzene-sulfonyl ester gramicidin C (PABS gramicidin C) was found to be 0.68 that of gramicidin A. In membranes containing a mixture of these 2 gramicidins, a hybrid channel was evident in addition to 2 pure channels. The hybrid channel conductance was 0.82 that of gramicidin A. Fluorescence energy transfer from dansyl gramicidin C to diethylamino-phenylazobenzene-sulfonyl ester gramicidin C (DPBS gramicidin C), provided an independent way to measure the fraction of hybrid channels on liposomes. For both techniques the fraction of hybrid channels was found to be 2ad where a^2 and d^2 were the fractions of the 2 kinds of pure channels. This result strongly supports a dimer channel and the hybrid data excludes the possibility of a

William Veatch is now at the Department of Pharmacology, Harvard Medical School, Boston, MA 02115.

tetramer channel. The study of hybrid species by conductance and fluorescence techniques should be generally useful in elucidating the subunit structure of oligomeric assemblies in membranes.

The various models which have been proposed for the conformation of the gramicidin transmembrane channel are briefly discussed.

Key words: gramicidin A, channel, fluorescence energy transfer, membrane fluorimeter, antibiotic, hybrid channels, gramicidin C derivatives

INTRODUCTION

Gramicidin A, a linear polypeptide antibiotic, renders biological membranes and synthetic lipid bilayer membranes permeable to alkali cations and protons (1—4). The amino acid sequence of valine gramicidin A is (5):

CHO-L-Val-Gly-L-Ala-D-Leu-L-Ala-D-Val-L-Val-D-Val-
1   2   3   4   5   6   7   8
L-Trp-D-Leu-L-Trp-D-Leu-L-Trp-D-Leu-L-Trp-NHCH$_2$CH$_2$OH
9   10   11   12   13   14   15

The distinctive features of this amino acid sequence are the alternation of D and L amino acids, the presence of hydrophobic side chains, and the absence of any charged groups. Gramicidin C is a naturally-occurring variant in which L-tryptophan at position 11 is replaced by L-tyrosine.

Gramicidin A induces cation permeability by forming transmembrane channels rather than by acting as a diffusional carrier (6). Synthetic bilayer membranes containing very small amounts of gramicidin A exhibit discrete changes in conductance which arise from the formation and breakdown of individual gramicidin channels (4). The conductance of a single channel depends on the concentration and type of ion but not on the thickness or viscosity of the membrane (6). It has been observed that the membrane conductance is approximately proportional to the square of the amount of gramicidin A added to the aqueous phase, which suggested that the conducting channel is a dimer (7—8). However, this inference is not unequivocal because gramicidin A has such a low solubility in water that it irreversibly adsorbs to the membrane, and so the actual amount incorporated in the membrane is uncertain. The order of the channel-forming reaction has been further studied by a voltage-jump approach (9), which is based on the finding that the number of channels increases as the membrane is thinned by an applied voltage (6). The results of these voltage-jump experiments are consistent with the hypothesis of an equilibrium in the membrane between a nonconducting monomer and a conducting dimer of gramicidin A (9), but these data do not strongly exclude the possibility that channel formation is a trimerization (10). Similar results have also been obtained from an autocorrelation analysis of the conductance fluctuations (10—11).

Clearly the most direct way to characterize the equilibrium between channel and nonconducting gramicidin in the membrane is to measure directly the surface density of gramicidin in the membrane. To this end Veatch and Blout (12) prepared dansyl gramicidin C, which is a highly fluorescent and fully active analog of gramicidin A. The preparation of the 3 gramicidin C derivatives used in this work are described below. First, we will develop the theoretical framework we need to analyze the simultaneous conductance and fluorescence measurements on planar bilayers containing dansyl gramicidin C. Later we will extend our analysis to predict the fraction of hybrid channels in mixtures of 2 different gramicidins. After we have described the results of the hybrid channel experiments, we will conclude by considering the various models that have been proposed for the conformation of the gramicidin channel.

PREPARATION OF GRAMICIDIN C DERIVATIVES

The 3 gramicidin C derivatives used in this study, shown in Fig. 1, were formed by reacting counter-current purified gramicidin C (the generous gift of Dr. Erhard Gross) with the corresponding sulfonyl chlorides. The reaction mixture was then chromatographed on a Sephadex LH-20 column to separate the gramicidin C derivative from the unreacted gramicidin. The elution profile for dansyl gramicidin C is shown in Fig. 2a (12). The ratio of the dansyl absorbance at 350 nm to the tryptophan absorbance at 290 nm showed that the retarded peak contained 1.0 mole of dansyl per mole of gramicidin C. Fraction CIII was estimated to be 90% pure, and has been further chemically and physically characterized by Veatch and Blout (12). PABS gramicidin C and DPBS gramicidin C are non-fluorescent and were prepared specifically to be used as acceptors of fluorescence energy transfer from dansyl gramicidin C. The details of their preparation are given by Veatch and Stryer (14).

STRATEGY FOR MAKING SIMULTANEOUS FLUORESCENCE AND CONDUCTANCE MEASUREMENTS

Consider the equilibrium between an ion-conducting channel containing n molecules, G_n, and nonconducting monomers, G_1:

$$n\,G_1 \rightleftharpoons G_n \tag{1}$$

$$[G_n] = K[G_1]^n \tag{2}$$

where K is the equilibrium constant. The channel surface density, $[G_n]$ (mole cm^{-2}), is readily calculated from the membrane conductance because we know the single channel conductance. The membrane fluorescence is, to a first approximation, proportional to the total amount of gramicidin on the membrane, $[G_t]$ (mole cm^{-2}), given by:

$$[G_t] = [G_1] + n\,[G_n] \tag{3}$$

Figure 3 is a plot of the solution of equation 2 and equation 3 for the dimer case (n = 2). Log $[G_2]$ is plotted as a function of log $[G_t]$ for various values of the dimerization

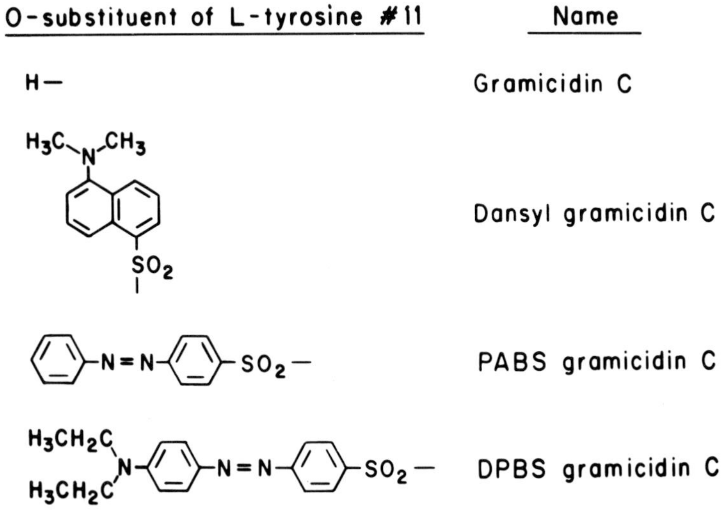

O-substituent of L-tyrosine #11	Name
H—	Gramicidin C
	Dansyl gramicidin C
	PABS gramicidin C
	DPBS gramicidin C

Fig. 1. Structure and nomenclature of derivatives of gramicidin C.

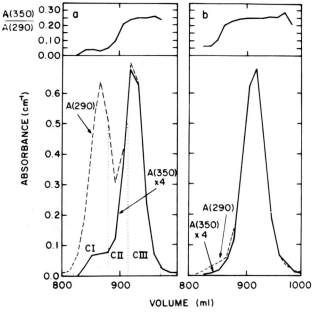

Fig. 2. (a) Elution profile of dansylation products of gramicidin C on Sephadex LH-20 column (150 cm × 4 cm) in methanol. (b) Rechromatography of fraction CIII from (a).

constant K. This solution takes on a simple mathematical form in 2 limiting cases which are of great interest to us. For sufficiently low values of $[G_t]$ and K, essentially all of the gramicidin is monomeric, $[G_t]$ closely approximates $[G_1]$, and the slope of the log-log plot is equal to the number of molecules in the channel, n, here equal to 2.

$$[G_n] \simeq K [G_t]^n \qquad \text{for } [G_t]^{n-1} K \ll 1 \tag{4}$$

The other limit of great interest occurs when $[G_t]$ and K are sufficiently high so that essentially all of the gramicidin is aggregated. In this case the conductance is not dependent upon the dimerization constant, and the log-log plot has a slope of unity.

$$[G_n] \simeq \frac{[G_t]}{n} \qquad \text{for } [G_t]^{n-1} K \gg 1 \tag{5}$$

To test our model and determine n and K for a single membrane, it is evident from Fig. 3 that one would have to measure $[G_2]$ and $[G_t]$ over many orders of magnitude. However, not all combinations of $[G_t]$ and $[G_2]$ are experimentally accessible. $[G_t]$ must be sufficiently high so that the fluorescence of dansyl gramicidin C in the membrane exceeds the background fluorescence due to the membrane lipids. In practice, this occurred when $[G_t]$ was greater than 10^{-14} mole cm^{-2}. In contrast, $[G_2]$ had to be less than about 4×10^{-14} moles cm^{-2} so that the membrane conductance could be measured accurately; at higher values of $[G_2]$, the resistance of the solution surrounding the membrane is much greater than that of the membrane itself. The experimental significance of these limits on the observable values of $[G_t]$ and $[G_2]$ can be appreciated by considering Fig. 3. For a single kind of membrane, it is not feasible to make simultaneous fluorescence and conductance measurements over a range of $[G_t]$ yielding mostly monomer ($[G_t] \ll 1/K$) to mostly dimer ($[G_t] \gg 1/K$). However, these limiting cases, which are most decisive

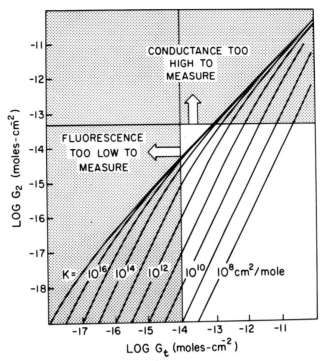

Fig. 3. Theoretical dimerization curves and feasibility region for simultaneous fluorescence and conductance measurements. The curves are plots of the dimer surface density, $[G_2]$, as a function of the total surface density, $[G_t]$, for values of the dimerization constant, K, ranging from 10^8 to 10^{17} $mole^{-1}$ cm^2, according to equations 2 and 3 for n = 2.

in testing the dimer model (equations 4 and 5), are experimentally accessible if membranes having very different values of K are used. This was achieved by using a series of glycerol-ester membranes differing in the thickness of their hydrocarbon core (6, 13) (Table I). The duration of single channels of gramicidin A in these glycerolester membranes (6) suggested that they have a wide range of dimerization constants, which is in fact the case. We will refer to these membranes by the thickness of their hydrocarbon core (e.g., 26 Å-glycerolester membrane).

Later, we will extend equation 4 and equation 5 to predict the fraction of hybrid channels in mixtures of 2 gramicidins for each of our 2 limiting cases; but first let us consider the results of the simultaneous conductance and fluorescence measurements on planar bilayer membranes containing dansyl gramicidin C.

SIMULTANEOUS CONDUCTANCE AND FLUORESCENCE MEASUREMENTS

Veatch et al. (15) have shown that dansyl gramicidin C is a fully active and fluorescent analog of gramicidin A. The fluorescence excitation and emission spectra of dansyl gramicidin C on liposomes are shown in Fig. 4. The quantum yield was found to be 0.45. The single-channel conductance for dansyl gramicidin C in 1M KCl was found to be 2.4 $\times$ 10^{-11} Ω^{-1}. The membrane fluorimeters used to measure the fluorescence from single planar lipid bilayer membranes, shown schematically in Fig. 5, have been described in detail by Veatch et al. (15).

TABLE I. Hydrocarbon Thickness of Bilayer Membranes Formed From Glycerol Monoester-Alkaline Mixtures

Glycerol monoester	Alkane	Hydrocarbon thickness (Å)
Glycerol-l-palmitoleate	n-hexadecane	26
Glycerol-l-oleate	n-hexadecane	31
Glycerol-l-oleate	n-tetradecane	40
Glycerol-l-oleate	n-decane	47

From Hladky and Haydon (6).

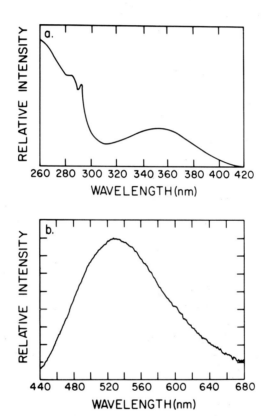

Fig. 4. Corrected fluorescence excitation and emission spectra of dansyl gramicidin C in vesicles. The vesicles contained a 1:50 mole ratio of dansyl gramicidin C to dioleoyl phosphatidyl choline in 0.16 M KCl (plus 4% ethanol). For the excitation spectrum in (a) the emission wavelength was 530 nm and for the emission spectrum in (b) the excitation wavelength was 350 nm. The slit widths were 4 nm and 2 nm, respectively. A red-sensitive photomultiplier tube (EMI 9658R) was used to obtain these spectra.

The conductance and fluorescence intensity of planar bilayer membranes containing dansyl gramicidin C were measured simultaneously to test directly the dimer model. As mentioned previously, such simultaneous measurements are feasible only if the fluorescence is sufficiently high and the membrane conductance is sufficiently low (Fig. 3). We found that simultaneous fluorescence and conductance measurements could be made over a 10-fold range in the concentration of dansyl gramicidin C in a thick 47 Å-glycerolester membrane. A plot of the logarithm of the conductance versus the logarithm of the fluorescence intensity (Fig. 6) has a slope of 2.0 ± 0.3. For a certain amount of dansyl gramicidin C fluorescence, the 47 Å-glycerolester membrane has about 10^3 lower conductance than the 26 Å-glycerolester membrane. Since gramicidin has the same single-channel conductance on all glycerolester membranes (6), this means that fewer than one gramicidin molecule per 1,000 is involved in channels under these conditions at any given time. Since $[G_t]$ K ≪ 1, the observed slope of 2.0 proves that the channel is a dimer of the nonconducting species.

Is Every Gramicidin Dimer a Conducting Channel?

The absolute surface density of gramicidin must be known to answer this question. Our task of converting the observed fluorescence intensity to the absolute surface density of gramicidin has been greatly facilitated by the work of Zingsheim and Haydon (16). They determined the surface density of 8-anilino-1-napthalene-sulfonic acid (ANS) adsorbed to a 47 Å-glycerolester planar bilayer membrane as a function of the concentration

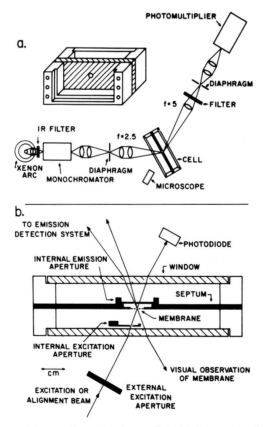

Fig. 5. Schematic diagram of the membrane fluorimeter. Part (a) shows a top view of the physical layout of the standard membrane fluorimeter with a xenon lamp and a monochromator as the excitation source. Part (b) shows a cross-section of a modification of the standard membrane fluorimeter in which an argon-ion laser was used with apertures inside the cell to eliminate the possibility of detecting torus fluorescence. The emission optics external to the cell were unchanged.

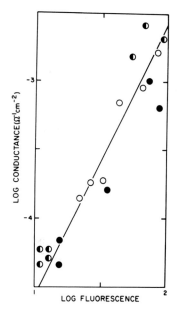

Fig. 6. Conductance as a function of fluorescence for dansyl gramicidin C in 47 Å-glycerolester membranes. The laser excitation modification was used to obtain 3 independent sets of points. These
fluorescence values were then normalized using membrane-bound ANS as a fluorescence standard. The
least-square slopes for these 3 sets of data are 2.0 ± 0.2 (open circles), 2.1 ± 0.2 (half-filled circles), and
1.7 ± 0.2 (filled circles).

of ANS in the ambient solution. We used a 47Å-glycerolester membrane in 0.1 M NaCl
containing 1.3×10^{-6} M ANS, which gives an ANS surface density of 7.1×10^{-13} mole
cm^{-2} (16), as a membrane fluorescence standard. The surface density of dansyl gramicidin C could then be calculated from the ratio of the fluorescence intensity of dansyl
gramicidin C to that of the ANS membrane standard, taking into account the relative
fluorescence parameters of the 2 chromophores (15).

The simultaneous conductance and fluorescence data for membranes of varying
thickness are shown in Fig. 7, superimposed upon the calculated dimerization curves of
Fig. 3. Note that the fluorescence has been converted to total surface density (mole cm^{-2})
and the conductance to channel surface density (multiplied by 2). For a fixed gramicidin
surface density, the membrane conductance increases dramatically as the thickness of the
glycerolester membrane decreases from 47 Å (open circles) to 40 Å (half-filled circles), to
31 Å (open square) and 26 Å (filled circle). The estimated dimerization constant, summarized in Table II, increases at least 1,000-fold for a thickness change from 47 Å to 31 Å.
However, the structure of the lipid also affects the dimerization constant. The 48 Å thick
phosphatidyl choline membrane (filled square) has a dimerization constant 200-fold
greater than the glycerolester membrane of the same thickness.

The last important conclusion to be drawn from Fig. 7 requires a quantitative comparison of the fluorescence and conductance found for the 26 Å-glycerolester membrane.
The average fluorescence value was about 30% less than that calculated from the average
conductance value, assuming that all of the gramicidin on this thinnest membrane was in
dimer channels. Because it is estimated that the gramicidin surface density calculated from

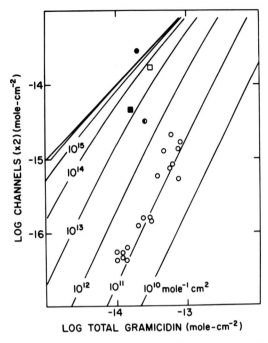

Fig. 7. Channel surface density as a function of total gramicidin surface density for planar bilayer membranes of different composition. The lines are theoretical dimerization curves like those in Fig. 3. The fluorescence has been converted to total gramicidin surface density, and the specific conductance has been converted to channel surface density. The single-channel conductance of the glycerolester membranes in 0.1 M NaCl was taken to be $4 \times 10^{-12} \Omega^{-1}$. For the phosphatidyl choline membrane in 1 M NaCl, the single-channel conductance was estimated to be $7 \times 10^{-12} \Omega^{-1}$. The laser excitation modification was employed for the 40 Å- and the 47 Å-glycerolester membranes and the standard membrane fluorimeter for the others. Open circles: 47 Å-glycerolester membrane; half-filled circle: 40 Å-glycerolester membrane; open square: 31 Å-glycerolester membrane; filled circle: 26 Å-glycerolester membrane; filled square: 48 Å-phosphatidyl choline membrane.

the fluorescence is correct within a factor of 2, these results strongly suggest that most, if not all, gramicidin dimers are conducting channels. Thus it should be possible to use spectroscopic techniques to study the structure of the dimer channel.

THE HYBRID STRATEGY FOR STUDYING OLIGOMERS

An alternative way to determine the number of gramicidin molecules in the transmembrane channel is to measure the fraction of hybrid channels in a mixture of 2 chemically different gramicidins. Figure 8 illustrates the result expected for a dimer. Let us denote the 2 gramicidins as "A" and "D". If the fraction of pure A dimers is a^2 and the fraction of pure D dimers is d^2, then the expected fraction of hybrid dimers is $2ad$. This is exactly the result obtained for the gramicidin channel. The results expected for the most simple trimer and tetramer models are summarized in Table III. Veatch and Stryer (14) have used 2 independent methods to measure the fraction of hybrid channels: single-channel conductance measurements and fluorescence energy transfer measurements on liposomes.

TABLE II. Dimerization Constants for Dansyl Gramicidin C Estimated From Simultaneous Fluorescence and Conductance Measurements

Membrane	Hydrocarbon thickness (Å)	Dimerization constant $(mol^{-1} cm^2)$
Glycerolester	47†	1×10^{11}
	40†	3×10^{12}
	31†	$\geqslant 10^{14}$
	26†	$\geqslant 10^{14}$
Phosphatidyl choline	48‡	2×10^{13}

†From Hladky and Haydon (6).
‡From Bamberg and Läuger (9).

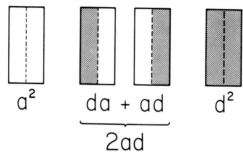

Fig. 8. In the dimer model, the relative proportion of the hybrid species is 2ad, where a and d are the mole fractions of the 2 kinds of gramicidin.

TABLE III. Calculated Probabilities of Pure and Hybrid Channels for Various Models

	Pure A	Hybrid	Pure D
Dimer	a^2	$2ad$	d^2
Trimer	a^3	$3a^2d + 3ad^2$	d^3
Tetramer	a^4	$4a^3d + 6a^2d^2 + 4ad^3$	d^4
n-mer	a^n	$(a + d)^n - a^n - d^n$	d^n

Single-Channel Conductance Measurements: Demonstration of Hybrid Channels

The single-channel conductance of PABS gramicidin C is 0.68 that of gramicidin A (Figs. 9a, b). An interesting result was obtained for membranes containing both PABS gramicidin C and gramicidin A. These membranes exhibited 3 kinds of channels: a pure PABS gramicidin C channel, a pure gramicidin A channel, and a hybrid channel with an intermediate conductance (Fig. 9c). A histogram of the frequency of occurrence of a conductance step as a function of the step size, measured from many records like the one in Fig. 9c, is shown in Fig. 10. The average single-channel conductance of the hybrid species is 0.82 that of gramicidin A. This value for the hybrid corresponds to the geometric mean of the values for the 2 pure species. The standard deviation of the single-channel conductance of the hybrid is not appreciably greater than that of the 2 pure channels. Thus, the hybrid channel appears to be a unique species.

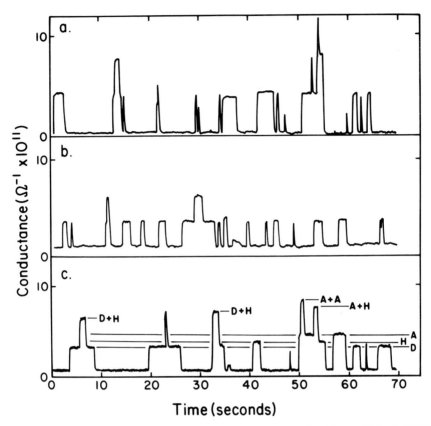

Fig. 9. Single-channel conductance fluctuations of membranes containing (a) gramicidin A, (b) PABS gramicidin C, and (c) a mixture of the 2. The horizontal lines in (c) indicate the conductance corresponding to pure PABS gramicidin C channels (labeled D), pure gramicidin A channels (labeled A) and hybrid channels (labeled H). The conductance levels arising from 2 channels are also shown.

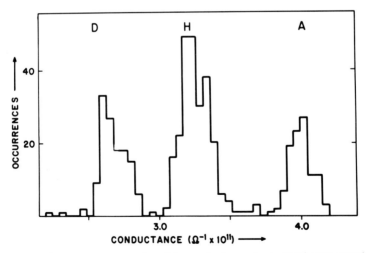

Fig. 10. Frequency of occurrence versus size of the conductance step in membranes containing a mixture of PABS gramicidin C and gramicidin A. The labels D and A refer to the pure species and H to the hybrid. The standard deviation is 2.8% for H, compared to 3.0% for D and 2.3% for A.

The frequencies of these 3 kinds of channels depended on the relative amounts of PABS gramicidin C and gramicidin A in the membrane-forming solution (Fig. 11). The frequency of the hybrid channel reached a maximum value of 0.5 when the frequencies of the pure channels were each about 0.25. This finding suggests that the hybrid channel is a dimer, which is predicted to have a hybrid frequency of $2ad = 0.5$ when $a^2 = d^2 = 0.25$. In the following discussion we will denote the concentrations of pure gramicidin A dimers by $[AA]$, of the pure PABS gramicidin dimers by $[DD]$, and of the hybrid dimers by $[AD]$.

Conductance Evidence That the Hybrid Channel is a Dimer

Because single-channel conductance measurements are made at very low surface densities, only a minute fraction of the gramicidin on these membranes will form channels at any given time. We need to extend our previous expression for the channel surface density in this limiting case, equation 4, rewritten below for $n = 2$:

$$[G_2] \simeq K[G_t]^2 \qquad \text{for } K [G_t] \ll 1 \qquad (4')$$

Let us denote the fraction of pure A channels by f_A, the fraction of pure D channels by f_D, and the fraction of hybrid channels by f_H.

$$f_A = a^2 \qquad (6)$$
$$f_D = d^2 \qquad (7)$$
$$f_H = 2ad \qquad (8)$$

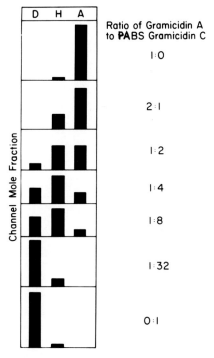

Fig. 11. Probabilities of the 3 kinds of channels (D, H, and A) as a function of the ratio of gramicidin A to PABS gramicidin C in the membrane-forming solution. Each histogram represents the average of several records accumulated by the probability-distribution analyzer (Saicor model 42A).

To understand the meaning of a and d in general, we must define a few more experimental parameters. Let us denote the pure A dimerization constant as K_A, the pure D dimerization constant as K_D, and the hybrid dimerization constant as K_H. The total monomer concentrations in the membrane-forming solution, denoted $[A_s]$ and $[D_s]$, are related to the total monomer surface densities $[A_t]$ and $[D_t]$ by empirical partition coefficients P_A and P_D. Note that all we can determine in this experiment are the concentrations in the membrane-forming solution $[A_s]$ and $[D_s]$, because we can not make fluorescence measurements at these very low surface densities. If the dimerization constants are all equal, and the partition coefficients are both equal as well, then a and d are the mole fractions calculated from the known concentrations in the membrane-forming solution, $[A_s]$ and $[Ds]$, and $a/d = [A_s]/[D_s]$. In general (as long as $K_H^2 = K_D K_A$) the ratio $a/d = \gamma \, [A_s]/[D_s]$ where

$$\gamma = \left[\frac{K_A P_A^2}{K_D P_D^2} \right]^{1/2} \tag{9}$$

The experimental results can be compared with predictions for the dimer model by casting equations (6) to (8) into a simple form. The ratio of the probability of each of the pure channels to that of the hybrid is directly proportional to the concentration of the 2 gramicidins in the membrane-forming solution.

$$\frac{f_H}{2f_D} = \frac{2f_A}{f_H} = \gamma \, \frac{[A_s]}{[D_s]} \tag{10}$$

A plot of log $[f_H/(2f_D)]$ and of log $(2f_A/f_H)$ versus log $([A_s]/[D_s])$ is shown in Fig. 12. Three conclusions can be drawn from these data. First, the experimental data for the ratio of $2f_A/f_H$ are approximately equal to those for $f_H/2f_D$, confirming the dimer model (equation 10). Second, the fit of these data to a line having a slope of 1.0 (the solid line in Fig. 12) indicates that the ratio of the 2 kinds of gramicidin in the membrane is in fact proportional to their ratio in the membrane-forming solution. This proportionality holds at low surface densities, but not at very high surface densities of gramicidin (15). Third, Fig. 12 shows that the factor γ in equation 10 is equal to 3.6. It is known that the dimerization constant for dansyl gramicidin C is not less than that for gramicidin A (15). Most likely, γ differs from unity because gramicidin A partitions more into the membrane than does PABS gramicidin C.

Another way of depicting the experimental data is shown in Fig. 13. The fractions of the 3 kinds of channels are plotted as a function of the effective mole fraction of gramicidin A, which is equal to $\gamma \, [A_s]/(\gamma[A_s] + [D_s])$. This quantity was calculated from $[A_s]$ and $[D_s]$ using the value of $\gamma = 3.6$ determined from Fig. 12.

Energy Transfer Evidence That the Hybrid Channel is a Dimer

Fluorescence energy transfer was used as a complementary means of ascertaining the frequency of hybrid channels. The strategy was to label one gramicidin with a fluorescent energy donor and another with a suitable energy acceptor. The donor-acceptor pair was chosen so that most of the donor fluorescence in a hybrid channel was quenched by energy transfer to the acceptor. The fluorescence intensity of the membranes containing both kinds of gramicidins then revealed the frequency of hybrid channels, which could be compared with predictions for various models.

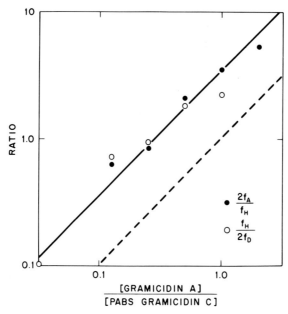

Fig. 12. The probabilities of the 3 kinds of channels (f_A, f_D, and f_H) are shown as a function of the ratio of gramicidin A to PABS gramicidin C in the membrane-forming solution. The ordinate is the ratio $2f_A/f_H$ (filled circles) or $f_H/2f_D$ (open circles). The approximate equality of these ratios supports the dimer model. The fit of these data to the solid line having a slope of 1.0 indicates that the ratio of the 2 kinds of gramicidin in the membrane is proportional to their ratio in the membrane-forming solution. The dashed line is calculated for the case in which the ratio of the 2 gramicidins in the membrane is the same as in the membrane-forming solution. The shift of the solid line from the dashed one indicates that gramicidin A partitions preferentially into the membrane by a factor of 3.6.

Dansyl gramicidin C (Fig. 1) was the fluorescent energy donor in these experiments. PABS gramicidin C (Fig. 1) was considered as a potential energy acceptor. However, it effectively quenches the dansyl fluorescence only at distances of less than about 20 Å because its longest wavelength absorption band is weak ($\epsilon = 500 \text{ cm}^{-1}\text{M}^{-1}$ at $\lambda_{max} = 460$ nm). The strength of this band was increased by preparing DPBS gramicidin C (Fig. 1), the diethylamino derivative of PABS. The resulting extinction coefficient of 33,000 $\text{cm}^{-1}\text{M}^{-1}$ markedly extended the range of efficient energy transfer, as calculated below. The overlap of the emission spectrum of dansyl gramicidin C and the absorption spectrum of DPBS gramicidin C is shown in Fig. 14.

In Förster's theory, the efficiency of singlet-singlet energy transfer E is:

$$E = r^{-6} / (r^{-6} + R_0^{-6}) \tag{11}$$

where r is the distance between the centers of the donor and acceptor chromophores, and R_0 is the distance at which the transfer is 50% efficient (17, 18). R_0 can be calculated from

$$R_0 = (Q_0 \, J \, n^{-4} \, K^2)^{1/6} \times 9.7 \times 10^3 \text{ Å} \tag{12}$$

where Q_0 is the quantum yield of the donor in the absence of the acceptor, J is the spectral overlap integral, n is the refractive index of the intervening medium, and K^2 is the dipole-dipole orientation factor. For transfer from dansyl gramicidin C to DPBS gramicidin C, $Q_0 = 0.45$ (15), $J = 5.1 \times 10^{-14} \text{ cm}^{-3}\text{M}^{-1}$ (Fig. 14), and n is about 1.4. K^2 is assumed to have a value of 2/3, which corresponds to rapid randomization of the orientations of the donor and the acceptor. The plausibility of this assumption is supported by examination of molecular models and by our nanosecond emission anisotropy measurements which show that the dansyl chromophore rotates over an angular range of about 25° in a time that is short compared to the excited state lifetime (19). These values give an R'_0 (20) of 39 Å for transfer from dansyl to DPBS.

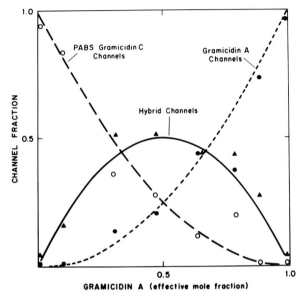

Fig. 13. The observed probabilities of the pure PABS gramicidin C channel (open circle), the pure gramicidin A channel (filled circle), and the hybrid channel (triangle) are plotted as a function of the effective mole fraction of gramicidin A. The calculated probabilities for the dimer model are shown by the dashed, dotted, and solid lines, respectively.

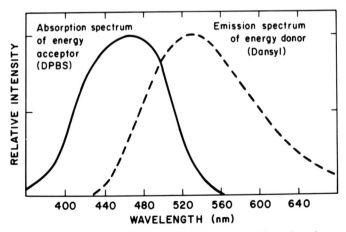

Fig. 14. The absorption spectrum of DPBS gramicidin C (in methanol) overlaps the corrected fluorescence emission spectrum of dansyl gramicidin C (excited at 350 nm) on phosphatidyl choline liposomes. The maximum extinction coefficient of DPBS is 33,000 $cm^{-1}M^{-1}$. The spectral overlap integral is 5 × 10^{-14} $cm^{-3}M^{-1}$.

Liposomes rather than planar bilayer membranes were used because more precise measurements of the fluorescence intensity of liposomes can be made. Also, the ratio of the mole fractions of the donor and acceptor gramicidins in the membranes of liposomes is in fact equal to the ratio at which they were added. Nearly all of the gramicidin is in the channel form in bilayer membranes having sufficiently short hydrocarbon chains and a high enough surface density of gramicidin (15). These 2 conditions are met in the liposomes used in this study. Hence, our fluorescence energy transfer measurements provide information about the structure of the channel.

Energy transfer measurements were carried out on di-(dihydrosterculoyl) phosphatidyl choline liposomes containing a fixed amount of dansyl gramicidin C and a variable amount of DPBS gramicidin C. The surface density of the total gramicidin was less than 1 gramicidin per 1,000 lipid molecules, which means that the mean distance between channels was greater than 250 Å, and so energy transfer between chromophores in different channels was negligible. As the mole fraction of DPBS gramicidin C, the energy acceptor, was increased from 0 to 0.8, the relative fluorescence quantum yield of the dansyl energy donor decreased from 1 to 0.4 (Fig. 15). This quenching of the dansyl fluorescence is due to efficient energy transfer from dansyl to DPBS within a hybrid channel. No quenching would have been observed if the gramicidins were monomeric in this membrane.

We will denote the pure dansyl gramicidin C dimers by [DD], the pure DPBS gramicidin C dimers by [AA], and the hybrid by [AD], where here D refers to the energy donor and A to the energy acceptor. Let us derive the dependence of Q/Q_0, the relative fluorescence quantum yield of the donor, on a, the mole fraction of the energy acceptor, for a dimer. First, we need to extend our previous expression for the channel surface density in the limiting case where almost all of the gramicidin is dimerized, equation 5, rewritten below for n = 2:

$$[G_2] \simeq \frac{[G_t]}{2} \qquad \text{for } K[G_t] \gg 1 \qquad (5')$$

We again obtain the results summarized in equations 6–8. Here a and d are the mole fractions calculated from the total membrane surface densities, $[A_t]$ and $[D_t]$, which we know directly on liposomes. These results are independent of any difference between the dimerization constants K_A and K_D (so long as $K_H{}^2 = K_D K_A$) because essentially all of the gramicidin is dimerized.

If the transfer efficiency within a hybrid dimer is E, then Q/Q_0 is

$$\frac{Q}{Q_0} = \frac{2[DD] + (1-E)[AD]}{2[DD] + [AD]} = 1 - \frac{E[AD]}{2[DD] + [AD]} \qquad (13)$$

Substituting equations 6, 7, and 8 into equation 13, one obtains the very simple expression for the quenching in a dimer

$$Q/Q_0 = 1 - Ea \qquad (14)$$

Thus, for a dimer channel, the relative quantum yield of the donor decreases linearly with the mole fraction of the acceptor. For the simplest trimer models in which all hybrid species are assumed to have the same transfer efficiency (see Table III), $Q/Q_0 = 1 - E + E(1-a)^2$, and for the simplest tetramer model, $Q/Q_0 = 1 - E + E(1-a)^3$.

The observed dependence of Q/Q_0 on a is shown in Fig. 15 with the least-squares fits of the dimer, trimer, and tetramer model to these data. The experimental results best

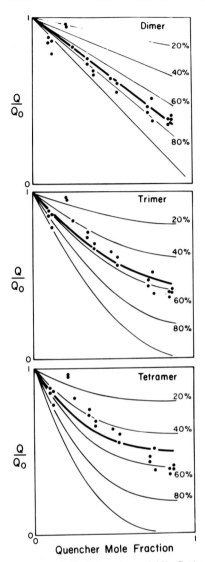

Fig. 15. Relative fluorescence quantum yield of dansyl gramicidin C, the energy donor, as a function of the mole fraction of DPBS gramicidin C, the energy acceptor. The experimental data (closed circles) are compared with light curves calculated assuming 20%, 40%, 60%, 80%, and 100% energy transfer for (a) dimer, (b) trimer, and (c) tetramer models. The bold curves are the least-squares best fits. The best fit standard deviation for the tetramer model is 90% greater than for the dimer model.

fit a dimer model (Fig. 15a). The trimer model cannot be excluded by these results alone (Fig. 15b). However, the trimer model is incompatible with the results of the simultaneous conductance and fluorescence study, which requires that the number of molecules in the channel be an even number, since we proved that the channel was a dimer of the non-conducting species. The tetramer model can be rejected in view of the poor fit of the experimental data to this model (Fig. 15c). The least-squares fit to the dimer model (Fig. 15a) shows that the efficiency of energy transfer within the hybrid channel is 75%. The apparent distance between the centers of the dansyl and DPBS chromophores is 33 Å for $E = 75\%$ and $R'_0 = 39$ Å.

DISCUSSION

Simultaneous Conductance and Fluorescence Measurements on Planar Bilayers

The structure of the gramicidin transmembrane channel is of interest as a model for the passive ion-pathways of cell membranes. The chromophores of the gramicidin C derivatives (Fig. 1) provide useful probes of that structure. The conductance properties of all of these derivatives are very similar to those of gramicidin A. The strong fluorescence of dansyl gramicidin C enabled us to measure its absolute surface density in planar bilayer membranes. In previous studies, the concentration of gramicidin A in the bilayer membrane was not directly measured. The number of active channels corresponding to a particular surface density of gramicidin was ascertained from simultaneous measurements of the membrane conductance. Three conclusions can be drawn from these experiments:

1) The slope of 2.0 ± 0.3 in the double logarithmic plot of the conductance versus the fluorescence intensity over a concentration range for which nearly all of the gramicidin is nonconducting (Fig. 6) proves that the channel is a dimer of the nonconducting species.

2) In the 26 Å-glycerolester membrane, nearly all of the dansyl gramicidin C was dimeric. The number of channels in this membrane was approximately equal to the number of dimers. Hence, not only are all the channels dimers, but all the dimers are channels.

3) The dimerization constant of dansyl gramicidin C increases 30-fold in going from a 47 Å- to a 40 Å-glycerolester membrane (Table II). The dimerization constant in a 48 Å-phosphatidyl choline membrane is 200 times larger than in a 47Å-glycerolester membrane. Thus, the dimerization constant depends markedly on both the type of lipid and on the thickness of the hydrocarbon core. Hladky and Haydon (6) found that the mean duration of a single channel increases monotonically the thinner the membrane. They attributed this effect to a variation in the extent of local thinning or dimpling of the membrane in the vicinity of the conducting channel. Our data are consistent with their proposal. The greater than 1,000-fold decrease in the dimerization constant in going from a 31 Å- to a 47 Å-glycerolester membrane corresponds to an increase in the free energy of dimerization of at least 4.5 kcal/mole. This free energy difference might represent the cost of deforming a small region of the 47Å membrane to match the length of the gramicidin channel.

We can detect the fluorescence of as few as 50 molecules per square μm on planar bilayer membranes. This surface density is comparable to that of many receptors in vivo. If these receptors can be reconstituted into planar membranes at these surface densities, then they can be studied using the fluorescence techniques which we have developed.

Single-Channel Conductance and Energy Transfer Measurements of Hybrid Channels

Our single-channel conductance and fluorescence energy transfer experiments show that hybrid channels are formed when two kinds of gramicidins are mixed. These hybrid channels differ from the pure species in 2 readily observable ways. First, hybrid channels have a single-channel conductance intermediate between those of the pure species. The relative conductance of the hybrid channel is 0.82, whereas those of pure PABS gramicidin C and of the pure gramicidin A channel are 0.68 and 1.00, respectively. Second, the efficiency of energy transfer between dansyl gramicidin C, the energy donor, and DPBS gramicidin C, the energy acceptor, in a hybrid channel is 75%. There is virtually no energy transfer between different channels if the surface density of gramicidin in the membrane is sufficiently low. In both the conductance and energy transfer experiments, the quantitative dependence of the fraction of hybrid channels on the ratio of the 2 kinds of gramicidin in the membrane reveals that the channel consists of 2 molecules of gramicidin. In particular, the possibility of a tetrameric channel of gramicidin in equilibrium with a nonconducting dimer is excluded by these hybrid studies.

The study of hybrid species should be generally useful in elucidating the subunit structure of oligomeric assemblies in biological membranes and in model membrane systems. This experimental approach requires that the hybrid species in the membrane have a distinctive property that is readily detected. Single-channel conductance and fluorescence characteristics are especially well-suited for such studies because they can be measured sensitively and precisely. In particular, fluorescence energy transfer is a useful indicator of a hybrid species, provided that the donor and acceptor chromophores are within about 40 Å of each other. The relative fluorescence yield of the donor as a function of the mole fraction of the acceptor can then be used to distinguish amongst various oligomeric models. Single-channel conductance measurements are ideal for the detection of hybrid channels, provided that the pure species have sufficiently different conductance values. This may be achieved by chemical modification, as in this study. Alternatively, it may be feasible to form distinctive hybrid channels in reconstituted membranes by mixing subunits of related, naturally-occurring molecules, such as acetylcholine receptors from different species.

What is the Conformation of the Gramicidin Channel Dimer?

Now that the dimeric nature of the channel is established, we can turn to these questions: What is the detailed conformation of the channel? How does it interact with ions and with membrane phospholipids? We know from the simultaneous conductance and fluorescence measurements that nearly all gramicidin dimers are channels, and we know from the fluorescence energy transfer measurements that nearly all of the gramicidin in liposomes is dimerized. Hence, spectroscopic studies of gramicidin in liposomes should provide information about the structure and dynamics of the transmembrane channel. It should be feasible to determine whether the conformation of the channel corresponds to the π_6 (L, D) helical dimer (Fig. 16a) proposed by Urry (21, 22), or to one of the parallel or anti-parallel-β double helices (Fig. 16b) proposed by Veatch et al. (23). All of these models provide a polar channel about 4 Å in diameter and about 25–30 Å in length. All have hydrophobic exteriors to interact favorably with the membrane interior and have more polar ends to stabilize the channel in the transmembrane configuration.

Urry et al. (22) have reported the preparation of a covalent gramicidin dimer in which the formyl group of each gramicidin has been removed and the 2 amino groups joined by a malonic acid linkage. This is equivalent to replacing the 2 formyl protons by a methylene bridge. This material does appear to have many of the membrane conductance characteristics expected for a unimolecular channel. However, I have used silica thin layer chromatography to fractionate samples of this material (kindly supplied by Dr. Dan Urry), and the membrane activity does not appear to comigrate with the major chemical component. Hence, there is some doubt as to the chemical identity of the membrane active species.

If the formyl groups are indeed very close together in the channel dimer, then the anti-parallel-β double helix (Fig. 16b) is ruled out. Both the parallel-β double helix (not shown) and the π_6 (L, D) helical dimer (Fig. 16a) place the formyl groups in close proximity. Further measurements will be required to distinguish between these possibilities.

a.   **b.**

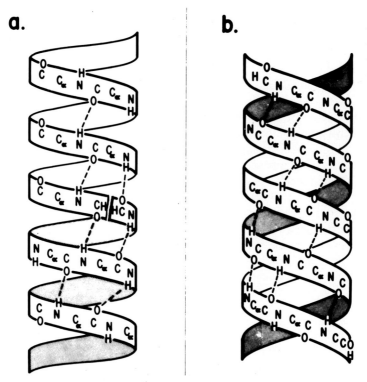

Fig. 16. Proposed models of the conformation of the gramicidin dimer channel. These schematic diagrams show the conformation of the polypeptide backbone with the side chains removed. Hydrogen bonds are shown as dashed lines and 1 chain is shown shaded. (a) Urry's π_6 (L, D) helical dimer. (b) The antiparallel-β double helix proposed by Veatch et al. (23). It is also possible to form a parallel-β double helix (not shown) in which the chains run in the same direction.

ACKNOWLEDGMENTS

I would like to thank Dr. Lubert Stryer of Yale University and Dr. Elkan Blout of Harvard University for their consistent encouragement and support. We thank Dr. Erhard Gross of the National Institutes of Health for providing the counter-current purified gramicidins, and Dr. Dan Urry of the University of Alabama for the samples of the covalent gramicidin dimer material. This work was supported by grants from the National Institute of General Medical Sciences (GM-16708, GM-21714, and GM-00167).

REFERENCES

1. Chappell, J. B., and Crofts, A. R., Biochem. J. 95:393 (1965).
2. Harris, E. J., and Pressman, B. C., Nature (London) 216:918 (1967).
3. Mueller, P., and Rudin, D. O., Biochem. Biophys. Res. Comm. 26:398 (1967).
4. Hladky, S. B., and Haydon, D. A., Nature (London) 225:451 (1970).
5. Sarges, R., and Witkop, B., J. Amer. Chem. Soc. 87:2011 (1965).
6. Hladky, S. B., and Haydon, D. A., Biochim. Biophys. Acta 274:294 (1972).
7. Tosteson, D. C., Andreoli, T. E., Tieffenberg, M., and Cook, P., J. Gen. Physiol. 51:373S (1968).
8. Goodall, M. C., Biochim. Biophys. Acta 219:471 (1970).
9. Bamberg, E., and Läuger, P., J. Membr. Biol. 11:177 (1973).

10. Zingsheim, H. P., and Neher, E., Biophys. Chem. 2:197 (1974).

11. Kolb, H. A., Läuger, P., and Bamberg, E., J. Membr. Biol. 20:133 (1975).

12. Veatch, W. R., and Blout, E. R., Biochemistry 15:3026 (1976).

13. Fettiplace, R., Andrews, D. M., and Haydon, D. A., J. Membr. Biol. 5:277 (1971).

14. Veatch, W. R., and Stryer, L., J. Mol. Biol. (in press).

15. Veatch, W. R., Mathies, R., Eisenberg, M., and Stryer, L., J. Mol. Biol. 99:75 (1975).

16. Zingsheim, H. P., and Haydon, D. A., Biochim. Biophys. Acta 298:755 (1973).

17. Förster, T., in "Modern Quantum Chemistry, Istanbul Lectures." O. Sinanoglú (Ed.). Academic Press, New York, section III-B, pp. 93–137 (1966).

18. Stryer, L., and Haugland, R. P., Proc. Nat. Acad. Sci. USA 58:719 (1967).

19. Yguerabide, J., Epstein, H. F., and Stryer, L., J. Mol. Biol. 51:573 (1970).

20. Wu, C-W., and Stryer, L., Proc. Nat. Acad. Sci. USA 69:1104 (1972).

21. Urry, D. W., Proc. Nat. Acad. Sci. USA 68:672 (1971).

22. Urry, D. W., Goodall, M. C., Glickson, J. D., and Mayers, D. F., Proc. Nat. Acad. Sci. USA 68:1907 (1971).

23. Veatch, W. R., Fossel, E. T., and Blout, E. R., Biochemistry 13:5249 (1974).

Journal of Supramolecular Structure 5:453 (57)–456 (60) (1976)

The Gating Currents of Sodium Channels: Pore-Population-Size Effects

M. D. Rayner, J. S. D'Arrigo, and L. L. Conquest

Departments of Physiology and Biostatistics-Epidemiology, University of Hawaii, Honolulu, Hawaii 96822

Sodium-channel behavior has been modeled in order to determine the answer to the following question: How large must a population of "on-off" sodium pores be before the inherently random behavior of the individual channels becomes smoothed to yield the expected gating current-conductance relationships which would be predicted from an infinite pore array? Results of this analysis show that for the "opening" situation, an excellent fit was obtained whenever more than about 10 pores were considered. Significant discrepancies were observed in the "closing" situation, however, for pore arrays of 50 or less. Marked hysteresis is apparent in the behavior of small pore populations.

Key words: gating currents, sodium channels, pore populations

INTRODUCTION

In their original presentation of the now classic Hodgkin-Huxley (H-H) hypothesis, these authors noted that observed changes in sodium and potassium conductance of nerve could be conceptualized as resulting from either 1) change of diameter in a fixed number of ion-selective membrane channels, or 2) from change in the proportions of these channels in a) "open," conducting, and b) "closed," nonconducting, states (1). Although the first concept contains the attractive element that, for example, all sodium pores could be considered to be in the same condition at the same time, it unfortunately also requires that pore selectivity [which apparently is fixed (2)] be maintained over a wide range of pore diameters. Hodgkin and Huxley, as well as later workers have, therefore, appeared to favor the second of these conceptualizations. Subsequently, evidence from studies of conductance "noise" in different excitable membranes (3, 4) has added strong support for the essentially "on-off" nature of individual conductance channels.

It follows, then, that there must be a necessary distinction between the behavior of individual channels and the behavior of the membrane as a whole. How large must a population of pores be before the inherently random behavior of the individual channels becomes smoothed to yield the expected relationships which would be predicted from an infinite pore array?

In seeking an analytical answer to this question, we chose to consider changes in "activation" of Na^+-selective channels as controlled by the m variable of the H-H equations.

Where h, the "inactivation" variable, is ignored:

$$\frac{dg_{Na}}{dt} = \frac{dg_{Na}}{dm} \cdot \frac{dm}{dt} \tag{1}$$

The fundamental relationship, dg_{Na}/dm, can thus be studied separately from the time-dependent process dm/dt. If we further state that it is only f, the fraction of pores in the open state, which truly concerns us, then:

$$\frac{dg_{Na}}{dm} = \frac{df}{dm} \tag{2}$$

where both f and m are simple functions varying between 0 and 1.

For an infinite pore array, the H-H formulation makes clear that f must always be equal to m^3, m being obtained from the kinetic relationship:

$$m' \underset{\beta_m}{\overset{\alpha_m}{\rightleftharpoons}} m \tag{3}$$

in which α_m and β_m are voltage-dependent rate constants. By contrast, for a single, isolated "on-off" pore (a 1-pore array), we can readily see that f is not equal to m^3 at all values of m. For such a pore to open, all 3 of its controlling "particles" must be in the m rather than the m' state. Thus as m rises from 0 to 0.33, 0.67, and 1, f remains 0 until m reaches 1. [Note that when m = 0.67, f is still 0, not $(0.67)^3$.]

The original question thus becomes: How large must the array of pores be before f comes to approximate m^3 at all values of m?

METHODS

The simplest model for the behavior of small pore arrays (up to n = 13, where n is the number of pores in the array) can be obtained by utilizing a deck of playing cards with 1 suit removed. The triplets with the same face value then represent the 3 m-gates associated with a single sodium pore. When the cards have been thoroughly and carefully shuffled, the f:m relationship can be studied either for pore opening (cards are dealt until full triplets are obtained, m = fraction of cards dealt, 1−f = fraction of triplets obtained) or for pore closing (m' = fraction of cards dealt, 1−f = fraction of pores closed, remembering that a pore is closed by the laying down of a single card from each potential triplet).

To verify results obtained by this method and to study larger pore arrays than can conveniently be modeled by direct methods, a probabilistic model was developed for computer use. We modeled only the pore-closing situation in this way, however, since for the pore-opening situation f rapidly approaches m^3 as n is increased, and becomes essentially equal to m^3 at all times, even in a 13-pore array.

For pore-closing, the question was posed in the form: How many gates are required to change from the m to the m' condition in order to close j pores? Our basic approach involved recognition that at any stage during the closing process, gates and pores may be separated into 3 subpopulations: firstly, the j−1 pores already closed by either 1 or more m to m' transitions; secondly, the single jth pore which will be next to close by a single such m to m' transition; and finally, there are those remaining gates (in the m state)

associated with either open or closed pores. Where q is the number of additional m to m'
transitions possible with respect to the already closed j−1 pores, and where r is the number
of pores in this first subpopulation closed by 3 gates in the m' state, then the number of
gates, E(j,n), required to close j pores is given by the following equation:

$$E(j,n) = \frac{3^j n!}{(3n)! \cdot (n-j)!} \sum_{q=0}^{2j-2} (j+q)! \cdot [3n-(j+q)! \cdot$$

$$\sum_{r=0}^{j-1} [r! (q-2r)! (j-1-q+r)!]^{-1} 3^{-r} \qquad (4)$$

In equation 4, $E(j,n) \equiv (1-m) = m'$, while $f = j/n$.

RESULTS

Results of this analysis are shown in Fig. 1. In this figure, the solid curve represents
the f−m relationship predicted from the infinite pore array, namely $f = m^3$. For the
"opening" situation (i.e., increasing m, increasing f), an excellent fit was obtained wherever
n was greater than about 10 pores. Significant discrepancies were observed in the "closing"
situation, however, for pore arrays of 50 or less. Marked hysteresis is apparent in the
behavior of small pore populations.

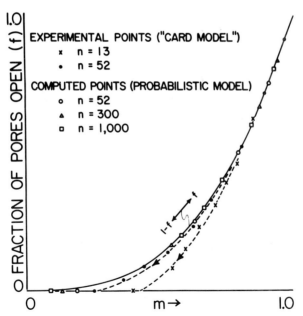

Fig. 1. Gating current-conductance relationships for pore populations of various sizes. The solid curve
refers to an infinite pore array; the curve reflects both the opening (f) and closing (1−f) of sodium
pores as a function of m-gate transitions (m' to m, and m to m', respectively). The dashed lines refer
to small pore populations; these curves reflect only the closing of sodium pores as a function of m-gate
transitions (m to m'). See text for further discussion.

DISCUSSION

The analysis presented here was undertaken, initially, because we had suspected that discrepancies between predicted results (from H-H equations) and observed sodium tail currents and associated gating currents (5—7) might perhaps arise from pore-population-size effects, i.e., from hysteresis of the type observed for very small pore arrays in Fig. 1. It is very clear that this could not be the case. In fact, there must be very few situations in which sufficiently small pore arrays could be encountered experimentally to produce hysteresis as a result of population size.

It is interesting to note, however, that the "kinetic formulation" of the H-H equations, as modified initially by Bezanilla and Armstrong (8), and more extensively by Moore and Cox (9), superimposes on the original H-H formulation just such a hysteresis between pore opening and pore closing as we had sought to uncover in this study.

ACKNOWLEDGMENTS

This work was supported in part by NSF Grant No. BNS76-02647, and by NOAA Office of Sea Grant, No. 04-5-158-17.

REFERENCES

1. Hodgkin, A. L., and Huxley, A. F., J. Physiol. 117:500 (1952).
2. Chandler, W. K., and Meves, H., J. Physiol. 180:788 (1965).
3. Anderson, C. R., and Stevens, C. F., J. Physiol. 235:655 (1973).
4. Begenisich, T., and Stevens, C. F., Biophys. J. 15:843 (1975).
5. Bezanilla, F., and Armstrong, C. M., Science 183:753 (1974).
6. Armstrong, C. M., and Bezanilla, F., J. Gen. Physiol. 63:533 (1974).
7. Keynes, R. D., and Rojas, E., J. Physiol. 239:393 (1974).
8. Bezanilla, F., and Armstrong, C. M., Phil. Trans. R. Soc. Lond. B 270:449 (1975).
9. Moore, J. W., and Cox, E. B., Biophys. J. 16:171 (1976).

Regulation of the Growth and Development of Sympathetic Neurons In Vivo

Ira B. Black

Laboratory of Developmental Neurology, Department of Neurology, Cornell University Medical College, New York, New York 10021

The superior cervical ganglion (SCG) in the neonatal mouse and rat has been employed as a model system to study the regulation of ontogeny of presynaptic cholinergic nerves and postsynaptic adrenergic neurons. During postnatal development presynaptic choline acetyltransferase (ChAc) activity increases 30- to 40-fold, whereas postsynaptic tyrosine hydroxylase (T-OH) activity rises 6- to 8-fold. Transection of the presynaptic cholinergic nerves innervating the SCG prevents the normal development of T-OH activity and the normal accumulation of T-OH enzyme molecules in each postsynaptic neuron. The trans-synaptic regulation of T-OH development is apparently mediated by acetylcholine and postsynaptic depolarization, since pharmacologic ganglionic blockade also prevents normal maturation. Ganglion decentralization also prevents the normal maturation of adrenergic nerve terminals, and the development of end-organ innervation by SCG. Consequently, trans-synaptic factors regulate the ontogeny of adrenergic terminals as well as perikarya. Moreover, normal efferent as well as afferent connections are apparently required for sympathetic development, since removal of salivary glands and orbital contents, target organs of the SCG, in neonates also prevents T-OH development in the ganglia.

The postsynaptic neuron contributes to the development of presynaptic cholinergic fibers in SCG. Selective destruction of adrenergic neurons in neonatal mice with either 6-hydroxydopamine or antiserum to nerve growth factor prevents the normal maturation of ChAc activity in presynaptic terminals of SCG. Thus, presynaptic and postsynaptic cells appear to exert reciprocal regulatory influences during ontogeny.

INTRODUCTION

Study of neuronal growth and development is essential for understanding mechanisms controlling orderly maturation and specialization within the nervous system. Such knowledge may, in addition, lead to a more precise definition of synaptic plasticity and elucidation of the biochemistry of communication between nerve cells. Although it has been established that development of innervation is necessary for normal maturation of organs such as skeletal muscles (1), little is known about mechanisms by which developing neurons interact to regulate the maturation of one another.

Developmental milestones in the mammalian central nervous system have been documented by anatomical (2, 3), ultrastructural (4), electrophysiological (5), and biochemical (6, 7) approaches. However, due to the complexity of the central nervous system, such studies have been largely descriptive. Even the simplest brain nuclei contain heterogeneous groupings of cells which differ morphologically, biochemically, and probably functionally.

Studies in the periphery (8, 9) provide simpler models of neural ontogeny. Sympathetic ganglia in mouse, rat, and cat contain primarily two neural elements in synaptic contact: presynaptic cholinergic nerve terminals and postsynaptic adrenergic neurons (8). Specifically, the well-defined, relatively noncomplex superior cervical ganglion (SCG) is ideal for the study of neuronal growth and development because the SCG is composed of biochemically distinct, well-defined neural elements consisting primarily of the cholinergic-adrenergic neural unit defined above. In addition, recent studies have indicated the presence of low numbers of small neurons (10), adrenergic fibers (11), and scattered cholinergic cells (12) in sympathetic ganglia. The SCG is anatomically discrete and easily accessible, and its bilaterally symmetric nature allows rigorously controlled experiments within a single animal (13). Ontogenetically and anatomically there is no fundamental difference between the autonomic and somatic systems, neurons of the latter arising un-interruptedly from the neural crest (14). Hence, while the SCG is less complex than central models, data derived from its study may define mechanisms governing growth and development throughout the nervous system.

In the present communication the maturation of mouse and rat SCG in vivo will be described utilizing a combination of biochemical and morphological parameters. Choline acetyltransferase (ChAc), the enzyme catalyzing the conversion of acetyl CoA and choline to the neurotransmitter acetylcholine, is used as a marker for the development of pre-synaptic cholinergic fibers. The enzyme is highly localized to these presynaptic terminals (15). Maturation of postsynaptic neurons is followed by measuring the activity of tyrosine hydroxylase (T-OH), the rate-limiting enzyme in the biosynthesis of noradrenaline (16), the postganglionic neurotransmitter. Visualization of ganglion synapses with the electron microscope is used to estimate the development of synaptic connections.

METHODS

Experimental Animals

Litters of Swiss Albino mice and Sprague-Dawley rats were housed with mothers which were fed Rockland Laboratories chow and water ad libitum. The animals were killed by exposure to ether vapor and ganglia were removed under a dissecting miscroscope.

Surgical Procedure

The ganglia were decentralized in 4-day-old mice or rats which were anesthetized with halothane (4% in 100% oxygen) blown over the nose through a rubber nose cone. The vagosympathetic trunk was transected unilaterally, 2—4 mm proximal to the ganglion, with a dissecting microscope. The wound was closed with celloidin and the animals were returned to their mothers. This procedure results in approximately a 2% mortality rate, due primarily to failure by the mother to accept the pups.

Enzyme Assays

Tyrosine hydroxylase, DOPA decarboxylase, and choline acetyltransferase activities were assayed by modifications of methods previously described (13, 17—19). Total protein was measured by a modification of the method of Lowry et al. (20).

RESULTS AND DISCUSSION

Biochemical Development of the Superior Cervical Ganglion

ChAc activity increases 30- to 40-fold during the course of development (13). From low levels on day 1, enzyme activity rises rapidly during the first 2 weeks of life, reaching a hyperbolic plateau by approximately 3 weeks (Fig. 1). This increase in enzyme activity may reflect either ongoing invasion of the ganglion by presynaptic nerve endings and/or transport of the enzyme to nerve endings already present in the ganglion.

The developmental curve for T-OH activity differs significantly from that of ChAc. T-OH activity increases six- to eight-fold from birth to adulthood (13). The major increase occurs during the 2nd week of development when enzyme activity undergoes nearly a three-fold rise with little subsequent elevation to the 38th day of life (Fig. 1).

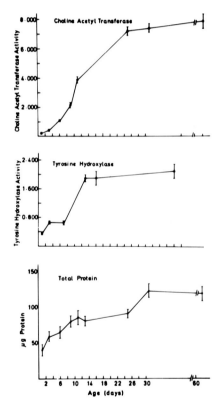

Fig. 1. Developmental increases of transmitter enzyme activities and total protein in mouse superior cervical ganglia. Groups of six mice were taken from litters of varying ages and ganglion pairs from each animal were assayed for enzyme activities and total protein. Choline acetyltransferase activity is expressed as mean (nanomoles product per ganglion pair) per hour ± SEM (vertical bars). Tyrosine hydroxylase activity is expressed as $(10^{-11}$ mol product per ganglion pair) per hour. Total protein is expressed as mean micrograms per ganglion pair ± SEM (13).

During development total ganglion protein increases only three-fold, rendering the rises in enzyme-specific activities highly significant (13) (Fig. 1). This relatively modest increase in total protein has been observed previously during the development of ganglia (21).

Mechanism of the Developmental Increase of Enzyme Activity

These increases in enzyme activity could be due either to the activation of pre-existent enzyme molecules or to the synthesis of new enzyme protein. To distinguish between these alternatives neonatal mice were treated with the protein synthesis inhibitor, cycloheximide. Such treatment prevents the normal developmental increase in T-OH activity (22), suggesting that the developmental T-OH rise is dependent on the ongoing synthesis of new enzyme molecules. Immunotitration studies employing a specific antibody to tyrosine hydroxylase enzyme protein confirmed this impression: the developmental increase in T-OH activity is entirely attributable to accumulation of increased numbers of enzyme molecules in each adrenergic neuron (23).

Trans-Synaptic Regulation of Sympathetic Development

To appreciate the functional significance of these biochemical correlates of maturation, their temporal relation to the development of interneuronal connections was defined (13). Synaptic junctions were identified and counted, as described by Bloom and Aghajanian (24) in ganglia of mice aged 1–60 days. During this period, total synapses per ganglion increase from approximately 8,000 on day 1 to 3,000,000 by day 60. The curve describing the developmental increase in synapse numbers closely approximated that for the development of T-OH activity. These observations suggested that the development of T-OH activity in postsynaptic neurons might be dependent on contact with presynapic nerve endings.

To determine whether presynaptic cholinergic nerve terminals regulate the development of T-OH activity in the postsynaptic neuron, ganglia were decentralized in neonatal mice. The preganglionic trunk was transected unilaterally in mice aged 5–6 days. The contralateral normal ganglion served as control. Mice were killed at varying times postoperatively, ipsilateral ptosis and reduced ganglion ChAc activity indicated success of the procedure. As expected, ChAc activity was reduced to less than 10% of control values. T-OH activity failed to increase above normal 7-day levels, remaining at approximately 30% of the activity of contralateral unoperated ganglia (13, 22) (Fig. 2). Moreover, immunotitration studies demonstrated that decentralization prevented the normal accumulation of T-OH enzyme molecules in each adrenergic neuron (23).

The Trans-Synaptic Message

Treatment of neonatal mice and rats with nerve growth factor (NGF) results in profound hyperplasia and hypertrophy of adrenergic neurons throughout the animal (25). Consequently, this substance was considered a prime candidate for the trans-synaptic message. However, treatment with NGF does not fully reverse the effects of decentralization on ganglion T-OH development (22), and therefore, NGF cannot completely replace presynaptic terminals during maturation. On this basis NGF cannot be considered alone as *the* presynaptic message.

Another approach to the problem of identifying the trans-synaptic factor(s) regulating adrenergic neuron development has involved the use of long-acting ganglionic blocking agents (26, 27). These compounds prevent depolarization of postsynaptic neurons

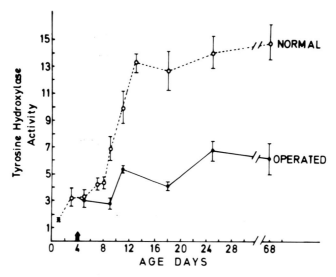

Fig. 2. Effect of surgical decentralization on development of tyrosine hydroxylase activity in mouse superior cervical ganglion. Groups of six mice were killed at various times postoperatively and tyrosine hydroxylase activity (picomoles per ganglion per hr) was measured in control and contralateral decentralized ganglia. The value obtained 1 day after surgery does not differ significantly from control; all other values are significantly lower than respective controls at $p < 0.01$ (22).

in sympathetic ganglia by competing with acetylcholine for receptor sites. Indeed, the structurally dissimilar, long-acting ganglionic blocking agents, chlorisondamine and pempidine, prevent the normal development of T-OH activity in postsynaptic neurons of the superior cervical ganglion (26, 27) (Fig. 3). The developmental curve obtained for T-OH maturation with ganglionic blockade (Fig. 3) was similar to that observed after surgical decentralization (Fig. 2). These observations suggest that acetylcholine itself may constitute one of the trans-synaptic messages.

Trans-Synaptic Regulation of the Development of Target Organ Innervation

To determine whether trans-synaptic influences regulate the development of nerve terminals as well as perikarya, the SCG and two of its target organs, the iris and pineal gland, were studied by biochemical and histofluorescent approaches. During postnatal ontogeny the activity of tyrosine hydroxylase increased 50-fold in iris and 34-fold in pineal nerve terminals of the rat. These increases paralleled the in vitro rise in iris [^{3}H] norepinephrine ([^{3}H] NE) uptake, a measure of the presence of functional nerve terminal membrane. These biochemical indices of end-organ innervation correlated well with developmental increases in density of innervation, adrenergic ground plexus ramification, and nerve fiber fluorescence intensity as determined by fluorescence microscopy (28).

Unilateral transection of the presynaptic cholinergic nerves innervating the ganglion in 2–3-day old rats prevented the normal development of ganglion innervation: T-OH activity failed to increase normally in irides innervated by decentralized adrenergic neurons (28) (Fig. 4). In addition [^{3}H] NE uptake, innervation density, plexus ramification, and fluorescence intensity did not mature normally in irides innervated by decentralized ganglia (28).

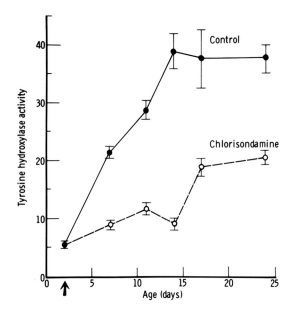

Fig. 3. Effect of chlorisondamine on the development of ganglion tyrosine hydroxylase activity: time course. Animals were treated with chlorisondamine 5 μg/g body weight subcutaneously every 12 hr beginning on day 2 of life (arrow). Each value represents the mean ±SEM (vertical bars) for from six to eight animals. Control animals (solid lines) were treated with saline at appropriate times. Dashed line indicates chlorisondamine-treated animals. Each value for chlorisondamine-treated animals differs from respective controls at p < 0.001 (27).

These investigations indicate that presynaptic cholinergic fibers in the ganglion have a generalized regulatory effect on the ontogeny of adrenergic neurons, regulating terminal as well as cell body maturation. Trans-synaptic influences govern end organ innervation, but not, apparently, end organ growth. Decentralization did not alter the developmental increases in iris (Fig. 4) and pineal (not shown) total protein (28), suggesting that trans-synaptic factors in the ganglion and distal adrenergic terminals do not regulate end organ growth.

We are presently studying the manner in which trans-synaptic influences interact with other factors such as NGF in the regulation of development of target-organ innervation.

The Role of Target Organs in the Development of Sympathetic Neurons

To define the effect of end-organ extirpation on the development of ganglion T-OH activity, salivary glands and orbital contents, targets of the SCG, were unilaterally removed from 3-day old rats. Six weeks after surgery, T-OH activity was examined in the ipsilateral and contralateral control ganglia from the operated rats. Enzyme activity was also determined in ganglia from unoperated littermate controls (Fig. 5).

End-organ removal prevented the normal developmental increase in ganglion T-OH activity (29). Enzyme activity was depressed whether compared to the contralateral ganglion within the same animal, or to ganglia from unoperated littermates (Fig. 5). T-OH activity was 61% of that in contralateral control ganglia, and 54% of that in ganglia from unoperated animals. There was no significant difference in activity between control

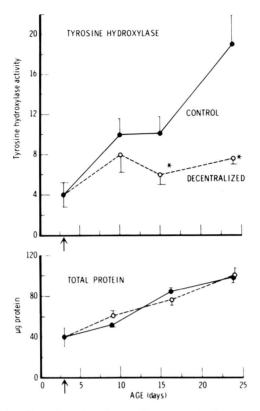

Fig. 4. Time course of the effect of ganglion decentralization on the development of tyrosine hydroxylase activity and total protein in the iris. Rats were treated as described in the text and killed at the indicated times after surgery which was performed on day 3 of life (arrow). Parallel determinations of tyrosine hydroxylase activity and total protein were performed on aliquots taken from the same iris homogenates. Results for tyrosine hydroxylase activity are expressed as picomoles/iris/hr, and total protein is expressed as microgram/iris for contralateral control irides (solid line) and ipsilateral decentralized irides. Each point represents the mean of determinations on six to eight irides. For total protein, none of the pairs of points differ significantly. *Differs from respective control at $p < 0.01$ (28).

ganglia from operated rats and ganglia from unoperated animals, suggesting that surgery per se did not alter development of T-OH activity (29).

To more fully document the effect of target organ removal on the development of ganglion T-OH activity, unilateral sialectomy and iridectomy were performed in neonatal rats, and the time course of development was examined. End-organ removal was associated with long-lasting inhibition of the normal development of T-OH activity (Fig. 6). One day after surgery there was no significant difference between experimental and contra-lateral control ganglia. By the 5th postoperative day, however, T-OH activity in the ex-perimental ganglia was significantly lower than that in the contralateral controls. At all subsequent times studied, activity in experimental ganglia remained significantly depressed at 60–75% of control levels. However, T-OH activity in the experimental ganglia never fell below the value observed one day postoperatively. Both experimental and control ganglia reached plateau levels of T-OH activity at approximately 14 days of age (29) (Fig. 6).

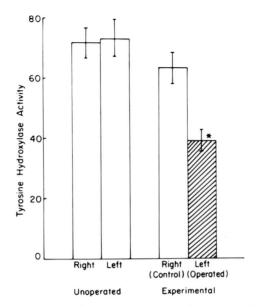

Fig. 5. Effect of end-organ removal on the development of ganglion tyrosine hydroxylase activity. Unilateral sialectomy and iridectomy were performed in eight 3-day old rats ("Experimental"), and eight littermates served as unoperated controls. All animals were killed at 3 weeks of age. Values are expressed as means picomoles/ganglion · hr ± SEM for "Right" and "Left" ganglia in each group. *Differs from contralateral "right (control)" group, and from "unoperated groups at p < 0.01. All other groups do not differ significantly from each other (29).

To determine whether inhibition of development was specific for T-OH or more generalized, altering other aspects of ontogeny, the development of total ganglion protein was also examined after surgery. The accretion of total ganglion protein was employed as an index of overall ganglion growth. In contrast to T-OH development, there was no significant difference in total protein until 40 days after surgery. Thereafter, protein was significantly lower in ganglia depreived of salivary glands and orbital contents (Fig. 6). Although total protein did not differ significantly at any single time before 43 days of age, the mean value was always lower in the experimental ganglia after the first post-operative day (29) (Fig. 6).

To determine whether the effect of target-organ removal on the ontogeny of ganglion enzyme activity was limited to T-OH or affected other enzymes as well, DOPA decarboxylase (DDC) activity was also measured. DDC, which catalyzes the conversion of L-DOPA to dopamine, is highly localized to adrenergic neurons in the SCG (30). Since the regulation of DDC activity is different from that of T-OH (30), it was of interest to ascertain whether end-organ extirpation similarly influenced the two enzymes.

Animals were subjected to unilateral sialectomy and iridectomy on day 3 of life, and the development of DDC activity was examined 16 days postoperatively. DDC activity failed to develop normally in ganglia deprived of normal target organs, remaining at 64% of that in contralateral control ganglia (29) (Fig. 7).

The precise mechanisms by which salivary glands and iris influence adrenergic maturation have yet to be elucidated. However, our studies are consistent with a growing body of evidence which indicates that target organs regulate neuronal development. Thus, for example, removal of the field of innervation prevents normal ontogeny of sensory

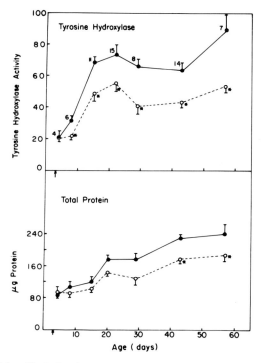

Fig. 6. Time course of the effect of end-organ removal on the development of ganglion tyrosine hydroxylase activity and total protein. Surgery was performed as in Fig. 5 (arrow) and groups were killed at the indicated times. Each value represents the mean ± SEM for contralateral control ganglia (solid line) and ganglia ipsilateral to end-organ removal (dashed line). Number of animals in each group is indicated next to each point in the top diagram. Tyrosine hydroxylase activity is expressed as in Fig. 1 and total protein as micrograms/ganglion. *Differs from respective control at $p < 0.05$ (29).

neurons (31), anterior horn motor neurons (32, 33), and neurons within the ciliary ganglion (34). Viewed in conjunction with the work described above, our studies suggest that, for normal growth and development, adrenergic neurons require normal efferent as well as afferent connections.

Regulation of Presynaptic Cholinergic Development by Postsynaptic Neurons

A number of the studies described in previous sections indicated that presynaptic cholinergic terminals regulate the growth of postsynaptic neurons in SCG. To determine whether, conversely, postsynaptic neurons regulate the development of presynaptic nerves, adrenergic cells were selectively destroyed in neonatal mice. Animals were treated with 6-hydroxydopamine (35) which resulted in a 94% decrease in ganglionic T-OH activity, and a 92% decrease in ganglion neuron numbers, indicating virtually complete destruction of adrenergic neurons in the SCG (35) (Fig. 8). In addition, presynaptic ChAc activity failed to develop normally (Fig. 8).

Destruction of adrenergic neurons in the superior cervical ganglion was also accomplished by immunological means. Four-day old mice were treated with a single injection of NGF antiserum and were killed at 28 days of age. A marked diminution of T-OH activity indicated the efficacy of this procedure. ChAc activity again failed to develop normally after destruction of postsynaptic neurons in this manner (35).

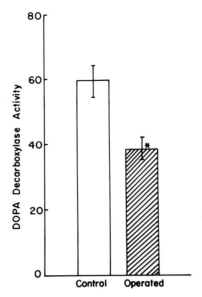

Fig. 7. Effect of end-organ removal on the development of ganglion DOPA decarboxylase activity. Unilateral surgery was performed on a group of eight rats as described in the text and they were killed at age 19 days. Enzyme activity is expressed as mean nanomoles/ganglion · hour ± SEM. *Differs from contralateral "Control" group at p < 0.005 (29).

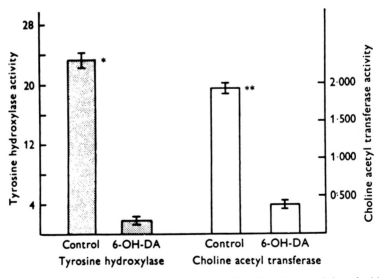

Fig. 8. Effect of 6-hydroxydopamine on the developing ganglion. Six mice were injected with 6-hydroxydopamine in 0.2% ascorbic acid, 150 mg/kg subcutaneously, on days 2, 4, 6, and 8 of life, and were killed on day 13. Six littermate controls were treated with vehicle at appropriate times. Ganglia pairs were removed and assayed as indicated in the text. Results are expressed as mean (nanomole product/ganglion pair)/hr ± SEM (vertical bars) for choline acetyltransferase and as picomole product/pair/hr for tyrosine hydroxylase. *, **Control differs from appropriate treated groups at p < 0.001 (35).

The precise nature of the developmental defect in the presynaptic neuron has not been identified. ChAc activity in presynaptic fibers in the developing ganglion may reflect enzyme synthesis and degradation in the preganglionic neuron perikarya in the spinal cord, axoplasmic transport of the enzyme to the ganglion terminals, degradation of the enzyme within the nerve endings, and invasion of the ganglion by cholinergic terminals. The decrease in ChAc activity observed in the present studies may reflect alteration of any or all of these processes. Alternatively, the failure of ChAc to develop normally in these ganglia may reflect a more generalized abnormality, or even absence, of presynaptic terminals.

ACKNOWLEDGMENTS

This work was supported by National Institutes of Health grants NS 10259, NS 11666, aided by a grant from the National Foundation—March of Dimes, and was made possible by a grant from the Dysautonomia Foundation, Inc. Ira B. Black is the recipient of the Teacher-Investigator Award of NINDS 11032.

REFERENCES

1. Guth, L., Physiol. Rev. 48:645 (1969).
2. Eayrs, J. T., and Goodhead, B., J. Anat. (Lond.) 93:385 (1959).
3. Peters, V. B., and Flexner, L. B., Am. J. Anat. 86:133 (1950).
4. Aghajanian, G., and Bloom, F. E., Brain Res. 6:716 (1967).
5. Deza, L., and Eidelberg, E., Exp. Neurol. 17:425 (1967).
6. Lognado, J. R., and Hardy, M., Nature 214:1207 (1967).
7. Hebb, C. O., J. Physiol. (Lond.) 133:566 (1956).
8. Giacobini, E., Biochem. of Simple Neuronal Models. Adv. Biochem. Psychopharmacol. vol. 2 (1970).
9. Giacobini, G., Marchisio, P. C., Giacobini, E., and Koslow, S. H., J. Neurochem. 17:1177 (1970).
10. Williams, T. H., and Palay, S. L., Brain Res. 15:17 (1969).
11. Hamberger, B., Norberg, K. A., and Sjoqvist, F., J. Neuropharmacol. 2:279 (1963).
12. Sjoqvist, F., "Cholinergic Sympathetic Ganglion Cells." (1962).
13. Black, I. B., Hendry, I. A., and Iversen, L. L., Brain Res. 34:229 (1971b).
14. Monnier, M., Autonomic Functions. Gen. Physiol. 1:91 (1968).
15. Hebb, C. O., and Waites, G. M. H., J. Physiol. (Lond.) 132:667 (1956).
16. Levitt, M., Spector, S., Sjoerdsma, A., and Udenfriend, S., J. Pharmacol. Exp. Ther. 148:1 (1965).
17. Black, I. B., and Geen, S. C., Brain Res. 63:291 (1973).
18. Black, I. B., Brain Res. 95:170 (1975).
19. Lamprecht, F., and Coyle, J. T., Brain Res. 41:503 (1972).
20. Lowry, O. H., Rosebrough, N. J., Farr, A. L., and Randall, R. J., J. Biol. Chem. 193:265 (1951).
21. Cohen, S., Proc. Nat. Acad. Sci. U.S.A. 46:302 (1960).
22. Black, I. B., Hendry, I. A., and Iversen, L. L., J. Neurochem. 19:1367 (1972b).
23. Black, I. B., Joh, T. H., and Reis, D. J., Brain Res. 75:133 (1974).
24. Bloom, F. E., and Aghajanian, G. K., J. Ultrastruct. Res. 22:361 (1968).
25. Levi-Montalcini, R., and Angeletti, P. U., Physiol. Rev. 48:534 (1968).
26. Hendry, I. A., and Iversen, L. L., Proceedings of the 5th International Congress on Pharmacology, San Francisco 100 (1972).
27. Black, I. B., and Geen, S. C., Brain Res. 63:291 (1973).
28. Black, I. B., and Mytilineou, C., Brain Res. 101:503 (1976).
29. Dibner, M. D., and Black, I. B., Brain Res. 103:93 (1976).
30. Black, I. B., Hendry, I. A., and Iversen, L. L., Nature 231:27 (1971a).
31. Detwiler, S. R., Biol. Rev. 8:269 (1933).
32. Prestige, M. C., The neurosciences: Second Study Program 73 (1970).
33. Prestige, M. C., Brit. Med. Bull. 30:107 (1974).
34. Landmesser, L., and Pilar, G., J. Physiol. (Lond.) 241:715 (1974).
35. Black, I. B., Hendry, I. A., and Iversen, L. L., J. Physiol. (Lond.) 221:149 (1972).

Biochemical Investigations of Retinotectal Specificity

Richard B. Marchase, Jean-Claude Meunier, Michael Pierce, and Stephen Roth

Department of Biology, The Johns Hopkins University, Baltimore, Maryland 21218

An in vitro assay for retinotectal specificity has been described. The results show that, in the chick embryo, cells dissociated from the dorsal retina preferentially adhered to ventral tectal surfaces while cells from the ventral retina preferentially adhered to dorsal tectal surfaces. These adhesive preferences thus mimic the retinotectal specificity observed in vivo. The assay has been extended for use with plasma membrane preparations from retinal cells.

Experiments in which retinal cells or tectal surfaces were treated with purified proteases and glycosidases have partially characterized the moieties responsible for the observed specificities. These results are consistent with a double gradient in the dorsal-ventral axis of complementary proteins and carbohydrates. The carbohydrate moiety would be expected to terminate in an acetylated hexosamine and to be more concentrated dorsally in both retina and tectum. A protein that is complementary to the hexosamine terminus would be localized in the ventral parts of retina and tectum.

INTRODUCTION

The visual system of submammalian vertebrates is a well-studied example of neuronal patterning in which a continuous spatial representation of the retina maps across the surface of the optic tectum. In this map, the dorsal and ventral portions of the retina project respectively to the ventral and dorsal portions of the tectal surface (1).

A possible mechanism for the continuous topographical relationship between retina and tectum was proposed by Sperry (2). He postulated the existence of two cytochemical gradients spreading at roughly right angles to each other across both the retina and the optic tectum. According to its location in the retinal gradients, any given ganglion cell would carry unique numbers or types of chemical groups on its surface and would connect exclusively with the tectal locus that possessed the complementary pattern.

To test this possibility, Barbera et al. (3) developed an in vitro assay that measured the adherence of ^{32}P-labeled cell bodies from either the dorsal or the ventral halves of chick embryo neural retinas to dorsal and ventral tectal halves. When a labeled, single-cell suspension was prepared from dorsal half-retinas, more cells bound to the ventral halves of the tecta. When the labeled cells were from ventral half-retinas, more bound to dorsal half-tecta. This preferential adhesion mimics the retinotectal projection found in vivo and is likely to be a result of the same molecular mechanisms as those responsible for neuronal recognition.

A subsequent paper (4) proposed cell surface glycosyltransferases and their oligosaccharide acceptors as potential candidates for the cytochemical gradients suggested by Sperry.

METHODS

Collection Assay

The collection assay has been described in detail previously (3, 5). Dorsal or ventral halves of neural retina from 7–10-day chick embryos were dissected and incubated for 2–5 hr in medium containing 0.5 mCi of ^{32}P. This suspension was added to a Petri dish containing both dorsal and ventral tectal halves pinned to a layer of paraffin in the bottom of the dish. The dish was reciprocated so that the cells in suspension washed across the tectal surfaces. After the collection, each tectal half was removed, gently rinsed, and counted to determine the number of adhering, radioactive retinal cells.

Retinal Membranes

Dorsal or ventral retinal thirds from 20–30 chick embryos 6–9-days old were incubated for about 16 hr in nutrient medium containing 50 μCi of ^{3}H-glucosamine. Suspensions enriched for plasma membranes were derived from the labeled neural tissue by a modification of the method of Merrell and Glaser (6). This method will be described in detail elsewhere (7). Flotation of the crude membrane suspension was carried out at 1.4×10^5 g for 150 min in a discontinuous gradient consisting of 60%, 37%, and 20% (wt/vol) sucrose at pH 7.2.

Degradative Enzyme Treatments, Ganglioside Preparations, and Galactosyl Transferase Assay Methods

All of these methods will be described elsewhere (8).

RESULTS AND DISCUSSION

The Collection Assay

A full treatment of the data and results from the collection assay concerning the adhesive specificities of retinal cells to tectal surfaces has been published previously (3, 5). A brief summary of these experiments will be presented.

Figure 1 shows the results of a typical experiment using labeled, dorsal retinal cells. As a function of collection time up to 6 hr, the dorsal retinal cells showed an adhesive preference for ventral tectal halves. When a similar experiment was performed with labeled ventral cells, a different result was obtained (Fig. 2). After short collection times, ventral retinal cells adhered preferentially to ventral tectal halves. After longer times, however, the preference was reversed: ventral retinal cells adhered preferentially to dorsal tectal halves. Together these results indicate that for collection times longer than 3 hr, the adhesive preference of dorsal and ventral retinal cells for ventral and dorsal tectal halves, respectively, mimics the specificity seen in vivo.

The change in adhesive preference by ventral retinal cells after 3 hr of collection was shown by preincubation experiments probably to be a function of the sensitivity of these cells to trypsinization and their subsequent recovery. That is, when ventral retinal cells were preincubated for intervals greater than 3 hr and then incubated with freshly dissected tectal halves, they immediately adhered preferentially to the dorsal tectal halves.

As controls, suspensions of labeled cells from embryonic chick liver, cerebellum, and cerebrum were tested in the collection assay. None of these cell suspensions showed preference for either tectal half.

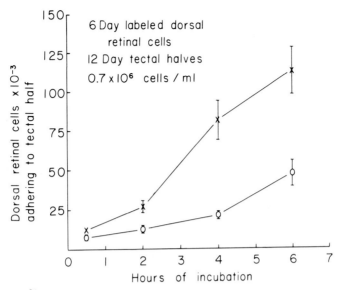

Fig. 1. Number of ^{32}P-labeled retina cells adhering to dorsal and ventral tectal halves as a function of incubation time. Cell suspension was prepared from 6-day dorsal half-retinas, 0.7 × 10^7 cells/ml. Four to six tectal halves of each type from 12-day old embryos were used for each data point. Standard error of the mean is shown for each point. O represents cells adhering to dorsal tectal halves. X represents cells adhering to ventral tectal halves.

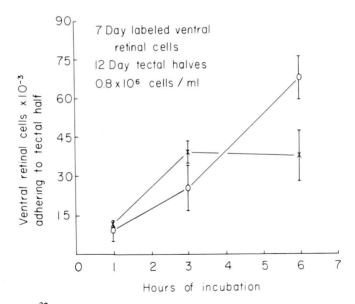

Fig. 2. Number of ^{32}P-labeled retina cells adhering to dorsal and ventral tectal halves as a function of time of incubation. Cell suspension was prepared from 7-day ventral half-retinas, 0.8 × 10^6 cells/ml. All other details are as described in the legend to Fig. 1.

When the collection assay was performed with tecta that had never been innervated by retinal axons, identical results were obtained. This ruled out the possibility that retinal axons on the tectal surfaces were solely responsible for the observed adhesive specificity.

Experiments were performed in which the developmental age of either the tectal halves or the retinal cells was varied. There was no change in the observed adhesive specificities when the age of the tectal halves was varied from 8 to 14 days. Further, dorsal retinal cells always showed adhesive preference towards ventral tectal halves when the retinal cell age was varied from 3 to 9 days. Ventral retinal cells, in contrast, did not show specificity toward dorsal tectal halves until after day 6.

In light and electron micrographs of innervated and noninnervated tecta that had collected retinal cells, no direct attachment of the collected cells to tectal cell bodies could be observed. The cells seemed to be bound to either tectal cell processes or an extracellular matrix.

It should be noted that this collection assay measures adhesive preferences of a heterogeneous population of retinal cell bodies to tectal surfaces. In vivo, however, only the axonal tips of the retinal ganglion cells are responsible for the retinal projection upon the tectum. If the adhesive specificities determined by the collection assay do play a role in the formation of the retinal projection, then some of the molecules responsible for recognition must be found on retinal cell bodies as well as on axonal tips.

Retinal Plasma Membranes

A plasma membrane (PM)-enriched fraction (0.1–0.3 mg protein) recovered from sucrose gradients at the 37–20% sucrose interface was identified by its increased specific radioactivity (2.5-fold) and alkaline phosphatase specific activity (3-fold) over the crude membrane fraction. Other commonly used PM markers, including 5'-nucleotidase, Na^+K^+-ATPase, and phosphodiesterase, were not useful in this system because of their exceedingly low activities. The collection assay described above was used to study the binding properties of the $[^3H]$-PM-enriched fractions to isolated tectal halves.

Preliminary results indicated that dorsal $[^3H]$-PM bound more readily to ventral than to dorsal tectal halves, the ventral to dorsal ratio being greatest (1.7) when PM derived from young (6–7-day old) retina were tested. Thus, dorsal $[^3H]$-PM showed the same adhesive preference to ventral tectal halves as the intact cells from which they were derived.

Ventral $[^3H]$-PM, however, regardless of developmental age and in spite of the fact that they are prepared from untrypsinized tissue, do not exhibit any increased binding rate to dorsal over ventral tectal halves. The reason for failure of ventral $[^3H]$-PM to exhibit adhesive properties complementary to those of dorsal $[^3H]$-PM is unknown at present.

Biochemical Approaches

Data that have been gathered in the chick retinotectal system (3, 5) show that in vitro rates of adhesion directly correlate with the morphogenetic patterns formed when retinal axons interact with the tectal surface in vivo. The simplest interpretation of these data is that the adhesive processes measured by the collection assay are the same as those responsible for the establishment of the retinotectal projection. If this supposition is valid, it follows that information about the biochemical nature of the in vitro adhesion will be directly applicable to the naturally occurring biochemistry of recognition. Also, if the importance of the recognition molecules implicated by perturbations of the collection assay could be verified in vivo, then the validity of applying collection techniques to biological problems would be strongly supported.

Initially, information about the nature of the molecules responsible for adhesive specificity in the retinotectal system came from dissociation of retinal tissue into single cells (3). Dorsal retinal cells adhered preferentially to ventral tecta immediately and retained this specificity for at least 8 hr. Ventral retinal cells, on the other hand, required 3 hr of incubation in nutrient medium before exhibiting specificity for dorsal tecta. In the complementary experiment (4), the tectal surfaces were lightly treated with proteases. The binding of ventral retina to dorsal tecta was unaffected, while the binding of dorsal retina to ventral tecta was greatly diminished.

These results suggested that the basic unit of adhesion in the retinotectal system is the interaction of a nonproteinacious moiety with a complementary protein, and that one of the molecules is located on the tectal surface and the other on the retinal cells. In addition, these results are consistent with a double gradient distribution of the two molecules in the dorsoventral axes of both retina and tectum (Fig. 3). The properties of such a model are discussed elsewhere (4, 8, 9).

Briefly, this model predicts adhesive preferences of a magnitude similar to those obtained in the collection experiments, provides a means of guiding axonal tips on the surface of the tectum to their appropriate final locuses and accounts for the continuous topography and 180° reversal that characterize many neural projections. Gottlieb et al. (10) found further experimental support for such a model when retinal-retinal adhesion was assayed. Dorsal retinal cells adhered preferentially to ventral retinal cells and vice versa.

Subsequent experiments used purified glycosidases to characterize the nonproteinacious molecule (4). When tecta were treated with hexosaminidase, only the binding of ventral retina cells to dorsal tecta was significantly decreased. Furthermore, when tecta were treated with galactosidase, the binding of ventral retinal cells to ventral tecta increased while their binding to dorsal tecta remained nearly constant. Other purified, degradative enzymes showed no such effects.

In accordance with these results, the model was more completely defined: a carbohydrate was implicated as a recognition molecule (8). The carbohydrate moiety involved in the binding might be expected to be terminated with an acetylated hexosamine and to

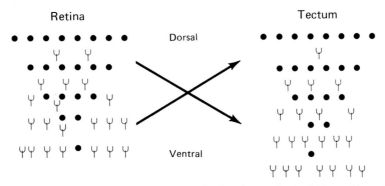

Fig. 3. A simple model of gradients of molecules in the dorsal-ventral axis which would provide adhesive connections similar to the observed retinotectal map. Cell from the dorsal region of the retina have many ●'s and few Ψ 's. The ventral part of the tectum would be its complement since it has few ●'s and many Ψ 's, thereby allowing the maximum number of bonds (Ψ) to be formed. In the same manner, processes from the ventral retina, rich in Ψ 's and poor in ●'s, would form the maximum number of connections with the dorsal tectum which is rich in ●'s and poor in Ψ 's.

be more concentrated dorsally in both the retina and the tectum. The same carbohydrate, but masked with a terminal galactose, would also be expected to be present in both retina and tectum. The protein involved in the binding, now thought to be complementary to a terminal hexosamine, would again be localized in the more ventral parts of both retina and tectum. This arrangement could lead to the observed retinotectal adhesive specificity and would also be consistent with the results obtained with the degradative enzymes.

Thus, one of the molecules implicated in the adhesive process was thought to be relatively insensitive to proteases, to be terminated with an acetylated hexosamine, and seemed, in some places, to be masked by a terminal galactose residue. One molecule that possesses these properties is the ganglioside GM_2 (Svennerholm notation, [11]). The structure of ganglioside GM_2 is:

$$\text{ceramide-glucose-gala} \overset{|}{\text{c}} \text{tose-N-acetylgalactosamine}$$

$$\text{N-acetyl-neuraminic acid}$$

By adding a galactose residue to the N-acetylgalactosamine, ganglioside GM_1 can be formed. This terminal galactoside on GM_1 and GM_2 should be insensitive to trypsin (8).

If this molecule were to participate in the formation of specific retinotectal adhesions as predicted by the double gradient model, it should be more concentrated on dorsal retinal cells than on ventral retina cells. This prediction is being tested.

The complementary recognition molecule predicted by the double gradient model would be expected to be sensitive to proteolysis. A potential candidate is the UDP-galactose:GM_2 galactosyltransferase. The feasibility of employing glycosyltransferases as recognition molecules has been discussed (4, 12, 13). Enzymes of this type have been shown to be present on the surface of retinal cell bodies (14) and in retinal synaptosomes (15). Their cell surface location, their complementarity to oligosaccharide chains, and a growing literature (16) implicating a role for them in recognition processes stimulated experiments to test for their distribution among the cells of the retina. Preliminary results suggest that they are more concentrated ventrally than dorsally. This distribution is consistent with their participation in the double gradient model for retinotectal specificity proposed above.

A number of other glycolipids, glycoproteins, and glycosyltransferases appear to show no such asymmetric localizations in the retina.

ACKNOWLEDGMENTS

This research was supported in part by research grants from the National Institutes of Child Health and Human Development. R.B. Marchase is supported by the Danforth Foundation. J.-C. Meunier is supported by the Anna Fuller Fund (grant no. 442) and the Centre National de la Recherche Scientifique (France). M. Pierce is a recipient of a Public Health training grant. This is communication #875 from the Department of Biology.

REFERENCES

1. Delong, G. R., and Coulombre, A. J., Exp. Neurol. 13:351 (1965).
2. Sperry, R. W., Proc. Nat. Acad. Sci. U.S.A. 50:703 (1963).
3. Barbera, A. J., Marchase, R. B., and Roth, S., Proc. Nat. Acad. Sci. U.S.A. 70:2482 (1973).
4. Marchase, R. B., Barbera, A. J., and Roth, S., in "Cell Patterning," CIBA Found. Symp. 29, ASP, Amsterdam 315–341 (1975).

5. Barbera, A. J., Dev. Biol. 46:167 (1975).

6. Merrell, R., and Glaser, L., Proc. Nat. Acad. Sci. U.S.A. 70:2794 (1973).

7. Meunier, J.-C., and Roth, S., manuscript in preparation.

8. Marchase, R. B., manuscript in preparation.

9. Roth, S., and Marchase, R. B., in "Current Topics in Neurobiology," S. H. Barondes (Ed.), New York: Plenum, II:227–248 (1976).

10. Gottlieb, D. I., Rock, K., and Glaser, L., Proc. Nat. Acad. Sci. U.S.A. 73:410 (1976).

11. Svennerholm, L., J. Lipid Res. 5:145 (1964).

12. Roseman, S., Chem. Phys. Lipids 5:270 (1970).

13. Roth, S., Q. Rev. Biol. 48:541 (1973).

14. Roth, S., McGuire, E. J., and Roseman, S., J. Cell Biol. 51:536 (1971).

15. Den, H., Kaufman, B., and Roseman, S., J. Biol. Chem. 245:6607 (1970).

16. Shur, B. D., and Roth, S., Biochim. Biophys. Acta 415:473 (1975).

Light-Dependent Proton Transport by Bacteriorhodopsin Incorporated in an Interface Film

S. B. Hwang, J. I. Korenbrot, and W. Stoeckenius

Departments of Physiology and Biochemistry, and Cardiovascular Research Institute, University of California, San Francisco, School of Medicine, San Francisco, California 94143

A mosaic monolayer of bacteriorhodopsin and lipid is formed at the air-water interface by spreading on the surface of water sonicated fragments of the "purple membrane" of Halobacterium halobium suspended in a hexane solution of purified soya phosphatidyl-choline. Surface potential and surface tension measurements confirm that the membrane fragments and lipids organize at the interface as a monolayer film. Freeze-etch and shadow-cast replicas of the film reveal that under appropriate conditions the fragments of purple membrane do not overlap at the interface and that they orient with their intracellular surface towards the aqueous phase. The spectrophotometric characteristics of the membrane fragments at the interface are identical to those in aqueous suspensions of the same fragments or of intact cells: the absorption spectrum in the visible range is typical of bacteriorhodopsin with a single absorption band with 570 nm λ_{max}. Furthermore, upon flash illumination the 570-nm peak undergoes a cyclic decrease in absorbance with the transient appearance of a blue-shifted photoproduct. Rapid positive changes in the monolayer surface potential are detected following illumination. These photopotentials are dramatically increased when the monolayer is covered with a thin layer (0.3 mm thick) of decane containing the hydrophobic proton acceptor FCCP. The action spectrum of the photopotential is identical to the absorption spectrum of bacteriorhodopsin in the purple membrane. The kinetics of the photoresponse is a function of the concentration of proton acceptor. The data indicate that bacteriorhodopsin acts as a light-driven proton translocator, transferring protons from the aqueous subphase across the interface to an acceptor in the organic phase.

INTRODUCTION

The plasma membrane of the cells in the nervous system is highly permeable to ions, and this ionic permeability plays a fundamental role in the function of the cell. The ionic permeability of the plasma membrane can increase, decrease, and/or change its ionic selectivity upon stimulation by an adequate stimulus. The ionic permeability of the plasma membrane and its change upon stimulation is now well understood, at least in terms of electrical equivalent circuits (1). However, the molecular mechanisms of this ionic permeability are not at all well understood. The introduction by Mueller et al. (2) of model lipid bilayers which simulate the basic structural characteristics of cell membranes has opened the possibility of developing our understanding of these molecular mechanisms.

As expected from simple thermodynamic considerations, lipid bilayers have extremely low ionic permeabilities (3). The high ionic permeabilities characteristic of nerve cell membranes must, therefore, arise from the protein or glycoprotein components of the membranes. High ionic permeabilities and even generation of action potentials can be induced in model membranes by incorporation of small peptide antibiotics into these membranes (4). These model ion translocators, discussed elsewhere in this conference, have been used to develop detailed molecular mechanisms for ion transport (4). This approach has been extended to study mechanisms of ion transport in biological membranes through attempts to isolate from these membranes putative ion translocators and to incorporate them into model lipid bilayers. The possible pitfalls of this approach are many. We do not yet understand in strict thermodynamic terms the energies involved in protein-lipid interactions in membranes, nor the details of the molecular assembly of most membranes (5). In trying to reconstitute functional model membranes we must therefore choose methods on a somewhat arbitrary basis. Nonetheless, successful reconstitution of some functional membrane lipid-protein complexes have been accomplished particularly through the pioneering methods of Racker and his collaborators (6, 7) (see also Segrest and Hubbell in this conference). Reconstitution, it must be remembered, should be considered successful only when the functional properties which can be measured in both the model and the biological system are the same.

We briefly report here on the ion translocating properties of bacteriorhodopsin incorporated in a novel model system. Bacteriorhodopsin is the only protein constituent of the "purple membrane" of Halobacterium halobium (8). Purple membrane consists of specialized patches in the plasma membrane of the bacteria which are synthesized by the bacterial cells only when grown at low oxygen tension (8). They mediate the ability of the cell to eject protons (9), synthesize ATP (10), and inhibit oxygen consumption upon illumination (11). Bacteriorhodopsin constitutes 75% of the dry weight of purple membrane and is organized as a two-dimensional crystalline array (12).

Analysis of electron diffraction patterns at 7-Å resolution (13) indicates that bacteriorhodopsin contains seven closely packed α-helical segments which extend roughly perpendicular to the plane of the membrane and span the bilayer. Bacteriorhodopsin contains a chromophore, retinal, covalently bound on a 1:1 mole ratio (8). This gives it a characteristic absorption spectrum with a 570 nm λ_{max}. Flash spectroscopy indicates that, in the light, bacteriorhodopsin undergoes a fast cyclic photoreaction (14, 15). A single photon absorbed induces a single protein molecule to undergo one cycle through at least five different spectroscopically recognizable intermediates, returning to the original state in about 8 msec at room temperature (20°C) (14). This fast cyclic photoreaction is accompanied by the release and uptake of a single proton (14, 16). When fragments of purple membrane are incorporated and oriented in a bilayer separating two aqueous compartments, the light-dependent uptake and release of protons by bacteriorhodopsin results in a net vectorial transport of protons from one compartment to the other, even against an electrochemical gradient. That is, bacteriorhodopsin functions as a light-driven proton pump (19).

The proton pump activity has been inferred from changes in extracellular pH detected upon illumination of intact bacteria (9), bacterial cell envelopes (17, 18), and model phospholipid vesicles containing bacteriorhodopsin as the only protein (19, 32). These systems, however, are of limited experimental value in trying to understand the mechanisms of the function of bacteriorhodopsin since only the outside compartment is accessible to direct measurements. To overcome these limitations, planar lipid films containing purple membrane and separating the large aqueous compartments have been developed by Drachev et al. (20). Also, Bogulavsky et al. (21) have formed films of purple membrane separating an aqueous from a nonaqueous compartment by adsorbing purple membrane fragments from water to an octane-water interface: Both of these systems, although promising, are limited by uncertainties in the amount of purple membrane at the interface and, more importantly, by the lack of control over the orientation of purple membrane in the films.

Amphiphilic molecules, that is, molecules whose structure includes both groups readily soluble in water (hydrophilic) and groups readily soluble in organic solvents (hydrophobic) (28) aggregate into micelles in the bulk of an aqueous solvent such that the hydrophobic groups segregate from the water. At the surface of the aqueous solvent, on the other hand, amphiphilic molecules form oriented monomolecular films (mono-layers) with their hydrophobic groups extended into the air and the hydrophilic groups oriented in the water. Formation of stable insoluble films at the air-water interface offers the possibility, therefore, of obtaining planar arrays of highly oriented molecules separating two compartments of very different dielectric constants. We have formed such insoluble films with fragments of purple membrane and have thus obtained planar films of known amounts of well oriented bacteriorhodopsin separating two compartments. We briefly present here some of the characteristics of the light-dependent proton translocation by bacteriorhodopsin in this model system.

METHODS

Insoluble films at the air-water interface were formed by spreading onto a clean water surface sonicated, delipidated fragments of purple membrane suspended in a hexane solution of purified soya phosphatidylcholine (Soya PC). These films are hereafter referred to as mosaic monolayers. The hexane suspension of purple membrane was prepared by the following standard procedure, developed on the basis of the experimental protocols of Das and Crane (22) and Gitler and Montal (23). Intact purple membrane fragments, prepared according to Oesterhelt and Stoeckenius (24), were suspended in 2 ml of basal salt solution (4.35 M NaCl, 0.275 M KCl, 0.080 M $MgSO_4$, 0.009 M Na citrate, pH 7) at a concentration of 0.56 mg/ml (1.15 OD at 570 nm). This suspension was sonicated for 30 sec in a bath sonicator (Model G-80-80-1, 80 W power: Laboratory Supply Co., Hicksville, N.Y.) 0.5 ml of a 0.32 mg/ml solution of Soya PC (purified according to Hanahan et al. [25]) in hexane was layered on top of the purple membrane suspension. This two-phase system was vigorously mixed in a vortex mixer (Vari-Whirl Mixer, VWR Scientific) for 5 sec. The immiscible phases were then separated by centrifuga-tion at 1,500 × g for 10 min in a clinical centrifuge, (Damon/IEC Division, Needham Hts., Mass.). After centrifugation, three phases were distinguished: a lower, clear aqueous phase; a middle, narrow turbid phase containing the purple membrane fragments and probably some water suspended in hexane; and an upper, clear hexane phase. The aqueous phase was carefully and completely removed with a Pasteur pipette. To the re-maining phases, 2.2 ml of hexane were added. Immediately before spreading, the sus-pension of purple membrane in hexane was sonicated for 60 sec in the bath sonicator. The timing of this sonication is critical, since long sonication periods (longer than 5 min) denature the protein. A fresh suspension was prepared in this way for every monolayer made.

The physical properties of the surface film were measured in a surface balance avail-able to us through the courtesy of Dr. J. Goerke who has described it in detail elsewhere

(26). Surface pressure was measured by the Wilhelmy plate method. Surface potential was measured with an ionizing surface electrode with 5 μCi of Ra^{226} as the source of α particles. Photopotentials were measured in a small fixed area trough made of Teflon with dimensions of 5 X 6 X 1 cm.

To measure photopotentials, a variable DC offset was used to null out the "dark" surface potential. Photopotentials were recorded as light-induced changes in surface potential.

Multilayer stacks of the mosaic monolayers were made by the classical technique of Blodgett and Langmuir (27). Clean glass slides were slowly (2 cm/min) inserted and withdrawn at right angles to the interface containing the mosaic monolayer. Material transferred from the surface to the solid support only as the slide was withdrawn from the interface. For electron microscopy, a single mosaic monolayer was transferred to a solid support, either glass or mica, and shadow-cast or freeze-etch replicas were made of the material. The replicas were observed with a Siemens 1A electron microscope with 80 kV accelerating voltage.

Absorption spectra of the multilayers were measured in either a Cary 118 C or a Cary 14 scanning spectrophotometer equipped with scattering transmission accessories.

To illuminate the mosaic monolayer, a 250-W quartz iodine lamp was used as a light source (Leitz Prado slide projector). Light was filtered through: 1) IR absorbing glass filters; 2) carefully calibrated neutral density filters; and 3) narrow band interference filters, as needed. A system of lenses and mirrors was used to produce an image which illuminated all of the surface of the trough (30 cm^2) from above. In the action spectrum experiments, the energy flow at each of the wavelengths tested was measured with a calibrated radiometer at the position of the water surface, and neutral density filters were used to obtain the same energy flux at all wavelengths.

Experiments were done with 4X distilled H$_2$O at pH 5.6–5.8 as the subphase. Water was distilled once from alkaline permanganate and once from acid. As in all surface chemistry work, extreme care must be taken to keep the troughs very clean and to purify and redistill organic solvents. All experiments were done at room temperature (20–22°C). Other methods are described in figure legends.

RESULTS AND DISCUSSION

To spread molecules into a film at an air-water interface, these molecules are usually dissolved in a "spreading solvent." Such a solvent should disperse the film-forming molecules at the interface and then evaporate while in no way chemically modifying these molecules. Low-boiling point organic solvents have been commonly used as spreading solvents in monolayer studies of phospholipids and fatty acids (29). We have used a suspension of sonicated purple membrane fragments in a solution of soya phosphatidyl-choline with hexane as the spreading solution.

The isolated purple membrane consists of sheet-like membrane fragments. In the PC-containing hexane phase one expects a disruption of the lipid bilayer structure of purple membrane fragments. Indeed, thin layer chromatography demonstrates that hexane extracts some of the endogenous lipids from the purple membrane. The modified membranes, however, remain as sheets and retain their normal structure. More importantly, bacteriorhodopsin does not appear to denature in the organic phase, at least as indicated by its absorption spectrum. Figure 1 illustrates the absorption spectrum of the purple membrane fragments before and after partition into the organic phase, followed by 5 min of sonication in the organic phase. The spectra are essentially identical, with only a slight blue shift in the λ_{max} ($\sim$8 nm) of the visible absorption band in the organic phase. With longer sonication times bacteriorhodopsin begins to denature in the hexane. Bacterio-rhodopsin in aqueous suspension in the dark reversibly blue-shifts its λ_{max} from 570 to 560 accompanied by an isomerization of its chromaphore from all-trans to 13-cis (33, 34). This reversible blue-shift is also seen in the organic phase.

When the hexane-PC suspension of purple membrane in hexane is spread at a clean water surface, insoluble surface films form. Characteristics of these films in the surface potential vs. area and surface pressure vs. area isotherms are shown in Fig. 2. Also illustrated are typical isotherms obtained when PC is spread alone. Purple membrane containing films show a more expanded surface pressure isotherm than PC monolayers. The collapse pressure however, is the same for both films. Surface potential isotherms also show the different compressibilities of the PC and purple membrane films. The observation that the surface potential of the purple membrane film is about 100 mV more negative (260 mV ± 20) than that of the PC film (380 mV ± 20) suggests that purple membrane has either a net negative change or a dipole oriented along a vector opposite to that of the dipole in the PC molecules, or both. The relatively negative surface potentials of the mosaic monolayer may arise at least in part from negatively charged purple membrane lipids incorporated into the lipid monolayer. The physical organization of the purple membrane film was studied

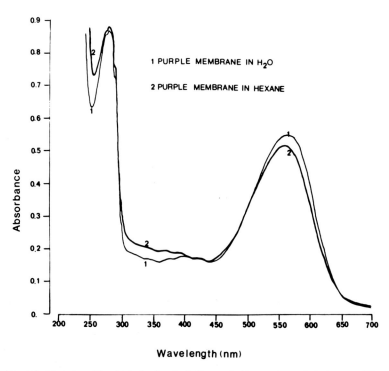

Fig. 1. Absorption spectra of bacteriorhodopsin before and after partition into hexane. The spectrum of a suspension of purple membrane fragments in 2 ml basal salt solution was recorded. The purple membrane fragments were partitioned into a solution of soy PC in hexane as described under Methods. After separation from the aqueous phase, the organic phase was continuously sonicated for 5 min and the absorption spectrum was then immediately recorded. The similarity of the two spectra indicates that bacteriorhodopsin is essentially intact in the organic phase.

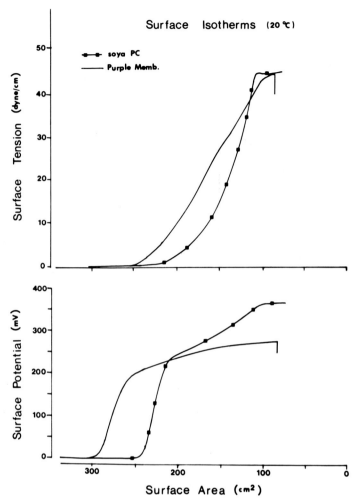

Fig. 2. Surface potential – area and surface pressure – area isotherms recorded in an automatic surface balance with a motor driven barrier. The mosaic monolayers are expanded and have a lower surface potential at collapse than soya PC monolayers.

by observing shadow-cast replicas of the monolayer in the electron microscope. A typical field is shown in Fig. 3. Small typically 0.1 μm diameter, fragments of purple membrane are seen. They are dispersed over a smooth background, which presumably represents the lipid monolayer. With the lipid to protein weight ratio used in these experiments, the fragments of purple membrane in the interface do not overlap and are homogeneously distributed. Approximately 36% of the water surface is covered by purple membrane fragments. Freeze-etch replicas of the mosaic monolayer show the same fracture faces as whole cells and they have been used to demonstrate the orientation of purple membrane at the interface. Only about 0.2% of the purple membrane fragments in the mosaic mono-layer fracture along their hydrophobic interior; the rest of the fragments show only the membrane surface. A typical freeze-fractured and etched replica is shown in Fig. 3. Most of the fragments appear to be "rough" and the hexagonal repeat unit of the crystalline array of proteins can be seen. This is the typical appearance of the cytoplasmic fracture face of whole cells. Few fractured fragments (arrow) are smooth. Non-fractured fragments are recognized by their thickness and smooth surface. A survey of many different fields suggests that about 85% of the purple membrane fragments are oriented such that the aqueous subphase is equivalent to the intracellular space in the bacteria.

One cannot assume that the bacteriorhodopsin protein will remain in its native structure when spread at an air-water interface, and preservation of structure at the interface must be demonstrated. We have investigated the structure of bacteriorhodopsin at the interface by studying the spectral characteristics of multilayers of mosaic monolayer both in the dark and following illumination. A typical absorption spectrum of a Langmuir-Blodgett multilayer formed by successive deposition of 80 monolayers is shown in Fig. 4. The absorption spectrum of bacteriorhodopsin in the multilayer is identical to that seen in aqueous suspension with a λ_{max} at 570 nm. The optical density at 570 nm for a single monolayer calculated from Fig. 4 is 3.75×10^{-4} O.D. Using a molar extinction coefficient of 63,000 (33) for bacteriorhodopsin and the known dimensions of the crystalline lattice of purple membrane ($63 \times 63 \times 50$ Å) which contains three single proteins, it is possible to calculate the fraction of the surface of a monolayer which must be occupied by purple membrane to account for the observed absorption. We obtain 41% which is in close agreement with the value of 36% estimated by electron microscopy. Further improvement on the agreement may result if the orientation of the chromophore in the multilayers could be accounted for. Figure 4 also illustrates that bacteriorhodopsin in the mosaic monolayer can undergo the "dark-adaptation" cycle seen in aqueous suspensions of purple membrane. The λ_{max} shifts from 570 to 560 after 3 hr in the dark. The λ_{max} returns to 570 after illumination. Flash spectroscopy of the multilayers has shown that bacteriorhodopsin after spreading still undergoes a photoreaction cycle similar to that seen in aqueous suspensions of bacteriorhodopsin if somewhat slower. Thus, we have formed planar film at the air-water interface which contain homogeneously distributed, highly oriented, and structurally intact bacteriorhodospin.

If bacteriorhodospin is functionally intact in the mosaic monolayer, and with its cytoplasmic surface towards the subphase, we would expect that, upon illumination, protons (positive charges) would be transported from the aqueous phase through the mosaic monolayer. We have tested this possibility by measuring light-induced changes in the electrical potential across the mosaic monolayer. This electrical potential, referred to as the surface potential, is defined as the difference in Volta potentials of the two phases, water and air, separated by the film. The surface potential, therefore, in addition to measuring the electrical properties of the film-forming molecules, such as their charge and dipole moments, also measures the distribution of charges between the two phases separated by the film. If charges move from one phase to another, this will result in a change in surface potential. In the convention used in these experiments positive potentials indicate transfer of positive charge from the aqueous to the air phase.

When the mosaic monolayer was illuminated, a small but consistent positive potential increase was detected (typically 1 mV), as shown in Fig. 5. This small photopotential could be caused by changes in the net charge or dipole moment of bacteriorhodopsin. However, if the photopotential were the result of charge transfer across the film, we would also expect it to be small because the Born charging energy of protons would make their transfer from H_2O to air most improbable (3). To minimize the Born energy difference for protons between the aqueous and nonaqueous phases we overlayed the mosaic monolayer with a thin layer of purified decane (0.3 mm thick) containing the lipid soluble proton acceptor FCCP (35) (carbonyl cyanide-P-trifluoromethoxy phenal

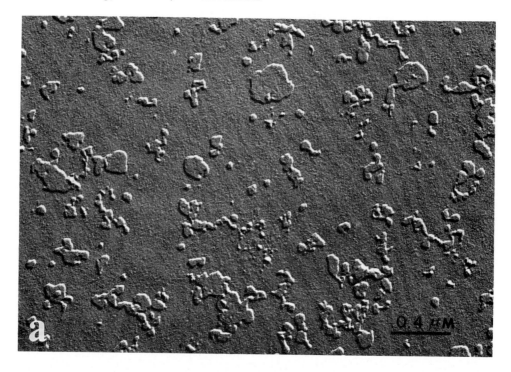

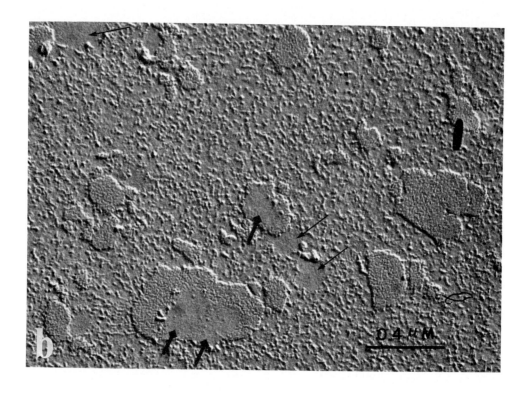

hidrazone). Decane has a dielectric behavior similar to that of air and would not be expected to disrupt the mosaic monolayer if carefully applied. When decane was gently applied drop by drop to the top of a collapsed mosaic monolayer, it slowly spread to a uniform layer in about 30 min and neither the surface pressure nor the surface potential of the film changed. As illustrated in Fig. 5, decane by itself had not effect on the surface photopotential. However, when the proton acceptor FCCP was present in the decane large photopotentials developed.

If the photopotential recorded is the result of the absorption of light by bacteriorhodopsin, then its action spectrum should be the same as the absorption spectrum of the protein. Fig. 6 illustrates that this indeed was the case. The photovoltage developed by mosaic monolayer as a function of wavelength matches the absorption curve of bacteriorhodopsin over the range tested.

The kinetic characteristics of the light response with 5×10^{-8} M FCCP are illustrated in Fig. 7. As light is turned on, a positive voltage develops which reaches a steady value maintained as long as the light is on. The surface potential returns to its original value when the light is switched off. The maximum voltage in the steady state is proportional to the logarithm of the light intensity. The "on" rate of the response, measured as the initial slope, increases steeply as light intensity increases. The "off" rate of the response, measured as the half-time of the voltage decay when light is switched off, is nearly independent of light intensity.

We have developed the following model to explain the observed characteristics of the surface photopotential. The acceptor is initially present in its protonated neutral form in the decane. When decane is layered on top of the mosaic monolayer, the acceptor partitions into the aqueous phase where it dissociates to an extent determined by the pH of the subphase. The negatively charged unprotonated form of the acceptor is a lipid soluble anion which partitions back into the decane until equilibrium is reached in the dark. When the mosaic monolayer is illuminated, bacteriorhodopsin absorbs a photon and translocates protons,* from the aqueous to the organic phase. This charge translocation produces the change in surface potential.

---

*That the positive charges transported are indeed protons is suggested by the facts that: 1)FCCP has been shown to be highly selective for protons (35) and 2) the subphase in all these experiments was unbuffered 4× distilled water in which concentration of cations other than H^+ would be expected to be extremely low. We can not, however, distinguish between H^+ moving into the decane and OH^- moving in the opposite direction.

Fig. 3. Electron micrographs of the mosaic monolayer. a) The shadow casted replica of a mosaic monolayer transferred to a mica support. The mosaic monolayer consists of non-overlapping homogeneously distributed fragments of purple membrane interspersed in a monolayer of lipid. b) Freeze-fracture etched replica of a monolayer transferred to glass and then covered with a soya PC monolayer and a copper plate applied to the surface. The resulting bilayer was frozen in Freon 22 and fractured in a Balzers BA510 unit. Fracture was followed by 5 min etching at $-100°C$. Shown is the replica from the glass side. The heavy arrow indicates a nonfractured surface. The light arrow indicates the smooth fracture face. The rest of the fragments in the micrograph reveal the rough fracture face.

Dark-Adaptation in multilayers

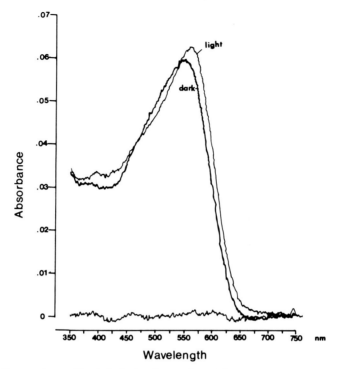

Fig. 4. Absorption spectrum of bacteriorhodopsin mosaic multilayers. Eighty monolayers were stacked successively on a glass slide by the method of Blodgett and Langmuir. The absorption spectrum recorded shows a λ_{max} at 570 nm, and it is indistinguishable from the spectrum recorded in aqueous suspensions of bacteriorhodopsin. The λ_{max} reversibly shifts to 560 nm during prolonged incubation in the dark.

Surface Photo-potential

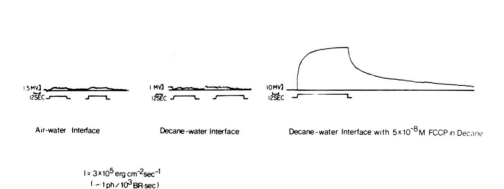

$$I = 3 \times 10^5 \, erg \, cm^{-2} sec^{-1}$$
$$(\sim 1 \, ph \, / \, 10^3 \, BR \cdot sec)$$

Fig. 5. Surface photopotential of the mosaic monolayer on unbuffered 4 times distilled water pH 5.6. A small positive change in surface potential is detected upon illumination. The photo-voltage is enhanced when a thin layer of decane containing the proton acceptor FCCP is layered on top of the monolayer. Decane without acceptor has no effect.

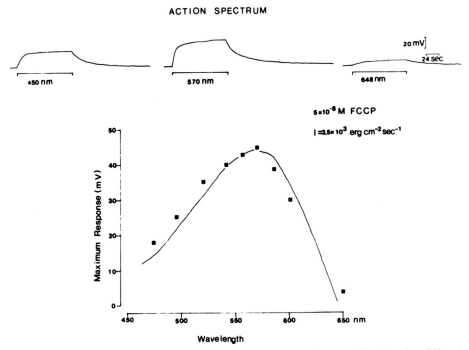

Fig. 6. Action spectrum of the surface photopotential. The monolayer was illuminated at different wavelengths with 96 sec light pulses of 3.5×10^3 erg cm^{-2} sec^{-1}. The steady-state photovoltage recorded at each wavelength is plotted as a function of wavelength. The decane phase contained 5×10^{-8} M FCCP.

The protons in the decane are accepted by the unprotonated form of the acceptor molecule and a protonated neutral form results, which partitions back into the water, creating a back-diffusion path for protons. The steady-state photovoltage observed in these experiments are therefore the balance of the light-dependent translocation of protons by bacteriorhodopsin from the aqueous to the organic phase and the light independent translocation of protons by FCCP$^-$ from the organic to the aqueous phase. As light intensity increases, more bacteriorhodopsin molecules are excited per unit time and this results in an increase both in the rate of proton transport and in the total amount of protons transported. This is reflected by the light dependence of both the "on" rate and the steady-state voltage of the photoresponse. The off-response results from the back-diffusion of protons mediated by the proton acceptor. The off rate, therefore, is determined by the concentration of the acceptor, since proton conductance induced by the acceptor is linearly proportional to its concentration (35).

This model for the mechanism of the observed photo response makes a few simple predictions: 1) photovoltages recorded in the steady state should be the same regardless of whether the FCCP$^-$ is initially added to the aqueous or the organic phase; 2) photovoltages with the same general characteristics observed should be obtained with other lipid-soluble proton acceptors; 3) the kinetics of the photovoltage should be a function of proton acceptor concentration. The steady-state voltage should increase in magnitude with proton acceptor concentration, reach a maximum, and then decrease. Furthermore, the steady-state photovoltage should begin to decrease in magnitude at concentration of

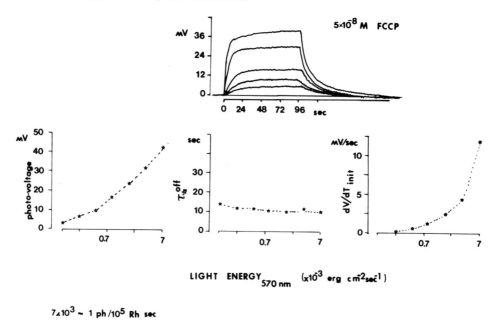

Fig. 7. Kinetics of the surface photopotential. The "on" rate is measured as the initial slope of the photo-response and the "off" rate is measured as the half-time of the return of the surface potential to its initial value after light is switched off. Steady voltage "on" rate and "off" rate are plotted as a function of light intensity. The light was filtered through a narrow band interference filter (15 nm half band width) centered at 570 nm.

acceptor that accelerate the rate of the "off" response. This is because the steady-state voltage is the result of a balance between the proton transport by bacteriorhodopsin into the decane and their back-diffusion mediated by the acceptor. As the concentration of acceptor increases, the number of negatively charged acceptor molecules in decane increases to a maximum amount limited by space charge considerations. This increases the steady-state concentration of protons in decane in the light because the Born energy difference for protons is being progressively decreased. At some concentration of acceptor, however, the back-diffusion rate which is proportional to acceptor concentration becomes comparable to the bacteriorhodopsin forward rate and the net proton accumulation in decane in the light is decreased; 4) the positive photovoltage should be cancelled in the presence of negatively charged lipid soluble anions such as tetraphenyl boron. This is because the positive voltage will force redistribution of lipid-soluble negative charges between the aqueous and organic phases to minimize changes in free energy. These predictions have all been confirmed experimentally (31).

In conclusion, we have developed a model system where intact and well-oriented bacteriorhodopsin molecules are increased between the two compartments, permitting us to measure the light driven translocation of protons by this protein.

ACKNOWLEDGMENTS

This research was supported by grants EY-01586 and HL-06285 from the National Institutes of Health and NGL-025-014 from the National Aeronautics Space Administration. We thank Knute A. Fisher for advice and help with the freeze-fracturing of the films, and Richard H. Lozier for the flash spectroscopy.

REFERENCES

1. Hille, B., in "Membranes – A Series of Advances," Vol. 3, A. Eisenman (Ed.). Marcel Dekker, Inc. (1975).
2. Mueller, P., Rudin, D. O., Tien, H. T., and Wescott, W. C., Nature 194:979 (1962).
3. Parsegian, A., Nature 221:844 (1969).
4. McLaughlin, S., and Eisenberg, M., Annu. Rev. Biophys. Bioengineer. 4:335 (1975).
5. Tanford, C., "The Hydrophobic Effect." New York: Wiley-Interscience Publication (1973).
6. Kagawa, Y., Biochim. Biophys. Acta 265:297 (1972).
7. Montal, M., Annu. Rev. Biophys. Bioengineer. 5:119 (1976).
8. Oesterhelt, D., and Stoeckenius, W., Nat. New Biol. 233:149 (1971).
9. Oesterhelt, D., and Stoeckenius, W., Proc. Nat. Acad. Sci. U.S.A. 70:2853 (1973).
10. Danon, A., and Stoeckenius, W., Proc. Nat. Acad. Sci. U.S.A. 71:1234 (1974).
11. Oesterhelt, D., and Krippahl, G., FEBS Lett. 36:72 (1973).
12. Blaurock, A. E., and Stoeckenius, W., Nat. New Biol. 233:152 (1971).
13. Henderson, R., and Unwin, P. N. T., Nature 257:28 (1975).
14. Lozier, R. H., Bogomolni, R. A., and Stoeckenius, W., Biophys. J. 15:955 (1975).
15. Dencher, W., and Wilms, M., Biophys. Struct. Mechanisms 1:259 (1975).
16. Chance, B., Porte, M., Hess, B., and Oesterhelt, D., Biophys. J. 15:913 (1975).
17. Kanner, B. I., and Racker, E., Biochem. Biophys. Res. Commun. 64:1054 (1975).
18. MacDonald, R. E., and Lanyi, J. K., Biochemistry 14:2882 (1975).
19. Racker, E., and Stoeckenius, W., J. Biol. Chem. 249:662 (1974).
20. Drachev, L. A., Kaulen, A. D., Ostroumov, S. A., and Skulachev, V. P., FEBS Lett. 39:43 (1974).
21. Boguslavsky, L. I., Kondrashin, A. D., Kozlov, I. A., Metelsky, S. T., Skulachev, V. P., and Volkov, D. G., FEBS Lett. 50:223 (1975).
22. Das, M. L., and Crane, F. L., Biochemistry 3:696 (1964).
23. Gitler, C., and Montal, M., Biochim. Biophys. Res. Commun. 47:1486 (1972).
24. Oesterhelt, D., and Stoeckenius, W., Methods Enzymol. 31:667 (1974).
25. Hanahan, D. J., Dittmer, J. C., and Warashina, E., J. Biol. Chem. 228:685 (1957).
26. Goerke, J., Harper, H. H., and Borowitz, M., "Surface Chemistry of Biological Systems," New York: Plenum Press (1970).
27. Blodgett, K. B., and Langmuir, I., Phys. Rev. 51:964 (1937).
28. Hartley, G. S., "Aqueous Solutions of Paraffin-Chain Salts," Paris: Hermann and Co. (1936).
29. Gaines, G. L., "Insoluble Monolayers at Liquid-Gas Interfaces," New York: John Wiley & Sons, Inc. (1966).
30. Miller, I. R., and Bach, D., Surface Colloid Sci. 6:185 (1973).
31. Hwang, S. B., Korenbrot, J. I., and Stoeckenius, W., manuscript in preparation.
32. Hwang, S. B., and Stoeckenius, W., unpublished results.
33. Oesterhelt, D., Meentzen, M., and Schuhmann, L., Eur. J. Biochem. 40:453 (1973).
34. Jan, L. Y., Vision Res. 15:1081 (1975).
35. Liberman, E. A., and Topaly, V. P., Biochim. Biophys. Acta 163:125 (1968).

The Role of Non-Neuronal Cells in the Development of Sympathetically Derived Neurons

Paul H. Patterson, Linda L. Y. Chun, and Louis F. Reichardt

Department of Neurobiology, Harvard Medical School, Boston, Massachusetts 02115

As the other speakers in this session have discussed, a variety of influences are brought to bear on presumptive sympathetic neurons during their migration and subsequent differentiation. Some of these influences, namely nerve growth factor (NGF) and electrical activity, continue to affect the functional state of these neurons even in the adult. These studies have involved axotomy, decentralization, transplantation in embryos, or explantation to the anterior chamber of the eye, to the chorioallantoic membrane, or to organ culture. Yet another approach has been to dissociate the neurons and grow them in cell culture. Investigation of their development in the absence of other cell types or in the presence of added cells of known origin then contributes information about the relative importance of such cellular influences as well as their mechanism of action. The potential for controlling the fluid environment as well as the substratum on which the cells are grown may also be exploited to yield information about normal development.

Such an approach presupposes the ability of neurons to differentiate after being dissociated, and to survive in the absence of other cell types. While there have been reports of difficulties along these lines (1—3), several culture systems are available which support the development of dissociated neurons and their growth in the virtual absence of other cell types, notably sympathetic (4—7) and sensory (8) neurons and neuronal tumor lines (9, 10). The ultimate in this type of system may be a study of the development of single isolated neurons so as to circumvent possible influences the neurons may have on each other. In such a situation the roles played by the fluid medium (hormones, growth factors, etc.) and the substratum (collagen, etc.) can be isolated and more effectively studied.

Considerable biochemical, electrophysiological, and morphological information is now available on the development of sympathetic neurons taken from neonatal rats and grown in the virtual absence of other cell types (Table I). Such neurons are mechanically dissociated and grown on collagen-coated dishes in media which are nonpermissive for the proliferation of the ganglionic non-neuronal cells, and which contain (among other ingredients) NGF, adult rat serum, and a polymer called methocel (6). Under these conditions they develop many of the properties expected for mature sympathetic neurons. They synthesize and accumulate the characteristic adrenergic neurotransmitters, norepinephrine (NE) and dopamine (DA), from the precursor tyrosine (6) and they develop this ability along a time course which at least qualitatively parallels that seen in in vivo studies of the catecholamine (CA)-biosynthetic enzymes and CA histofluorescence (11). This development in culture appears to be a real differentiation in that it differs in both magnitude and

TABLE I. Properties of Sympathetic Neurons Grown in the Absence of Other Cell Types

(A)	Synthesis and accumulation of DA and NE.
(B)	Development of this ability parallels in vivo time course and is different in magnitude and time course from overall neuronal growth.
(C)	No detectable synthesis and accumulation of GABA, 5-HT, or histamine, and little or no acetylcholine.
(D)	Storage of NE in vesicles.
(E)	Release of NE by depolarization which is Ca^{++}-dependent and blocked by Mn^{++}, Mg^{++}, or Co^{++}.
(F)	NE uptake system which is saturable, has high affinity, and is blocked by the appropriate drugs.
(G)	Generation and conduction of action potentials and sensitivity to acetylcholine.
(H)	EM evidence of adrenergic synapses between the neurons.

time course from overall neuronal growth as measured by synthesis and accumulation of protein, lipid, and RNA from radioactive precurors (11). As was expected, the neurons do not synthesize and accumulate detectable quantities of the transmitter candidates gamma-amino butyric acid (GABA), serotonin (5-HT), or histamine from their respective labeled precursors. However, very small amounts of acetylcholine (ACh) are made from radio-active choline in older cultures (6) and the significance of this observation will be con-sidered in more detail later. Evidence that the cells can store NE as well as synthesize it is of three types (12): (1) pharmacological — reserpine almost completely blocks the ability of the neurons to accumulate NE; (2) biochemical — ^{3}H-NE can be found in osmotically labile subcellular particles; and (3) morphological — recent autoradiographic studies done in collaboration with S. Rowe and P. Claude (unpublished observations) using ^{3}H-NE indicate that most of the NE is stored in vesicles. The visualization of large numbers of small granular vesicles with permanganate fixation may also be taken as evidence of NE storage (Ref. 7, and S. Landis, unpublished observations). The accumulated NE can also be released by depolarizing agents, that is, elevated KCl or veratridine. The release of ^{3}H-NE is rapid, is Ca^{++}-dependent, and is blocked by Mn^{++}, Co^{++}, or Mg^{++} (12, 13). Finally, the cultured neurons are able to take up NE. The uptake is saturable, has an apparent K_m of 1 μM, and is blocked by cocaine and desmethylimipramine (12).

Electrophysiological examination of the neurons has shown that they can generate and conduct action potentials and are sensitive to iontophoresed ACh as are their counter-parts in vivo (P. O'Lague, E. Furshpan, D. Potter, and K. Obata, unpublished observations). Finally, these neurons grown in the absence of other cells form morphological synapses with one another and these synapses have the fine structure expected of adrenergic cells: they have numerous small granular vesicles, occasional large granular vesicles, and both pre- and postsynaptic membrane specializations (Ref. 7, and S. Landis, unpublished observations).

In summary, then, the neurons grown in the virtual absence of non-neuronal cells develop, so far as is now known, in a fashion appropriate for sympathetic neurons in vivo. There are, of course, questions still unanswered: are the neuron-neuron synapses functional? Do similar synapses occur in the ganglion in vivo (e.g., Refs. 14, 15) or are they peculiar to the culture system, perhaps the result of the absence of any normal adrenergic target in the dish? Are CA enzyme levels or NE content increased in the cultured neurons in the presence of spinal cord explants or simply by making the sympathetic neurons electrically more active? (See I. Black, this volume.) Do NE uptake, synthesis, storage, and release appear in a defined sequence or simultaneously? These and other questions are now being investigated.

These studies form the foundation for the next series of experiments concerning the role of non-neuronal cells in neuronal development. The rationale was to investigate changes brought about in the neurons by coculturing them with ganglionic non-neuronal cells (a few of which are initially present and proliferate in permissive medium) or with non-neuronal cells from other sources.

An early and startling finding in mixed cultures of neurons plus ganglionic non-neuronal cells was that they could synthesize and accumulate as much as 1,000-fold more ^{3}H-ACh from ^{3}H-choline than did the neuron-only cultures which produced very little ACh (16). Furthermore, the ACh was not a minor by-product but rather was used as the neurotransmitter in functional cholinergic synapses between the neurons themselves (17, 18) and between the neurons and skeletal myotubes (19). Table II summarizes biochemical data from four typical culture preparations. Neurons can be grown alone either by using a medium which lacks bicarbonate and thereby does not permit growth and proliferation of non-neuronal cells ("L-15 Air," Ref. 6) or by using a medium with bicarbonate ("L-15 CO_2," Ref. 6) but containing a mitotic poison (cytosine arabinoside, "ARA-C," or fluorodeoxyuridine). Under these conditions, the neurons synthesize and accumulate substantial radioactive DA and NE from ^{3}H-tyrosine but little ^{3}H-ACh from radioactive choline. On the other hand, if ganglionic non-neuronal cells are grown with the neurons, the cultures produce significant amounts of ACh in addition to the catecholamines. In the course of his study on the development of synapse formation (18), P. MacLeish found that cholinergic synapses between neurons were detected earlier and to a greater extent by plating the neurons on a preformed monolayer of heart cells (both fibroblasts and muscle cells) rather than by simply allowing the ganglionic non-neuronal cells to reach confluency in 2–3 weeks. The procedure involves initially seeding dishes with dissociated cells from newborn rat heart and, when these cells reach confluency, the cultures are irradiated with ^{60}Co to block further cell division and prevent the overgrowth and rolling up of the cell mass (a technique introduced in our laboratory by P. O'Lague); neurons added at this stage develop from the outset in the presence of a substantial, constant number of non-neuronal cells. This procedure results in even higher ACh production (line 4, Table II); in fact, the cultures now produce more ACh than CAs. (Both the CA and the ACh values are lower in Table II than in the other data to be presented here; a consequence of assaying the cultures at a younger age: 10 days vs. 20–30 days.)

Since the neurons and the appropriate non-neuronal cells, when grown separately, produce little ^{3}H-ACh from ^{3}H-choline but do so when cocultured, it is natural to wonder what other biochemical changes occur when the cells get together. One change is the

TABLE II. The Effect of Non-Neuronal Cells on Neurotransmitter Production

Medium	Cells present	CA/N (fmol)	ACh/N (fmol)	ACh/CA
L-15 Air	Neurons	0.50 ± 0.06	0.005 ± 0.001	0.007 ± 0.006
L-16 CO_2 + ARA-C	Neurons	0.71 ± 0.08	0.010 ± 0.001	0.015 ± 0.012
L-15 CO_2	Neurons + non-neuronal cells	0.58 ± 0.02	0.336 ± 0.007	0.581 ± 0.009
L-15 CO_2	Neurons on heart cells	0.63 ± 0.03	1.636 ± 0.094	2.581 ± 0.100

appearance of an enzyme activity with the expected properties of choline acetyltransferase (CAT) which catalyzes the formation of ACh from choline and acetyl coenzyme A. Assays of homogenates of neuronal/non-neuronal mixed cultures show levels of CAT activity which can be $>$ 1,000-fold that seen in homogenates of either rat heart cells or neurons cultured separately (12). Other changes also occur since, as previously noted, the neurons form functional cholinergic synapses in mixed cultures.

The emergence of this new enzyme activity could be the result of an influence of the appropriate non-neuronal cells on the neurons or vice versa. Since, in the mixed cultures, the neurons formed cholinergic synapses, it seemed likely that the neurons themselves were capable of synthesizing, storing, and releasing ACh and would, therefore, be the site of the CAT activity. One method of demonstrating this would be to grow the non-neuronal cells and the neurons in separate dishes, transfer the culture medium from the former to the latter, and determine if an increase in ACh synthesis occurs in the neuronal culture, virtually free of non-neuronal cells. This experiment also bears on the question of whether CAT induction involves diffusable molecules or requires cell-cell contact between the neurons and non-neuronal cells. The results of such experiments are positive. That is, when neurons are grown in the virtual absence of non-neuronal cells but in medium "conditioned" by cardiac cells (fibroblasts and muscle cells) there is $>$ 100-fold increase in ACh synthesis and accumulation from ^{3}H-choline (12). A variety of controls have ruled out the possibility that the conditioned medium (CM) is acting by inducing the proliferation of non-neuronal cells in the neuronal cultures; thus, the non-neuronal cells can induce ACh synthesis in neurons via the extra-cellular medium.

What other changes does the CM induce in the neuronal cultures? It was previously reported that certain types of non-neuronal cells induce ACh production without appreciably affecting CA synthesis and accumulation by the same cultures (12, 16). However, more recently it has been found that as the magnitude of the ACh effect is increased, CA production actually decreases significantly. That is, by (1) employing L-15 CO_2 as the medium to be conditioned, which is better for non-neuronal cell proliferation than is L-15 Air, and (2) by analyzing older cultures (20–30 days rather than 10–15 days), the adrenergic or cholinergic character is more completely expressed and differences become larger. The inverse relationship between ACh and CA production is most apparent in the concentration dependence of the CM effect shown in Fig. 1. In this experiment neurons were grown in L-15 CO_2 but ganglionic non-neuronal cells were killed by treatment with cytosine arabinoside. Groups of 4 sister cultures were fed with CM from flasks of rat heart cells (and mixed with fresh L-15 CO_2 medium in the percentages shown) every 2 days for 20 days. At the end of this time all cultures were assayed for their ability to synthesize and accumulate both ACh and CA from the radioactive precursors. ACh production depends on the concentration of CM in the growth medium in a complex way and is still rising exponentially at the highest level of CM used, 62.5%. The increase over the control at this point is $>$ 40-fold. The ability to synthesize and accumulate CA is also exponentially, but inversely, related to the percent CM in which the neurons were grown. At the highest level CM shown, CA production is down nearly 30-fold from the control. As previously reported (12), the number of neurons is not greatly affected by CM treatment. These observations are relevant for the question of whether single neurons express both adrenergic and cholinergic properties. The inverse relationship of ACh and CA may also be taken as indirect support for the idea that single neurons can, in fact, express both properties, and this will be discussed in more detail later.

It is worth pointing out that it is possible to obtain sympathetically derived neuronal cultures virtually free of non-neuronal cells which 1) display adrenergic properties

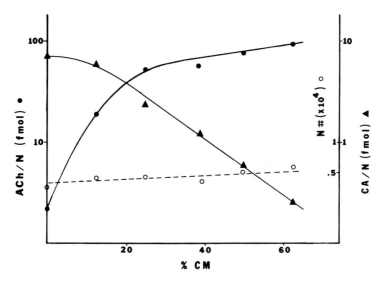

Fig. 1. The neuronal cell number (○), and the synthesis and accumulation of acetylcholine (●), and catecholamines (▲) are plotted as a function of the percent conditioned medium (CM) that the cells were grown in. The ordinate scales are logarithmic and the experimental protocol is given in the text.

almost exclusively (0% CM or Table I); 2) display striking cholinergic properties and have greatly diminished adrenergic properties (in 62.5% CM the synthesis and accumulation of ACh is > 1,000-fold more than the CA production); or 3) display hybrid properties (20% CM), all by simple manipulation of the medium. Recent electrophysiological experiments in collaboration with P. MacLeish have further emphasized the change brought about by CM in that cholinergic synapses between the neurons are very frequent in the 62.5% CM-treated cultures, infrequent in 25% CM-treated ones, and not detectable in the 0% CM-treated cultures. Thus, while in 0% CM the neurons form what appear morphologically to be adrenergic synapses with each other and can synthesize, store, and release CAs (Table I), in high concentrations of CM they form functional cholinergic synapses. The absence of non-neuronal cells will, of course, greatly aid biochemical analyses of these three conditions, e.g., membrane properties, immunological differences, etc., and perhaps yield information regarding different types of synapse formation.

One question which is important for understanding of the relevance of this cholinergic effect for normal autonomic development is what types of non-neuronal cells are able to induce ACh synthesis in these neurons? A number of such cell-specificity studies have been carried out and the results are briefly summarized here. Initially, it was found that when neurons were grown with ganglionic non-neuronal cells or C6 rat glioma cells high ACh production resulted, while 3T3 mouse fibroblasts did not cause a significant increase (16). An ambiguity in this type of experiment is that the particular non-neuronal cell type added (i.e. C6 cells) could act by causing an increased proliferation of ganglionic non-neuronal cells and thus cause an increase in ACh production without itself directly affecting the neurons. With the advent of CM, however, it is possible to grow and assay the neurons in the absence of ganglionic non-neuronal cells, making the interpretation much clearer. A variety of primary cells and cell lines have been tested as follows: a monolayer of non-neuronal cells is grown up in a flask, fresh medium is placed in the flask for 2 days (in the controls, medium is incubated in a flask without cells), then taken off and mixed with fresh medium to a concentration of 25% CM. This process is repeated every 2 days until the neurons are about 20 days old, at which time they are assayed for both CA and ACh production. On days 2–4 and 8–10 neurons are also treated with 10^{-5} M cytosine arabinoside to kill any proliferating non-neuronal cells. In some experiments the CM is also put through a 0.2 μm filter to ensure that it contains no non-neuronal cells. The first result of interest is that CM from primary cultures of several tissues taken from the new-born rat induced neuronal ACh synthesis. These tissues included heart, blood vessel, skeletal muscle, liver, and brain, and the ACh/CA values ranged from a control of < 0.1, to liver = 0.8 and skeletal muscle = 15.5. Since primary rat embryo fibroblasts were also positive (ACh/CA = 21.0), it is possible that the results from the primary tissues are all attributable to the fibroblasts in these tissues. This would be of interest not only because not all fibroblasts are the same (20) but because they produce a variety of developmentally important molecules such as NGF (21, 22), collagen (20), and hyaluronic acid (20). The fibroblasts do not lose the ability to induce ACh production after being carried in culture because a rat embryo fibroblast cell line (Microbiological Associates) was also positive. The L8 rat skeletal muscle cell line was also positive, but the steroid-secreting R_2 C Leydig cell rat tumor line was negative, indicating that not all rat cell types possess the cholinergic inductive capacity. In this series of experiments, the positive cell types not only increased the ACh/neuron values from 1.5 fmol to as high as 190 fmol, but they decreased the CA/neuron values from 28 fmol to as low as 8 fmol. The R_2 C line, which did not increase ACh levels, did not decrease the CAs.

Interestingly, three other fibroblast lines, all from non-rat sources (3T3 and L929 mouse fibroblasts, and BHK hamster fibroblasts) were very poor at inducing ACh (ACh/CA = 0.1–0.3). To test whether this is a species-specific phenomenon, CM was tested from primary chick and mouse heart flasks as well as rat. The rat neurons responded very poorly to the non-rat CM (ACh/CA = 0.01–0.04 vs. 2.37). These results indicate that the non-rat heart cells did not appropriately condition the medium, which may be because: 1) they do not have the capacity to do so; 2) they were adversely affected by the rat serum in the medium (although they grew well and beat vigorously); or 3) the neurons or the serum responded in a species-specific manner to the heart cells. These possibilities are being tested through various combinations of mouse neurons and mouse serum in addition to the usual cultures.

The finding of substantial ACh synthesis and cholinergic synapse formation in cultures of neurons taken from sympathetic ganglia requires comment. At least two hypotheses can be offered in explanation of these observations: 1) the neurons are behaving just as they do in vivo; or 2) the neurons are reacting appropriately to developmental cues they normally do not receive in vivo. In support of the first possibility is the evidence for the presence of cholinergic postganglionic sympathetic neurons in certain sympathetic ganglia including the superior cervical ganglion (SCG) of the rat (e.g., 23–25). Yamauchi et al. (25) obtained histochemical evidence consistent with the possibility that about 5% of the principal neurons in the adult rat SCG may be cholinergic. Such conventional cholinergic neurons might be responsible for the observed ACh synthesis (12) and formation of cholinergic synapses (18), and express these functions only in the presence of non-neuronal cells or CM. There are several observations which bear on this possibility. For instance, the neurons which form cholinergic synapses are not a small minority: they can make up more than half the neuronal population of mixed neuron/non-neuronal cultures. Moreover, treatment with high concentrations of CM does not cause large increases in the number of neurons (Fig. 1), which suggests that the neurons capable of making cholinergic synapses are also present in the neuron-only cultures but do not express this property. This argues against a selection hypothesis and favors a population of neurons reacting to changed culture conditions by modifying their differentiated fate. Consistent with this idea are recent observations that the best period for ACh induction is the second 10 days in vitro, rather than the first 10 days, and that ACh can still be induced in the neurons by CM addition from the 20th to the 30th day (Fig. 2). These experiments involve plating a large number of cultures and feeding them with either 0% or 25% CM every 2 days from day 0 to day 10, day 10 to day 20, or day 20 to day 30, and assaying all cultures at day 30. The results shown in Fig. 2 demonstrate that while addition of CM from day 10 to day 20 is clearly the optimal period for inducing ACh production, the effect is not due to an increase in the number of neurons nor does this feeding schedule result in increased CA production. Furthermore, this treatment gives the largest ACh effect even though the neurons were without CM for the final 10 days. These results not only argue against a selection phenomenon, but taken together with the high incidence of electrophysiologically demonstrated cholinergic neurons, support the idea that individual sympathetically derived neurons are capable of expressing cholinergic or adrenergic properties, depending on their environment. Currently, experiments are underway to study this question more directly. It is possible to grow single neurons in small wells with heart cells and assay them biochemically for transmitter synthesis and accumulation. The preliminary results using this technique have confirmed the electro-physiological findings of widespread cholinergic function in that > 80% of the single

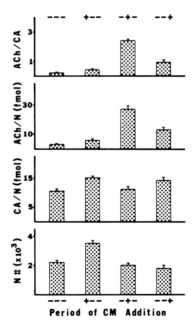

Fig. 2. The susceptibility of neurons of different ages to the presence of conditioned medium is shown for the parameters of neuronal cell number, and acetylcholine and catecholamine synthesis and accumulation. – – – refers to the neuronal cultures which were grown without CM for all three 10-day periods; + – – were cultures receiving CM from day 0 to day 10 but then grown without it from day 10 to day 20 and from day 20 to day 30; –+– were cultures receiving CM from day 10 to day 20 only. – –+ were cultures receiving CM only from day 20 to day 30. All cultures were assayed at day 30. Further details are given in the text. The small bars represent the SEM.

neurons thus far assayed have synthesized and accumulated significant levels of ACh. Control wells with heart cells but no neurons do not show ACh production. Furthermore, > 80% of the single cells assayed have shown significant ^{3}H-NE uptake. As expected from these two results, single neurons have been found which both synthesize and accumulate ACh and take up NE as well. Studies of CA production by individual neurons are in progress.

As J. Weston described earlier, the importance of the environment in controlling development of transmitter metabolism in vivo has been demonstrated by transplantation of neural crest cells to abnormal sites (26–28). Cells from the presumptive adrenergic crest (giving rise normally to sympathetic neurons or adrenal medulla) can be made to differentiate into parasympathetic cholinergic neurons by transplantation to the presumptive cholinergic region of the crest (28). It will be of interest to determine if the cholinergic induction by the non-neuronal cells in culture can be related to the influences brought to bear on presumptive parasympathetic neurons during their migration from the neural crest and/or at their final sites in their ganglia. Concerning potential influences within autonomic ganglia, the question arises, why, if sympathetic ganglionic non-neuronal cells can induce ACh synthesis in sympathetically derived neurons, do the neurons in situ remain primarily adrenergic? Of course the answer to this puzzle will not become clear until the nature of the inductive effect is understood, but several hypotheses can be offered at this point: 1) principal neurons are normally ensheathed by a special cell type (satellite cells) in vivo and they are "protected" from the non-neuronal cholinergic influence (and the minority of cholinergic sympathetic neurons are not?); 2) the ganglionic cell type which flourishes in culture (fibroblasts?) thereby greatly outnumbers the other cell types, is not so numerous within the ganglion in vivo; 3) the cholinergic induction may involve the serum in the culture medium and in vivo the neurons are not directly in contact with the serum; or 4) the cholinergic influence is present normally in vivo but is counterbalanced by an adrenergic influence not yet added to the cell cultures such as a normal sympathetic target tissue without fibroblasts.

Also of interest in this regard are the reports that non-neuronal cells influence growth and/or differentiation in a variety of neurons. Among these are a neuronal tumor line (29), sympathetic and parasympathetic ganglia explants (30–31), and dissociated sensory and sympathetic neurons (32–34). Similar techniques have also been applied to central nervous system cells in culture and these findings are of particular relevance in the present context. There is evidence consistent with CAT induction by non-neuronal cells in surface cultures from rat brain (35). Furthermore, Giller et al. (36) have reported that skeletal muscle cells increase CAT activity in spinal cord cultures. This effect is also transmitted via the medium (37). Characterization of the active factor(s) and the non-neuronal cells that produce it in this system as well as in the sympathetic system should provide information about the selectivity or generality of the cholinergic effect. In sum, it is clear that the opportunity for identifying normal developmental cues through control of the environment is being explored in a variety of culture systems and will no doubt eventually be combined with the in vivo embryological experiments in a synergistic fashion.

ACKNOWLEDGMENTS

It is a pleasure to acknowledge the able assistance of Doreen McDowell, Karen Fischer, and Kathy Birmingham with the culturing. We also thank Eleanor P. Livingston and Joe Gagliardi for excellent help with the manuscript. This work was supported by an American Heart Association Grant-in-Aid (73-877) and a United States Public Health

Service Grant (1 RO1 NS 11027) from the National Institute of Neurological and Communicable Diseases and Stroke. Paul H. Patterson is a Research Career Development Awardee of the N.I.N.C.D.S. (1 K04 NS 70806); Louis F. Reichardt has been a post-doctoral fellow of the N.I.N.C.D.S. (1 F22 NS 01784), Jane Coffin Childs Memorial Fund for Medical Research, and the Medical Foundation; and Linda L. Y. Chun is a Public Health Service Trainee (TO1 NS 05731).

REFERENCES

1. Moscona, A., in "Cells and Tissues in Culture," B. M. Willmer (Ed.). New York: Academic Press, p. 483 (1965).
2. Seeds, N,, Proc. Nat. Acad. Sci. 68:1858 (1971).
3. Varon, S., Raiborn, C., and Burnham, P., Neurobiology 4:231 (1974).
4. Levi-Montalcini, R., and Angeletti, P. U., Dev. Biol. 7:653 (1963).
5. Bray, D., Proc. Nat. Acad. Sci. 65:905 (1970).
6. Mains, R. E., and Patterson, P. H., J. Cell Biol. 59:329 (1973).
7. Rees, R., and Bunge, R. P., J. Comp. Neurol. 157:1 (1974).
8. Okun, L., J. Neurobiol. 3:111 (1972).
9. Schubert, D., Heinemann, S., Carlisle, W., Tarikas, H., Kimes, B., Patrick, J., Steinbach, J. H., Culp, W., and Brandt, B. L., Nature 249:224 (1974).
10. Nelson, P., Physiol. Rev. 55:1 (1975).
11. Mains, R. E., and Patterson, P. H., J. Cell Biol. 59:361 (1973).
12. Patterson, P. H., Reichardt, L. F., and Chun, L. L. Y., Cold Spring Harbor Symp. Quant. Biol. 40:389 (1975).
13. Burton, H., and Bunge, R. P., Brain Res. 97:157 (1975).
14. Elfvin, L.-G., J. Ultrastruct. Res. 37:411 (1971).
15. Elfvin, L.-G., J. Ultrastruct. Rev. 37:432 (1971).
16. Patterson, P. H., and Chun, L. L. Y., Proc. Nat. Acad. Sci. 71:3607 (1974).
17. O'Lague, P. H., Obata, K., Claude, P., Furshpan, E. J., and Potter, D. D., Proc. Nat. Acad. Sci. 71:3602 (1974).
18. O'Lague, P. H., MacLeish, P. R., Nurse, C. A., Claude, P., Furshpan, E. J., and Potter, D. D., Cold Spring Harbor Symp. Quant. Biol. 40:399 (1975).
19. Nurse, C., and O'Lague, P. H., Proc. Nat. Acad. Sci. 72:1955 (1975).
20. Schubert, M., and Hamerman, D., in "A Primer on Connective Tissue Biochemistry," Philadelphia: Lea & Febiger (1968).
21. Levi-Montalcini, R., and Angeletti, P. U., in "Regional Neurochemistry," S. Kety, and J. Elkes (Eds.), New York: Pergamon Press, p. 362 (1961).
22. Young, M., Oger, J., Blanchard, M., Asourian, H., Amos, H., and Arnason, B., Science 187:361 (1975).
23. Sjöqvist, F., Acta Physiol. Scand. 57:339 (1963).
24. Aiken, J., and Reit, E., J. Pharmacol. Exp. Ther. 169:211 (1969).
25. Yamauchi, A., Lever, J., and Kemp, J., J. Anat. 114:271 (1973).
26. Cohen, A., J. Exp. Zool. 179:167 (1972).
27. Norr, S., Dev. Biol. 34:16 (1973).
28. LeDouarin, N., Renaud, D., Teillet, M., and LeDouarin, G., Proc. Nat. Acad. Sci. 72:728 (1975).
29. Monard, D., Solomon, F., Rentsch, M., and Gysin, R., Proc. Nat. Acad. Sci. 70:1894 (1973).
30. Chamley, J., Campbell, G., and Burnstock, G., Dev. Biol. 33:344 (1973).
31. Coughlin, M., Dev. Biol. 43:140 (1975).
32. Varon, S., and Raiborn, C., J. Neurocytol. 1:211 (1972).
33. Burnham, P., Raiborn, C., and Varon, S., Proc. Nat. Acad. Sci. 69:3556 (1972).
34. Varon, S., Raiborn, C., and Burnham, P., Neurobiology 4:231 (1974).
35. Schrier, B., and Shapiro, D., J. Neurobiol. 5:151 (1974).
36. Giller, E., Schrier, B., Shainberg, A., Fisk, H., and Nelson, P., Science 182:588 (1973).
37. Nelson, P., Cold Spring Harbor Symp. Quant. Biol. 40:(1975).

Calcium Channels in Paramecium Aurelia

Stanley J. Schein

Departments of Molecular Biology and Neuroscience, Albert Einstein College of Medicine, Bronx, New York 10461

Reversal of swimming direction in paramecium is dependent on the calcium influx through the excitable-membrane calcium channels. Several mutants of Paramecium aurelia have been selected on the basis of their resistance to the paralyzing effect of barium. The mutants have reduced reversal behavior and are in the same three pawn genes as discovered by Kung (16, 17). Also, in barium solutions, the pawns live longer than the wild-type; however, pwB mutants are more resistant to barium toxicity than pwA mutants. These results suggest that the selection picked up mutants in the calcium channel. Electrophysiological studies demonstrate this point directly, showing defective calcium activation in all pawns, but also defective anomalous rectification in pwB mutants. A model is presented which accounts for the differences between pwA and pwB mutants. It ascribes the depolarization-sensitive "gate" function to the pwA gene product and the "pore" function to the pwB gene product. Additionally, the stability of the channel structure is demonstrated, channel half-life being from five to eight days.

Key words: calcium, excitability, paramecium, channels

INTRODUCTION

In recent years genetic techniques have been applied to a variety of neurobiological problems. The systems studied range in complexity from cerebellar mutants of mice (1) to chemotaxis mutants of bacteria (2). In the present paper I wish to discuss a genetic approach to the events underlying electrical excitability in membranes. In 1952 Hodgkin and Huxley (3) characterized excitability in terms of voltage-dependent conductances. Recent work has proceeded to the molecular level. Several lines of evidence, including the density of tetrodotoxin-binding sites (4), noise analysis (5), and the magnitude of the gating current (6, 7), indicate that the unit size of the voltage-dependent sodium conductance is several picomho, implicating ion flux through channels instead of via a carrier mechanism. Studies of ion selectivity, notably Hille's work on the permeability of the sodium channel of frog node of Ranvier to organic cations (8, 9), point to an oxygen-lined 3×5-Å pore. The movement of charge associated with the opening of the sodium channel (gating current), which Hodgkin and Huxley predicted, has now been measured (6, 7). While attempts at purification of the sodium channel have been made (10, 11), little progress has followed.

Dr. Schein is now at The Department of Psychology, Massachusetts Institute of Technology, Cambridge, Massachusetts 02139.

The ciliated protozoan Paramecium aurelia has a well-described excitable membrane, calcium carrying the inward current (12). Behavior, in the form of a reversal of swimming direction, is dependent on the "excitable" calcium influx (13). The genetic system is nearly ideal, involving both a "haploid" and a diploid life-style (Fig. 1) (14). Additionally, the protozoan may be grown in pure culture and would appear suitable for the biochemical approach to excitable membrane function. Finally, it is likely that the voltage-dependent calcium and potassium channels are located in ciliary membrane (15).

This report describes the results of investigations involving pawns, the name originally given by Kung (16, 17) for behavioral mutants of paramecia which are unable to reverse. A new selection was used to generate the pawns described here. Appropriate solutions of barium quickly paralyze wild-type paramecia. It was thought that a selection based on resistance to the paralyzing effect of barium would focus on mutants with defective calcium activation, and this reasoning appears to be valid. Results of behavioral study, genetic analysis, and electrophysiology, as well as some other related work, is presented, and a hypothesis which ascribes the gate and the pore (or channel wall) functions of the voltage-dependent calcium channel to different gene products is discussed. Additionally, phenotypic lag has been investigated with a variety of techniques, yielding a measure of channel stability.

MATERIALS AND METHODS

Culture Conditions

Cells were grown as in Sonneborn (18) except that the medium is richer (5 gm cerophyl/liter) and supports growth of cells to more than 5,000/ml (19).

Cell Strains

All strains described in the report were derived from a culture of wild-type, syngen 4, stock 51-s (non-kappa bearing), from Dr. C. Kung. The markers used were sp (spinner) and po (polyene resistance). Instead of swimming backward during reversal behavior, cells with the sp trait spin in place. Exposure to chlorpromazine (400 μM) permits observation of backward swimming or spinning in pawn mutants which normally do not

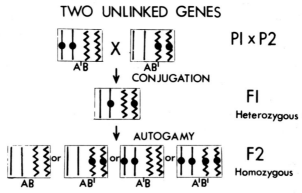

Fig. 1. When two (homozygous) paramecia with unlinked markers are crossed, P1 (genotypically A'/A' B/B) with P2 (A/A B'/B'), the resulting F1 is heterozygous (A/A' B/B'). After about 20 divisions, starvation will induce autogamy in the F1, each individual giving rise to one of the four listed homozygous F2.

reverse. Polyene resistance is tested by exposing cells to amphotericin B at 25 μg/ml; the wild-type are dead within 10 min, while cells in po-marked clones live more than 24 hr.

Life-Cycle: Mating and Autogamy

Figure 1 illustrates the life-cycle of P. aurelia, syngen 4. The product of a mating between homozygous parents with complementing recessive marker mutations is a heterozygous (phenotypically wild-type) F1. After growth through about 20 divisions, starvation induces autogamy in the F1 culture, each individual then giving rise to a homozygous F2 with genes which are the product of random segregation of the F1 characters. Details of induction of mating reactivity and autogamy may be found in Schein (19).

Mutagenesis

Four mutageneses with a 1-hr treatment of 75, 50, 75, and 100 μg/ml nitroso-guanidine (NTG) were performed and the mutants which resulted labeled as the 100, 200, 300, and 400 series, respectively. Mutagenesis followed the method reported by Kung (17). Exautogamous death ranged from 30% to 60%.

Selection for Mutants in Excitability: Barium Paralysis

Mutants were selected on the basis of their resistance to the paralyzing effect of barium. Cells were concentrated in growth medium to 2×10^4/ml, and 1 ml of 100 mM $BaCl_2$ was added to 9 ml of cells. The mixture was vortexed for 5 sec, spread in a trough, and any cells still swimming between 30 and 120 sec later were picked out and cloned. Several mutant, 202, 214, 314, 320, 325, 414, and 419 were isolated. Mutant 202 and 325 were lost and slow growing, respectively. Another mutant, 100, was isolated by chemotactic inhibition of galvanotaxis, a modification of Kung's chemotactic inhibition of geotaxis (17).

Reversal Behavior

The swimming behavior of cells, transferred in a micropipette from growth medium to Test-solutions-S and -P, was observed under a stereomicroscope.

Test-solutions-S (for stimulating: 1 mM NaH_2PO_4, 1 mM Na_2HPO_4, 2 mM Na-citrate, 1.5 mM $CaCl_2$, 2.0 mM $BaCl_2$) induces frequent reversals in the wild-type.

Within 15 sec of transfer to Test-solution-P (for paralyzing: 1 mM NaH_2PO_4, 1 mM Na_2HPO_4, 2 mM Na-citrate, 0.1 mM $CaCl_2$, 10 mM $BaCl_2$, 15 mM NaCl), wild-type cells are paralyzed.

Barium Toxicity

Cells were adapted in 1 mM Na_2HPO_4, 1 mM NaH_2PO_4, 2 mM Na-citrate, 0.33 mM $CaCl_2$ for 4 hr, followed by addition of $BaCl_2$ to 1 mM. At each time point, a sample of each tube was removed and the number of motile paramecia were counted. Motile and nonmotile cells were nearly equivalent to alive and dead cells.

Electrophysiology

Electrophysiological methods are described in detail in another report (20). The cells were impaled with a current-passing and a voltage-monitoring micropipette and then stimulated with rectangular 60 msec pulses of current. The oscilloscope records show, from top to bottom, current, voltage, and the derivative of voltage. Computation of active inward current is described in Results.

RESULTS

The seven mutants generated by the selection based on resistance to paralysis by barium were tested behaviorally, since defective calcium activation should be reflected in altered behavior. The mutants display a wide range of phenotypes, from nearly wild-type behavior to no reversal behavior at all. Observation of the effect of the two solutions (-S for stimulating, -P for paralyzing) permits sorting of mutants into Type 1 (wild-type) through Type 4 (a complete lack of reversal) behavior, using the classification scheme described in Table I. pwB(314) and pwC(320) display Type 2 behavior. I will refer to them as "partial" pawns, because reversal behavior can easily be elicited. The identification of these mutants is usually made not by behavioral tests, but instead by their resistance to the paralyzing effect of barium (Test-solution-P). pwA(214) is classified Type 3, since it is possible to observe hesitation of the cells upon exposure to the stimulating Test-solution-S. This mutant, as well as pwA(414), pwA(419), and pwB(100), which show no reversal behavior at all, are termed "extreme" mutants.

The mutants derive from three genes, pwA, pwB, and pwC, the same three genes represented in Kung and his associates' collection (17, 21), isolated on a behavioral basis. The form of the data which place mutants into particular genes is illustrated in Fig. 1. Assume that A' is a pawn mutation in the pwA gene, B' is a pawn mutation in the pwB gene. The product of conjugation, the "F1 generation," has a wild-type allele at both loci and is phenotypically wild-type, since the pawn mutations are all recessive. After growth through about 20 divisions, the F1 cells will undergo autogamy upon starvation, each individual F1 becoming, with equal probability, one of the four homozygous geno-types shown in the figure. One-quarter of the products will be wild-type, one-quarter pwA, one-quarter pwB, and one-quarter will have both mutations. Table II, Part a, de-monstrates the recessive character of the pawn mutations. The cross listed in Part b illustrates the above description and also shows the usefulness of pawns which retain some reversal behavior. In this case, the double mutant can be distinguished because it has a more extreme phenotype than either of its singly mutated sibs, a consistent obser-vation in all crosses between pawns in different genes (complementing mutations). Had the mutants been derived from the same gene, as in the case of pwB(314) and pwB(100), then the F1 would be pawn, and each F2 would necessarily become either pwB(314) or pwB(100) (Table II, Part c). The same reasoning may be applied to crosses which prove the genotype of the suspected double mutant described above. More extensive genetic data may be found in another report (19).

TABLE I. Levels of Reversal Behavior

Type	1	2	3	4
Response to solution -P	paralyzed within 15 sec	swims very slowly	swims slowly	swims normally
Response to solution -S	vigorous reversal response	vigorous reversal response	weak reversal response;* insufficient for an sp determination.	no reversal response
Summary of reversal	normal (wild-type)	slightly reduced: "partial" pawn	considerably reduced: "extreme" pawn	absent: extreme pawn

*The spinners do not, of course, reverse; however, the reversal response may be vigorous.

TABLE II. Genetics of Pawns

Cross					
P1	P2	F1 Phenotype	F2 pw/not pw	sp/not sp	po/not po
A) pwA(214)	sp	WT	14/10*	24/24	
pwB(314)	WT	WT	45/52		
B) pwA(214)-sp	pwB(314)	WT	WT/pwA/pwB/pwA-pwB 22 26 23 20	19/16†	
C) pwB(100)-sp	pwB(314)-po	partial pawn	60/0	33/27	27/33

*The presence of the pawn trait was determined only in spinners.
†Only the 314 and non-pawn F2s were classified with respect to the spinner trait.

Resistance to Barium Toxicity

In addition to paralysis, barium causes cell death. Mutants with defective calcium channels would be expected to withstand the toxicity of barium longer than the wild-type, and this is indeed the case. What is surprising, however, is that pwB mutants are superior to pwA mutants in this regard. Figure 2 illustrates differential killing by barium. A population of a "nearly extreme" pawn, pwA(214), is reduced by one log in 300 min (compared with 150 min for the wild-type), while a pwB (partial) mutant (314), which shows considerable reversal behavior, requires 1,600 min. The greater resistance of pwB over pwA mutants to barium toxicity is the first evidence that the pwA and pwB mutations have distinct effects.

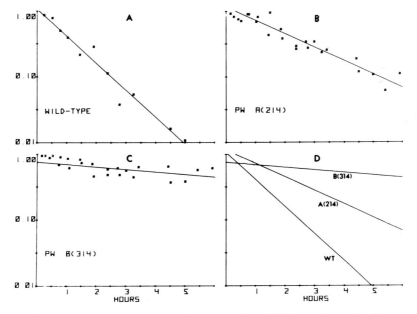

Fig. 2. Fig. 2A shows the result of one experiment; Figs. 2B and 2C show the results of two separate experiments. To cells adapted in 1 mM Na_2HPO_4, 1 mM NaH_2PO_4, 2 mM Na-citrate, 0.33 mM $CaCl_2$ for 4 hr, $BaCl_2$ was added to 1 mM. The number of motile cells (ordinate) were counted at each time point (abscissa). The lines were computed to give a least-squares fit, and all are plotted together in Fig. 2D.

Electrophysiological Characterization

 P. aurelia is relatively large (120 μm long, about 40 μm in diameter) and may be impaled with two micropipettes. Recordings were made using an active current source (or "current clamp"). If the membrane is modeled as in the circuit in Fig. 3, then the applied current may be divided into capacitative current (CdV/dt), ionic current through the resting conductance ($I_{passive} = V/R_p$), and (active) ionic current through the voltage-dependent conductance, the sum of the inward calcium current (early) and outward potassium (late) currents.

 Records from the wild-type (Fig. 4a), a partial mutant pwB(314) (Fig. 4b), and an extreme mutant pwA(414) (Fig. 4c) are shown. Resting potential, resting resistance, membrane time constant, and delayed rectification are all normal. The lesion is therefore rather specific.

 Computation of active inward current provides a quantitative measure of the decrease in excitability which is apparent in the actual records. The peaks of tracings of active inward current, such as those shown in Fig. 5a and 5a′, approach a maximum of 2.8 nA for the wild-type (Fig. 5b) and 0.7 nA for the partial mutant pwB(314) (Fig. 5b′). Tracings of active inward current in the case of the extreme mutant pwA(414) show only outward current (Fig. 5a″). While the decrease in active inward current might be due to defective calcium activation, it could also be due to faster turn-on of potassium conductance. It is noteworthy, therefore, that the outward currents in the extreme mutant pwA(414) (Fig. 5a″) do not commence until after the inward (calcium) current would normally reach its peak. In fact, the timing of the outward currents in the extreme mutant is consistent with what one would expect for wild-type potassium activation. Only calcium activation is affected by the pw mutations.

 A second difference between pwA and pwB mutants may also be noted in the electrophysiological study. Anomalous rectification, the "relaxation" of the voltage during hyperpolarizing current stimuli, like the wild type, is first observed in pwA mutants when the cell is hyperpolarized by about 15 mV from the resting potential (already 20–25 mV inside negative). However, anomalous rectification is first observed in pwB mutants at 35 mV [in the case of the partial pwB(314)] and 50 mV [in the case of

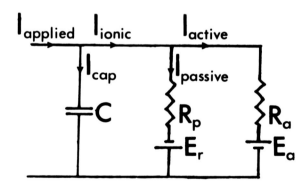

Fig. 3. Electric circuit model used for the computation of active inward current. The applied current may be divided into capacitative current (CdV/dt), ionic current through the resting conductance ($I_{passive} = V/R_p$) and (active) ionic current through the voltage-dependent conductance, the sum of inward calcium current (early) and outward potassium (late) currents.

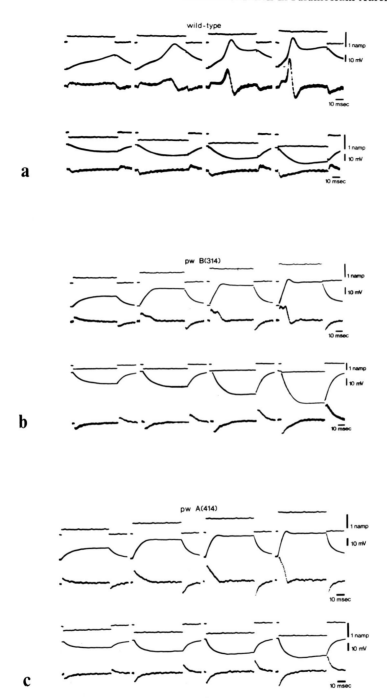

Fig. 4. The electrical response of (a) the wild-type, (b) the partial mutant pwB(314), and (c) the extreme mutant pwA(414). The changes in potential (middle traces) in a cell are produced by applied currents (top traces). The bottom trace in each picture is the time-derivative of voltage. The applied (stimulus) current increases from left to right, in the depolarizing (upper row of pictures) and the hyperpolarizing (lower row of pictures) directions.

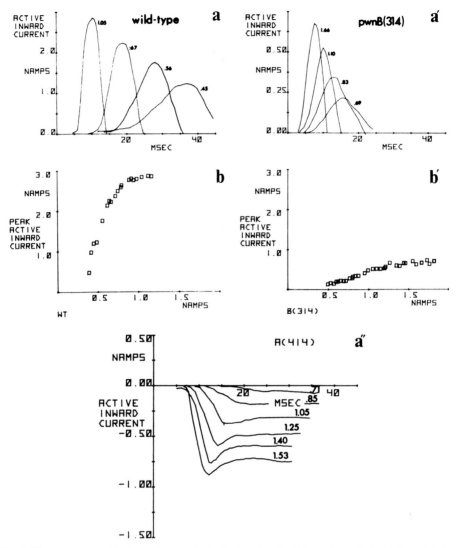

Fig. 5. The computed active inward current, obtained as described in the legend of Fig. 3, of (a) the wild-type, (a′) pwB(314), and (a″) pwA(314). In 5a and 5a′ the left-most curve was chosen because the peak active inward current is very close to the maximum for that cell. The peak active inward current (ordinate) is plotted vs applied current (abscissa) for (b) the wild-type and (b′) pwB(314).

the extreme pwB(100)] hyperpolarization from the resting potential. The electrical properties of all the mutants are summarized in Table III.

As expected, the double mutants are all less excitable than their single mutant parents. A particularly good illustration is the double mutant pwB(314)-pwC(320). The parents have, respectively, 25% and 50% of the wild-type active inward current. The records of the double mutant show little, if any, excitability.

TABLE III. Summary of Active Electrical Properties of Pawns

(1)	(2)	(3)	(4)
Cell type	Maximum active inward current	Presence of delayed rectification	Absolute activation voltage of anomalous rectification
Wild-type	2.8 (nA)	+	−40 mV
pwA(214)	0.13	+	−40
414	< 0.1	+	−40
419	< 0.1	+	−40
pwB(314)	0.7	+	−57
100	<0.1	+	−72
pwC(320)	1.3	+	−40

The Half-Life of the Channel

The life-cycle of P. aurelia permits exploitation of a phenomenon known as phenotypic lag. A delay in the full-fledged phenotypic expression of the genotype was clearly described in bacteria by Davis (22). His study, using penicillin selection of auxotrophs, led him to suggest that the wild-type enzyme had to be diluted out by growth before the auxotrophic genotype could be expressed.

The life-cycle of P. aurelia (Fig. 1) involves a "sudden" change in genotype at autogamy. The behavior and electrophysiology of cells switched by autogamy from heterozygous [+/pwB(100)] (phenotypically wild-type) to homozygous [pwB(100)/pwB(100)] pawn was followed through several divisions. Table IV shows the progress of cells from wild-type behavior (the F1) to Type 2 behavior after just one division following autogamy, to Type 3 by four divisions (16 cells/clone) and finally Type 4 by five divisions (32 cells/clone). The same results obtained with pwA(419). Electrophysiological measurements of the F1 [+/pwB(100)] show that the F1 has wild-type excitability. Recordings from individual cells when the exautogamous homozygous pwB(100)/pwB(100) clone has reached four and eight cells (Fig. 6) show that the active inward current approaches a maximum which halves with each division (Fig. 7), consistent with dimple dilution of the channels by each division. The electrophysiological results also establish the behavioral classification as a quantitative assay.

Since channel dilution, but apparently no channel decay, was observed in the 40 hr between autogamy and three divisions (eight cells/clone), phenotypic lag was followed in cells allowed to go through few divisions in a much longer time. Cells were fed sparingly and tested at 11 days (after two to three divisions) and at 20 days (after three to four divisions). When the clone size reached eight, after 11 days, the slowly grown pwB(100) showed Type 3 behavior. The data presented in Table IV show that the phenotype of the normally grown pwB(100) mutants appears as Type 3 when the clone has reached from 16 to 32 cells. If, after 11 days, an "8-cell-stage" paramecium behaves like a 16–32-cell-stage paramecium grown rapidly, then the effect of channel loss is to decrease excitability by an additional factor of 2 to 4 in those 11 days. The half-life is therefore between 11 and 5.5

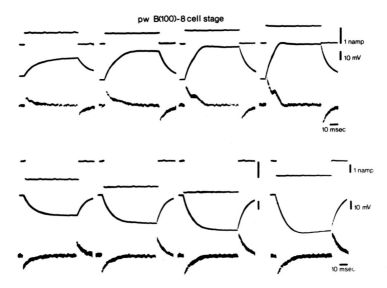

Fig. 6. Response of the pwB(100) at 40 hr postautogamy, when the clone had reached 8 cells, displayed as in Fig. 4.

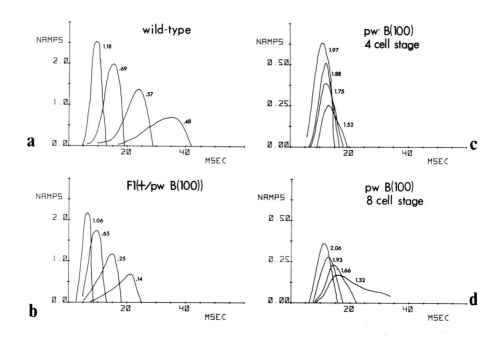

Fig. 7. The computed active inward current, obtained as described in the legend of Fig. 3, of (a) the wild-type, (b) the F1 [+/pwB(100)], (c) the pwB(100) at the 4-cell stage, and (d) the pwB(100) at the 8-cell stage. In each plot, the left-most curve was chosen because the peak active inward current is very close to the maximum for that cell.

TABLE IV. Phenotypic Lag in pwB (100)

Cells/clone	Number of clones tested	Number of spinners[2]	Behavioral phenotype[1]		
			Type 2	Type 3	Type 4
2	104	56[4]	51 (18, 22, 24, 27 hr)[3]	0	0
4	41	21	18 (27, 31 hr)	0	0
8	20	10	10 (41, 48 hr)	0	0
16[5]	44	14/23[6]	2(48 hr)	21 (48, 53 hr)	0
32	32	8/18	0	0	14 (53 hr)

[1] See Table I for summary of classification scheme.

[2] Spinning (or not spinning) is observed following transfer of individual paramecia to solution -S.

[3] All of the 2-cell stage pawn determinations were checked after the cultures had grown to more than 64 cells. Of the 104 2-cell cultures tested, 1 pawn culture was mistaken for a wild-type and 1 wild-type culture was mistaken for a pawn.

[4] The spinner genotype can be distinguished by the 2-cell stage, but only with difficulty. By the 4-cell stage and beyond, the determination becomes easy.

[5] Not all 16 and 32 cell cultures had exactly 16 or 32 cells. More than 8 was considered 16; more than 16 was considered 32.

[6] By this stage, none of the pawns could be classified as to the spinner trait, so column 4 now shows the number of spinner clones over the total number of clones which could be classified with respect to the trait.

days. Similar characterizations at different clone sizes and with pwA(419) give nearly identical limits for channel half-life, between 5.5 and 9 days in the case of pwB(100), and between 5.5 and 8 days in the case of pwA(419). Detailed data will be presented elsewhere (23).

DISCUSSION

The selection based on resistance to paralysis by barium was designed to focus specifically on mutants with defective calcium channels by taking advantage of the ion-specific properties of the channel. The behavioral results and the resistance to the toxic effects of barium indirectly demonstrate the success of the strategy. Electrophysiological recordings directly demonstrate the defectiveness of calcium activation in the mutants.

The use of phenotypic lag provided an unusual opportunity to measure physiologically the half-life of a membrane system, which in this case is quite long (5.5–8 days), especially compared to the approximately 8-hr generation time. Finally, the stability of the wild-type product in the mutant cell is also consistent with the idea that the target of the action of the pawn gene products is the calcium channel.

A Model

A model which attempts to explain the phenotypic differences between pwA and pwB mutants demonstrated in this paper (anomalous rectification, barium toxicity) is shown in Fig. 8. The important features of the model are: 1) a "pore" common to both

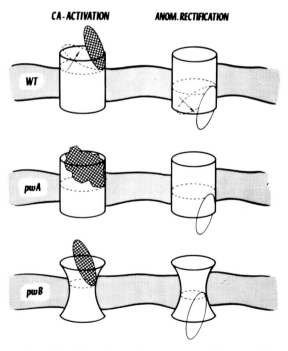

Fig. 8. The "garbage can" model of the calcium channels responsible for calcium activation and anomalous rectification. The 'pore' and the 'gates' are normal in the wild-type. The depolarization-sensitive 'gate' is defective in the pwA mutants, leaving normal anomalous rectification. The 'pore' is defective in pwB mutants, causing parallel effects on calcium activation and anomalous rectification.

calcium activation and anomalous rectification; 2) separate depolarization- and hyper-polarization-sensitive "gates;" and 3) for ease of visualization, separate structures for calcium activation and anomalous rectification.

Since both calcium activation and anomalous rectification are affected in parallel in pwB mutants, then it is likely that anomalous rectification is also due to a calcium conductance, and that the common element, the wall of the channel (or "pore"), is involved. The pwB gene product is therefore supposed to be the pore. Since pwA mutants have normal anomalous rectification, their pores must be normal; calcium activation is abnormal because the depolarization-sensitive gate is defective.

The model is also consistent with the differential resistance to barium toxicity. A defective gate might open, though less frequently than the wild-type, whereas a defective pore would never admit barium. Thus, pore mutants (pwB) should be more resistant to barium than gate mutants (pwA).

Finally, the model accounts for a curious frequency distribution of partial pawns in the pawns collected by Kung and his associates (17, 21) and myself (19). On the one hand, the severity of gate defects should span a wide range: the number of gating charges could be decreased, or the fraction of the transmembrane potential which is traversed when the gating charges move could be decreased. Both sorts of mutations would change voltage-sensitivity to varying degrees. Indeed, many partial mutants have been isolated in the putative gate gene, pwA. On the other hand, the channel displays ion-selectivity, and if it is anything like the sodium channel, which Hille (8, 9) suggests on the basis of selectivity studies is an oxygen-lined 3×5-Å pore, then a change of even a single Ångstrom unit would be enough to completely close the channel. In fact, very few partial mutants have been isolated in the putative pore gene, pwB.

While the model is rather speculative, it is amenable to experimental test. First, voltage clamping will permit measurement of voltage-sensitivity and time course of calcium activation as well as maximum active calcium conductance. The model predicts that voltage-sensitivity or time course will be altered in pwA mutants. While these quantities should be unchanged in pwB mutants, total active calcium conductance should be decreased. Second, it may be possible one day to incorporate the channel into planar artificial membranes, where single channel conductance and channel number could also be directly measured (24). The model predicts that either of these quantities will be decreased in pwB mutants. Conversely, should in vitro methods become available, the pawn channels will serve as a useful control (much like tetrodotoxin binding by the sodium channel), as well as a powerful probe into the mechanism of excitable membrane operation.

ACKNOWLEDGMENTS

I would like to thank Drs. Charles David and M. V. L. Bennett for advice and understanding during most of this study. I would also like to thank Drs. Mel Cohn and Tom August for encouragement in the early phase of the investigation. The work was supported by grants from the National Institutes of Health (GM 11301 and 5T5 GM 1674).

REFERENCES

1. Mullen, R. J., Eicher, E. M., and Sidman, R. L., Proc. Nat. Acad. Sci. U.S.A. 73:208 (1976).
2. Springer, M. S., Kort, E. N., Larsen, S. H., Ordal, G. W., Reader, R. W., and Adler, J., Proc. Nat. Acad. Sci. U.S.A. 72:4640 (1975).

3. Hodgkin, A. L., and Huxley, A. F., J. Physiol. 117:500 (1952).

4. Keynes, R. D., Ritchie, J. M., and Rojas, E., J. Physiol. 213:235 (1971).

5. Conti, T., DeFelice, L. J., and Wanke, E., J. Physiol. 248:45 (1975).

6. Armstrong, D. M., and Bezanilla, F., J. Gen. Physiol. 63:533 (1974).

7. Keynes, R. D., and Rojas, E., J. Physiol. 239:393 (1974).

8. Hille, B., J. Gen. Physiol. 58:599 (1971).

9. Hille, B., Fed. Proc. 34:1318 (1975).

10. Benzer, T. I., and Raftery, M. A., Proc. Nat. Acad. Sci. U.S.A. 69:3634 (1972).

11. Barnola, F. V., and Villegas, R., J. Gen. Physiol. 67:81 (1976).

12. Naitoh, Y., Eckert, R., and Friedman, K., J. Exp. Biol. 56:667 (1972).

13. Machemer, H., and Eckert, R., J. Gen. Physiol. 61:572 (1973).

14. Beale, G. H., "The Genetics of Paramecium aurelia." London: Cambridge University Press (1954).

15. Hyams, J. S., and Borisy, G. G., J. Cell Biol. 67:(2, Pt.2) 186a (Abstr.) (1975).

16. Kung, C., Z. Vergl. Physiol. 71:142 (1971).

17. Kung, C., Genetics 69:29 (1971).

18. Sonneborn, T. M., in "Methods in Cell Physiology," Vol. 4, 241–339. New York: Academic Press (1970).

19. Schein, S. J., Genetics (in press).

20. Schein, S. J., Bennett, M. V. L., and Katz, G. M., J. Exp. Biol. (in press).

21. Chang, S.-Y., van Houten, J., Robles, L. J., Lui, S. S., and King, C., Genet. Res. 23:165 (1974).

22. Davis, B. D., J. Am. Chem. Soc. 70:4267 (1948).

23. Schein, S. J., J. Exp. Biol. (in press).

24. Schein, S. J., Colombini, M., and Finkelstein, A., J. Memb. Biol. (in press).

Acetylcholine Receptors and Myasthenia Gravis: The Effect of Antibodies to Eel Acetylcholine Receptors on Eel Electric Organ Cells

Jon Lindstrom, Brett Einarson, and Murray Francy

The Salk Institute for Biological Studies, San Diego, California 92112

Antisera to acetylcholine receptors purified from Electrophorus electricus were tested for their ability to bind to receptors on electric organ cells, block the depolarizing response of the cells to carbamylcholine, and inhibit binding of ^{125}-I-α-bungarotoxin to the cells. It was found that although antibodies could bind to most of the receptors, resulting in substantial inhibition of the depolarizing response, binding of ^{125}-I-α-bungarotoxin to the cells was only slightly inhibited. This was consistent with the observation that these antibodies did not compete for the toxin binding site on detergent-solubilized receptor. These results suggest that the antibodies inhibited receptor activity primarily by interfering with the ionophore of the receptor or its regulation by the acetylcholine binding site. However, the possibilities could not be completely eliminated that blockage of a small fraction of the binding sites caused a large inhibition of the depolarizing response or that bound antibody allosterically reduced binding affinity for carbamylcholine without completely inhibiting toxin binding.

Key words: acetylcholine receptors, electrophorus electricus, electric organ cells, electroplax, ^{125}Iαbungarotoxin, neuromuscular transmission, myasthenia gravis, experimental autoimmune myasthenia gravis

INTRODUCTION

Antibodies to purified acetylcholine receptor (AChR) inhibit carbamylcholine-induced depolarization of the electric organ cells from which the AChR was purified (1–3). These antibodies are directed at an unknown, but probably large number of determinants on the AChR, but few (1) or none (4) of these antibodies are directed at the binding site for acetylcholine binding on detergent-solubilized AChR. However, the question remained whether binding of antibody to AChR in the membrane would allosterically block the acetylcholine binding site.

Abbreviations used in this paper: AChR, acetylcholine receptor; αBGT, α-bungarotoxin; MG, myasthenia gravis; EAMG, experimental autoimmune myasthenia gravis.

Animals immunized with AChR also develop antibodies which recognize AChR on skeletal muscle, and neuromuscular transmission is impaired in these animals (1—7). Because of the detailed similarities between animals immunized with AChR and humans with myasthenia gravis (MG), this model disease has been termed experimental autoimmune myasthenia gravis (EAMG) (3,4,6). The importance of antibodies to AChR in the pathology of these diseases is shown by the observations that both MG (8) and EAMG (9) can be passively transferred to normal recipients by injection of sera containing anti-AChR. However, although sera from animals with EAMG do inhibit AChR activity on muscle (7, 10), it is known that anti-AChR antibodies function in the disease process other than just as antagonists of AChR. In fact, antibodies bound to AChR on the postsynaptic membrane induce destruction of the membrane by macrophages (9). Antibody-induced modulation of AChR also appears to be important (11). But, although much of the impairment of neuromuscular transmission in EAMG and MG (12—14) can be accounted for by decreases in AChR content, a large fraction of the AChR remaining in the muscle have antibodies bound (11,14), and it is important to determine how this effects their activity.

Finally, there is the problem of relating structure of the AChR molecule to its function. If antibodies to AChR could be found which bound to determinants on AChR other than the acetylcholine binding site, yet which still affected AChR activity, then these antibodies could be used to determine functional roles of structural determinants defined in the purified AChR protein.

In this paper we report the effects of goat antiserum to AChR purified from electric eels on the activity of AChR in cells from eel electric organ assayed in vitro. By contrast with in vivo studies of the effects of antibodies by passive transfer (9), no macrophages were involved. Complement activity was also prevented. We found that, by contrast with the effects of antisera on cultured muscle cells (15), no substantial modulation of AChR was induced by antibody binding. Therefore, we were directly measuring only the effects of antibody binding on AChR activity. By studying AChR in eel cells rather than muscle, we had the additional advantage that all of the antibodies in the sera were directed at the AChR in our preparation rather than only a few percent of cross-reacting antibodies (3,4,6). The antiserum used was known to contain no detectable antibodies which interfered with binding of toxin to detergent-solubilized AChR (4). Our results suggest that antibodies can bind to AChRs in the cell membrane and block their activity without blocking their acetylcholine binding sites.

METHODS

Electrophysiological Studies

Single electroplax were dissected from the organ of Sachs in the caudal portion of large E. electricus (16). In order to maximize accessibility of antibody molecules to the innervated membrane of the electroplax, cells were pretreated with collagenase (Sigma type I, 2 mg/ml for 90 min). This did not result in disjunction of nerve endings, since endplate potentials could still be elicited after collagenase treatment. Cells were mounted between two pools of Ringer's solution in an apparatus resembling that used by Schoffeneils et al. (16). The noninnervated side of the cell was exposed to one pool of Ringer's and the innervated to the other. Nylon netting across the non-innervated side of the cell pressed the cell against a Vaseline-coated Mylar sheet with a 1-mm diam hole in it that exposed part of the innervated face to the other pool. Calomel electrodes (Corning

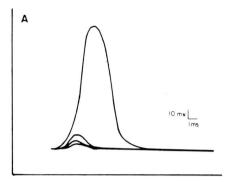

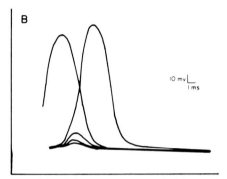

Fig. 1. Endplate and action potentials of electroplax recorded with extracellular electrodes. A) Tracing of response to indirect stimulation of collagenase-treated electroplax. Starting about 1 msec after the stimulus at the beginning of the trace, a subthreshold endplate potential develops. With increasing stimulator voltage (10–30 V) the amplitude of the endplate potential increases to a maximum of about 18 mV before an action potential of 130 mV amplitude is triggered. B) Tracing of superimposed response to direct stimulation (3 V). There is no delay between stimulus and onset of the action potential which reaches an amplitude of 120 mV.

476015-17) in each pool were used to measure potential across the cell. The electrodes were connected to a Grass P18 amplifier and thence to a storage oscilloscope and chart recorder. Chlorided silver wires in each pool connected in series with a $10^4 \Omega$ resistor to a Grass SD9 stimulator were used for electrically stimulating the cell. Another chlorided silver wire electrode connected the pool bathing the innervated face of the cell to the input ground of the amplifer. The use of extracellular electrodes permitted four cells to be mounted in separate apparatuses simultaneously and then be tested individually from time to time. Because the standard method for studying electroplax involves the use of intracellular electrodes, some of the results obtained with these extracellular electrodes are presented in Methods.

No potential was recorded across a resting cell, but action potentials of $\geqslant 120$ mV could be elicited by direct electrical stimulation of the cell (0.1 msec ~5 V innervated side +). Endplate potentials and indirect action potentials could be elicited by electrical stimulation of the opposite polarity (0.1 msec ~ 30 V innervated side −) (Fig. 1). Since resting membrane potential could not be measured with extracellular electrodes, action potential amplitude was used to determine the health of the cells. Cells exhibiting action potentials of amplitude less than 100 mV at any time during an experiment were discarded.

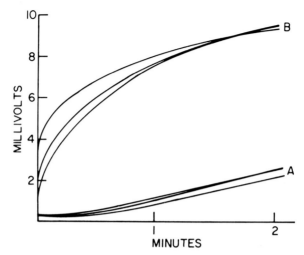

Fig. 2. Carbamylcholine response of electroplax measured with extracellular electrodes. A) An extreme example of a slow response to 3×10^{-5} M carbamylcholine in a cell not treated with collagenase. B) Successive responses at 30-min intervals to 3×10^{-5} M carbamylcholine in collagenase-treated cells.

Carbamylcholine (3×10^{-5} M) added to the pool exposed to the innervated face caused a potential difference to develop between the electrodes of 5–30 mV (Fig. 2). The absolute value of this potential depended on the particular cell, but was quite reproducible with a given cell. The absolute value probably depended partially on how well the cell was mounted. The resistances of the electroplax membranes are very low (the resting resistance of the innervated face is about 2–5 Ω cm^2, decreasing to about 1 Ω cm^2 during activity, and the resistance of the non-innervated face is about 0.3 Ω cm^2 [17]). Thus, sustained exposure to carbamylcholine might also result in a net change in internal ion composition (18). The time required for the carbamylcholine response to reach a maximum decreased with increasing carbamylcholine concentration, and at high concentrations ($> 10^{-4}$ M) the response rapidly desensitized. The relatively slow onset of the carbamylcholine response with use of low concentrations probably resulted from significant diffusion barriers to even this small molecule, since the onset of blockage of endplate potentials by low concentrations of benzoquinonium was also quite slow (Fig. 3).

In studies of the effects of antibodies to AChR on the carbamylcholine response, carbamylcholine was usually used at 3×10^{-5} M. At half-hour intervals two initial responses to carbamylcholine were determined. Then diluted serum was added to the pool bathing the innervated face and magnetically stirred. At 30-min intervals the serum was removed and the response to carbamylcholine was again determined. Before the carbamylcholine response was tested, action potential amplitude was measured. Cells with significantly reduced amplitudes were discarded.

Sera Used

A goat was immunized with AChR purified from E. electricus. The goat was bled out when it showed obvious muscular weakness due to EAMG. Reaction of this antiserum with AChR from Electrophorus and Torpedo has been previously described (4). Some sera from rats immunized with AChR from Electrophorus as previously described (6) were also used. Complement activity in all sera was inactivated by heating at 56°C for 30

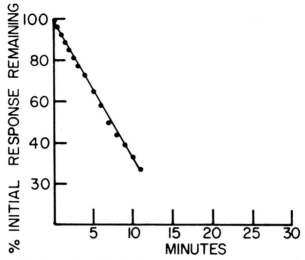

Fig. 3. Time course of blockage of a subthreshold endplate potential response by 10^{-6} M benzo-quinonium.

min. This had no effect on the activity of the goat serum, but did prevent blockage of the action potential response by high concentrations of rat serum. High titer goat anti-human gamma globulin serum was used as a control for goat anti-AChR serum. Serum from rats immunized only with adjuvant was used as a control for rat anti-AChR serum.

Biochemical Studies

α-Bungarotoxin (αBGT)[1] was labeled with ^{125}I to specific activities of $2-4 \times 10^{17}$ cpm/mol by the chloramine T procedure previously described (3).

Collagenase-treated electroplax were divided into two groups containing size-matched cells: 1) those treated with anti-AChR; and 2) those treated with control serum. After incubation at room temperature for 1 hr in a 3-ml vol of the appropriate serum dilution, the cells were washed with 3×10 ml of Ringer's. Then each group of cells was divided in two — one-half in Ringer' containing 10^{-3} M benzoquinonium to prevent binding of ^{125}IαBGT to AChR, the other half in Ringer's alone. All groups were then incubated for 1 hr with 3×10^{-8} M ^{125}IαBGT. This time was sufficient for maximal labeling. Groups were then washed with 6×10 ml Ringer's over 1 hr, and then the cells were individually counted in a γ counter. ^{125}IαBGT bound in the presence of benzoquinonium was subtracted to correct for nonspecific labeling. Labeling was 80–90% specific.

Cells were then homogenized individually in 0.5 ml of 0.5% Triton buffer (0.5% Triton X-100, 0.1 M NaCl, 0.01 M Na phosphate pH 7.0, 0.01 M NaN$_3$). After extraction overnight at 4°C on a rocker table, the cell debris was pelleted, and the supernatant removed and counted in a γ counter. The supernatants were then tested for antibody-AChR complexes by sucrose gradient centrifugation and immunoprecipitation.

In order to increase solubilization of AChR from electroplax treated with high concentrations of anti-AChR, electroplax were treated successively with dithiothreitol and iodoacetamide before labeling with ^{125}IαBGT. Dithiothreitol was used at a concentration of 10^{-3} M for 10 min, and then iodoacetamide was added to a concentration of 10^{-2} M for 10 min. Cells were then rinsed with 3×10 ml of Ringer's before labeling with ^{125}IαBGT.

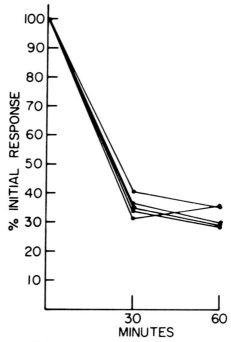

Fig. 4. Time course of blockage of the response to 3×10^{-5} M carbamylcholine by goat antiserum to AChR. Blockage is nearly maximal by 30 min. Data from five cells (two at serum/5, two at serum/10, one at serum/25).

^{125}IαBGT-labeled AChR solubilized from single cells in a volume of 0.5 ml was layered on 10.5 ml 5–20% sucrose gradients in 0.5% Triton buffer and centrifuged for 9 hr at 37,000 rpm in a Beckman-Spinco SW40.1 rotor. Thirty drop fractions were collected through a needle perforating the bottom of the tube and counted in a scintillation counter.

Antibody-AChR-^{125}IαBGT complexes in Triton X-100 extracts of single electroplax were quantitated by immunoprecipitation. In microfuge tubes, 0.5-ml extracts from single electroplax were mixed with 5 μl of normal goat serum as carrier and 100 μl of rabbit anti-goat IgG. After incubation at 4°C for 4 hr, precipitates were pelleted by centrifugation (2 min in a Brinkman microfuge), washed once with 1 ml 0.5% Triton buffer, and counted in a γ counter.

RESULTS

Exposure of the innervated face of eel electroplax to goat anti-AChR serum blocks the response to 3×10^{-5} M carbamylcholine. The degree of blockage at low dilutions of antiserum is near maximal in 30 min (Fig. 4). About 30% of the initial response remained after exposure to even very high serum concentrations, yet even quite low concentrations of serum could produce significant blockage (Fig. 5). The serum used could bind 2.8 $\times$ 10^{-6} mol ^{125}IαBGT labeled AChR per liter. The average number of ^{125}IαBGT binding sites on these cells was 6.9×10^{10}. Thus, at any serum dilution we tested, the cell was exposed to huge excesses of antibody. For example, at a 1:10 dilution of serum, enough antibody is present in the pool bathing the cell to bind 2.3×10^{14} AChR, and this is exposed to an area comprising only perhaps 10% of the innervated face of the cell. Thus, at a 1:10 dilution of serum, antibodies are in 3×10^4-fold excess over AChRs.

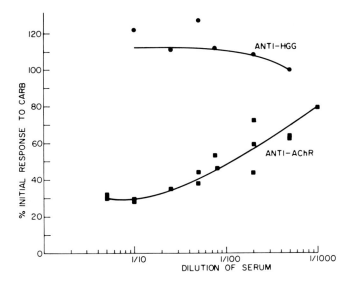

Fig. 5. Extent of blockage of the response to 3×10^{-5} M carbamylcholine by various dilutions of goat anti-AChR serum. Goat anti-human gamma globulin serum does not block AChR activity.

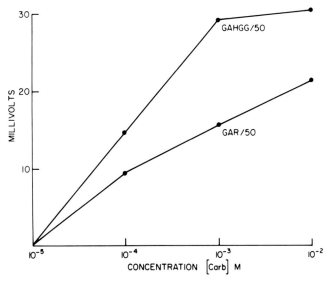

Fig. 6. Dose-response curves for carbamylcholine after treatment of electroplax for 1 hr with goat anti-AChR/50 or goat anti-human gamma globulin/50.

The effect of anti-AChR treatment on the response to other concentrations of carbamylcholine was tested (Fig. 6). Cells treated with control serum gave a near-maximal response at 10^{-3} M carbamylcholine, whereas cells treated with anti-AChR had not plateaued in their response at 10^{-2} M carbamylcholine.

TABLE I. Effect of Anti-Receptor Antibody of Receptors in Electroplax

	Serum dilution	Titer*	AChR bound by Ab (%)	Toxin binding sites blocked (%)	Carb. response blocked (%)
goat	1:10	2.8×10^{-7} M	70 (16 cells)	17 (27 cells)	69 (2 cells)
serum	1:50	5.6×10^{-8} M	56 (12 cells)	20 (18 cells)	59 (2 cells)
1 hr	1:200	1.4×10^{-8} M	30 (6 cells)	10 (10 cells)	42 (3 cells)
rat serum 1 hr	1:10	1.67×10^{-7} M		18 (3 cells)	62 (2 cells)
rat serum 19 hrs	1:10	1.67×10^{-7} M		29 (3 cells)†	

*Titer is expressed as moles ^{125}IαBGT binding sites precipitated per liter of diluted serum.
†No collagenase.

After exposure of electroplax to even very high concentrations of anti-AChR, which resulted in extensive blockage of AChR activity, binding of ^{125}IαBGT to the cells was inhibited only slightly (Table I). The fraction of the AChRs labeled with ^{125}IαBGT which had antibodies attached was determined by precipitating them with antibodies to goat IgG (Table I). Even at serum dilutions of 1:10, some of the AChR on the cells remained unbound by antibody, probably indicating the presence of a substantial diffusion barrier hindering the access of antibodies to membrane bound AChRs. However, totaling the fraction of AChR inhibited from binding toxin and the fraction of the AChR which bound both toxin and antibody showed that at 1:10 serum about 90% of AChR had at least one antibody bound. The fraction of total AChR bound with antibody was roughly proportional to the extent of blockage of the response to 3×10^{-5} M carbamylcholine (Fig. 7). Rat anti-AChR serum also produced substantial inhibition of AChR activity without extensive blockage of the ^{125}IαBGT binding.

The fraction of ^{125}IαBGT-labeled AChR which could be solubilized from electroplax treated with anti-AChR serum (46% of total) was substantially lower than that from electroplax treated with control serum (73%) (Table II). Since this might be due to crosslinking of AChR by antibodies into an insoluble matrix, antibody-treated electroplax were treated successively with dithiothreitol and iodoacetamide before labeling with ^{125}IαBGT. It was thought that this might reduce and alkylate some inter-H chain disulfide bonds on the crosslinking antibodies, permitting some of them to be cleaved into monomers. After reduction and alkylation, solubilization of AChR from electroplax treated with anti-AChR (86% of the total) was nearly equal to that from electroplax treated only with control serum (92% of total) (Table II).

In some experiments AChR content was measured by adding ^{125}IαBGT to the detergent extracts of cells and then precipitating ^{125}IαBGT-labeled AChR by successive additions of anti-AChR and anti-goat IgG. In two of five experiments no additional AChR which had not been labeled on the intact electroplax were detected in this way, but in three experiments an average of 45% ± 30% additional AChRs were detected. We do not know if this was due to a pool of AChR not accessible to ^{125}IαBGT on the cell surface in some eels or to some other factor.

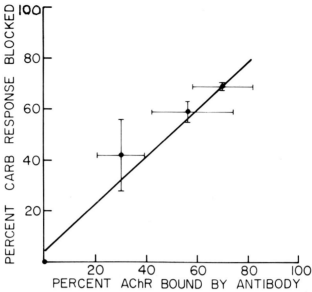

Fig. 7. Relationship between binding of antibodies to AChR in electroplax and blockage of AChR activity. Data is from Table I. Bars indicate standard deviation.

TABLE II. Effect of Reduction and Alkylation on Solubilization of AChR and Antibody-AChR From Electroplax

Treatment of cells	$^{125}I\alpha BGT$ per cell $\times 10^{10}$		
	Bound to intact cell	In Triton extract	Precipitated from the extract by anti-IgG
1) goat anti HGG serum/10 1 hr	7.24 ± 1.3 (n = 8)	5.26 ± 0.99 (n = 8)	0.27 ± 0.51 (n = 8)
2) goat anti HGG serum/10 1 hr, reduced and alkylated before being labeled with $^{125}I\alpha BGT$	6.57 ± 1.4 (n = 12)	6.06 ± 1.22 (n = 8)	0.55 ± 0.90 (n = 8)
3) goat anti-AChR serum/10 1 hr	5.19 ± 1.1 (n = 7)	$2.36 \pm .69$ (n = 8)	1.62 ± 1.2 (n = 8)
4) goat anti-AChR serum/10 1hr, reduced and alkylated before labeling with $^{125}I\alpha BGT$	6.56 ± 1.2 (n = 13)	5.62 ± 1.2 (n = 13)	5.41 ± 1.7 (n = 13)

Toxin-labeled AChR extracted from electroplax after treatment with anti-AChR sedimented on sucrose gradients as aggregates larger than the single 9.5S component observed in extracts of cells treated with control serum (Fig. 8). The smallest of these aggregates may correspond to complexes of one antibody molecule ($\sim$ 150,000 daltons) with one AChR molecule ($\sim$ 250,000 daltons). After reduction and alkylation the yield of this large component is increased, but still larger aggregates, probably containing several antibody molecules, are also observed (Fig. 9).

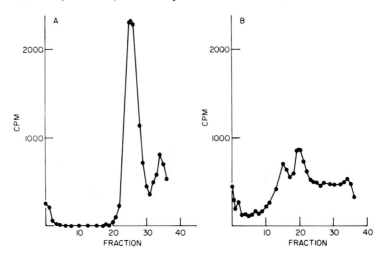

Fig. 8. Sucrose gradient sedimentation of ^{125}IαBGT-labeled AChR extracted from single electroplax. A) AChRs extracted from a cell treated with control serum/10 sediment as a single component ~9.5S. The small peak at the top of the gradient is free toxin. B) AChRs extracted from a cell treated with anti-AChR serum/10 sediment in two peaks and other aggregates, all larger than the 9.5S component.

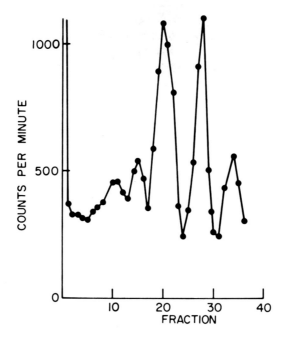

Fig. 9. Sucrose gradient sedimentation of ^{125}IαBGT-labeled AChR extracted from an electroplax treated with anti-AChR/10, and then reduced and alkylated. The peak at the top of the gradient shown on the right is free toxin. The next larger component is free AChR. The next three peaks and pellet contain antibody-AChR complexes of increasing size.

DISCUSSION

Goat anti-eel AChR serum does not interfere with toxin binding to solubilized AChR (4) and only slightly inhibits binding of toxin to AChR in membranes. The antibody to human AChR found in the serum of patients with myasthenia gravis (3,19–25) appears to behave similarly (23). The observation that the degree of blockage of the response to 3×10^{-5} M carbamylcholine was roughly proportional to the fraction of AChR on the electroplax bound by antibody suggests that binding of an antibody molecule to an AChR in the membrane at a site other than the binding site for acetylcholine inhibits the activity of that AChR. Antibody bound to the AChR might allosterically inhibit carbamylcholine binding without preventing αBGT binding. More likely, bound antibody interferes with regulation of ionophore or the ionophore itself. Many of the AChRs extracted from electroplax treated with anti-AChR are in aggregates larger than can be accounted for by units of one antibody and one AChR. Several antibodies may bind to one AChR, and/or antibodies may crosslink AChR. AChR are thought to be closely packed in areas of the postsynaptic membrane (26). Observation that reduction and alkylation greatly increases solubilization of antibody-AChR complexes is compatible with the idea that this treatment partially breaks up insoluble matrices of antibody crosslinked AChRs by splitting some of the antibodies into monovalent fragments, but solubilization might be increased through some other mechanism.

How an antibody bound to an AChR effects its activity is difficult to determine in detail. The number or fraction of active AChRs required to produce a given carbamyl-choline depolarization response is unknown. Studies of acetylcholine noise are the best way to determine the properties of individual active AChRs (27). Although quite elegant electrophysiological studies of electroplax have been made (28,29), noise studies of AChRs on electroplax have not yet been reported. In muscle, both the duration of ionophore opening and its conductance when open can be altered by small disturbances of the AChR. Binding of atropine decreases duration of channel opening (30). Reduction of the disulfide bond near the acetylcholine binding site of AChR (31) reduces affinity for ACh and decreases both amplitude and duration of the elementary conductance events (32). Agonists differ both in duration of ionophore opening and conductance when open (33). Even membrane potential effects AChR activity (34). Thus it is not surprising that binding to AChR of an antibody molecule of molecular weight comparable to the AChR should inhibit its activity, but whether ionophore opening is completely prevented or simply less effective is unknown. The antiserum used contains antibodies specific for a number of different determinants on the AChR. For example, antibodies are present against at least one site on each of the polypeptide chains composing AChR (35). The effects of antibodies bound to these different determinants is not likely to be equivalent. In other systems antibodies have been found which stimulate receptors (36), block ligand binding (37), or have no effect (38). Antibodies prepared against specific parts of the AChR molecule and tested for their ability to alter AChR activity may provide a method for determining the functional role of these structures in the AChR molecule.

REFERENCES

1. Patrick, J., Lindstrom, J., Culp, B., and McMillan, J. Proc. Natl. Acad. Sci. U.S.A. 70:3334, 1973.
2. Sugiyama, H., Benda, P., Meunier, J., and Changeux, J. FEBS Lett. 35:124, 1973.
3. Lindstrom, J., Lennon, V., Seybold, M., and Whittingham, S. N.Y. Acad. Sci. 274:254, 1976.
4. Lindstrom, J. J. Supramol. Struct. 4:389, 1976.

5. Patrick, J., and Lindstrom, J. Science 180:871, 1973.
6. Lennon, V. A., Lindstrom, J., and Seybold, M. E. J. Exp. Med. 141:1365, 1975.
7. Green, D. P. L., Miledi, R., and Vincent, A. Proc. R. Soc. Lond. Ser. B Biol. Sci. 189:57, 1975.
8. Toyka, K. V., Drachman, D. B., Pestronk, A., and Kao, I. Science 190:397, 1975.
9. Lindstrom, J. M., Seybold, M. E., Lennon, V. A., Engel, A. G., and Lambert, E. H. J. Exp. Med. 144:739, 1976.
10. Bevan, S., Heinemann, S., Lennon, V. A., and Lindstrom, J. Nature 260:438, 1976.
11. Lindstrom, J. M., Einarson, B., Lennon, V. A., and Seybold, M. E. J. Exp. Med. 144:726, 1976.
12. Fambrough, D., Drachman, D., and Satyamurti, S. Science 182:293, 1973.
13. Engel, A. G., Lindstrom, J. M., Lambert, E. H., and Lennon, V. A. Neurology, In press, 1976.
14. Lindstrom, J., and Lambert, E. H. Manuscript in preparation.
15. Lindstrom, J., and Heinemann, S. Manuscript in preparation.
16. Schoffeniels, E., and Nachmansohn, D. Biochim. Biophys. Acta 26:1, 1957.
17. Bennett, M. V. L. Annu. Rev. Physiol. 32:471, 1970.
18. Karlin, A. Proc. Natl. Acad. Sci. 58:1162, 1967.
19. Lindstrom, J. M., Seybold, M. E., Lennon, V., Whittingham, S., and Duane, D. Neurology, In press, 1976.
20. Lindstrom, J. Clin. Immunol. Immunopathol. In press, 1976.
21. Almon, R., Andrew C., and Appel, S. Science 186:55, 1974.
22. Appel, S. H., Almon, R. R., and Levy, N. N. Engl. J. Med. 293:760, 1975.
23. Mittag, T., Kornfeld, P., Tormay, A., and Woo, C. Natl. J. Med. 294:691, 1976.
24. Aharonov, A., Abramsky, O., Tarrab-Hazdai, R., and Fuchs, S. Lancet I:340, 1975.
25. Bender, A., Ringle, S., Engel, W., Daniels, M., and Vogel, Z. Lancet I:607, 1975.
26. Cartaud, J., Benedetti, L. L., Cohen, J. B., and Meunier, J. C. FEBS Lett. 33:109, 1973.
27. Katz, B., and Miledi, R. J. Physiol. 224:665, 1972.
28. Lester, H. A., Changeux, J. P., and Sheridan, R. E. J. Gen. Physiol. 65:797, 1975.
29. Sheridan, R. E., and Lester, H. A. Proc. Natl. Acad. Sci. U.S.A. 72:3496, 1975.
30. Katz, B., and Miledi, R. Proc. R. Soc. Lond. Ser. B Biol. Sci. 184:221, 1973.
31. Karlin, A. J. Gen. Physiol. 54:245, 1969.
32. Ben-Haim, D., Dreyer, F., and Peper, K. Pflügers Arch. 335:19, 1975.
33. Colquhoun, D., Dionne, V. E., Steinbach, J. H., and Stevens, C. F. Nature 253:204, 1975.
34. Anderson, C. R., and Stevens, C. F. J. Physiol. 235:655, 1973.
35. Lindstrom, J. Unpublished observations.
36. Adams, D. D., and Kennedy, T. H J. Clin. Endocrinol. 33:47, 1971.
37. Shiu, R. P. C., and Friesen, H. G. Science 192:259, 1976.
38. Kyte, J. J. Biol. Chem. 249:3652, 1974.

Cellular Neurobiology 131–137

Interactions of Autonomic Nerves and Smooth Muscle In Vitro

Geoffrey Burnstock

Department of Anatomy and Embryology, University College London, Gower Street, London, England

Interactions are described between autonomic nerves and both explants and single smooth muscle cells grown in culture.

Sympathetic nerves delay the process of dedifferentiation of cultured smooth muscle cells. Sympathetic chain extract and dibutyryl cyclic AMP (together with theophylline) mimic this effect, but noradrenaline, acetylcholine, and spinal cord extract do not. It is suggested that sympathetic nerves may release a trophic factor that acts on adenylate cyclase receptors leading to the production of cyclic AMP, which promotes differentiation; in this way dedifferentiation and the subsequent proliferation are delayed. However, further factors seem likely to be involved in the regulation of smooth muscle proliferation in vivo.

The presence of sympathetic nerves is not necessary for muscle effector bundle or gap junction (nexus) formation, but their presence accelerates the process. Cyclic AMP may also be involved in this process.

Sympathetic nerves are 'attracted' over distances of up to 2mm to normally densely-innervated (but not sparsely-innervated) smooth muscle. It is suggested that nerve growth factor (NGF) is produced by these explants and is responsible for this effect. In normal development in vivo, it is possible that programmed production of NGF in potentially densely-innervated effector tissues is one of the factors contributing to the establishment of differences in density of sympathetic innervation.

Sympathetic nerves form long-lasting, intimate, functional relationships with smooth muscle cells cultured from potentially densely-innervated tissues, but not with smooth muscle cells from potentially sparsely-innervated tissues or with fibroblasts. The nature of this 'recognition' system is unknown. Once this relationship is established, long-lasting associations with further nerve fibres are inhibited.

Fibres from cultured sympathetic ganglia form functional cholinergic excitatory junctions with sphincter pupillae. It is not yet clear whether this is due to selective growth of a small population of cholinergic neurons, to the absence of a 'trophic' trigger for noradrenaline synthesis in sympathetic neurons or to the presence of a 'trophic' trigger for acetylcholine synthesis.

Key words: tissue culture, smooth muscle, development, autonomic nerves, cyclic AMP, nerve growth factor

INTRODUCTION

Studies of the interaction of autonomic nerves with smooth muscle have in general lagged behind those of motor nerves with skeletal muscle. This was mainly because the skeletal neuromuscular junction is well defined and because a brilliant series of studies was carried out to analyse the process of short-term interaction or transmission between these two cell types (1, 2). Clarification of the nature of the autonomic neuromuscular junction followed (3) and short-term transmission was described in which emphasis was placed on muscle effector bundles with electrotonic coupling between neighbouring smooth muscle cells and "en passage" release of transmitter from extensive varicose terminal autonomic nerve fibres (4).

When interest turned to long-term or 'trophic' interactions between nerves and muscles, i.e., the influence of nerves on the development of muscle and conversely the influence of muscle on the pattern and orientation of growth of nerves, again the motor nerve-skeletal muscle model system was favoured first for in vitro studies (5, 6). However, there are certain unique advantages of the autonomic nerve-smooth muscle system for studying long-term interactions. Muscles with different well-defined innervation can be selected for particular study, such as vas deferens with high-density innervation, ureter with low-density innervation, arteries with nerves confined to one side of the muscle coat, and umbilical artery with no innervation. Thus, interactions of autonomic nerves with smooth muscle have been observed in vitro, both with explants and isolated muscle cells (7, 8, 9). A brief account of these studies follows.

INFLUENCE OF SYMPATHETIC NERVES ON THE DEVELOPMENT OF SMOOTH MUSCLE

Development of Cultured Smooth Muscle

Spontaneous contractions have been recorded in cultures of both explants of smooth muscle (10–14) and of isolated smooth muscle cells (9, 15–19). These cells exhibit electrical activity comparable to that recorded in adult animals (21) and show positive reactions with fluorescent antibodies to smooth muscle myosin (19, 22).

The behaviour of single smooth muscle cells in culture is complex (Fig. 1). Undifferentiated smooth muscle cells (e.g., from 10-day embryo chicken gizzard) divide and proliferate in culture until a confluent monolayer is formed within 36 hr (23). In contrast, differentiated smooth muscle cells from more mature animals (e.g., from newborn guinea pig vas deferens, taenia coli, ureter and rabbit aorta) dedifferentiate before proliferation and confluence takes place (9, 18, 19, 20, 24). As soon as a confluent monolayer is formed, differentiation occurs and is associated with appearance of myosin immunofluorescence and thick filaments. The cells then aggregate into either clumps or chains. Spontaneous contractions develop, which become synchronous as gap junctions (nexuses) form low-resistance pathways between neighbouring cells.

This sequence of changes in smooth muscle cells in culture is comparable to that described during normal development in vivo (25, 26), in anterior eye chamber transplants of smooth muscle (27) and in cultured explants of aorta (28).

Delay in Dedifferentiation of Smooth Muscle in the Presence of Sympathetic Nerves

In cultures of smooth muscle from guinea pig vas deferens the cells maintain their differentiation for 4–5 days before undergoing dedifferentiation and subsequent pro-

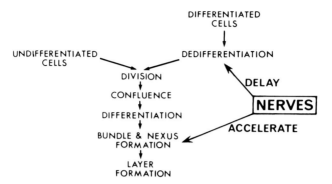

Fig. 1. The behaviour in culture of undifferentiated smooth muscle cells (e.g., from 10-day embryo chicken gizzard) and differentiated smooth muscle cells (e.g., newborn guinea pig vas deferens).

liferation. The presence of sympathetic nerves (but not necessarily long-lasting associations) delays this process by 2–7 days (18). Sympathetic chain extract and dibutyryl cyclic AMP (together with theophylline to prevent cyclic AMP breakdown) mimic this effect, but noradrenaline, acetylcholine, and spinal cord extract do not (29). These results could be explained by the release of a trophic substance from sympathetic nerves that acts on adenylate cyclase receptors in the smooth muscle cells, resulting in the production of cyclic AMP. The cyclic AMP might then act as a "second messenger" that promotes differentiation, thereby delaying dedifferentiation and proliferation.

A comparable result has been obtained with cultured vascular smooth muscle cells (9, 30, 31). However, Bevan (32) has shown that sympathetic denervation of the ear artery in the young rabbit results in fewer dividing cells than on the control side, suggesting that the presence of nerves enhances proliferation. Further factors may therefore be involved in the regulation of smooth muscle proliferation in vivo.

Acceleration of Muscle Bundle and Nexus Formation in the Presence of Sympathetic Nerves

Muscle effector bundle and nexus formation occurs in culture in the absence of sympathetic nerves, but is accelerated by their presence (18). In small clumps of muscle supplied by nerves, foci of synchronous contraction appear much earlier (3–5 days) than in similar clumps without nerves (8–12 days). An approximately 50% increase in gap junctions was seen in the muscle clumps associated with nerves. The mechanism by which nerves influence muscle development in this way is not known, but cyclic AMP has been shown recently to increase the formation of gap junctions in culture preparations (Sheridan, personal communication).

INFLUENCE OF SMOOTH MUSCLE ON THE DEVELOPMENT OF SYMPATHETIC NERVES

Development of Cultured Autonomic Neurons

Two types of neurons have been identified in cultures of sympathetic ganglia of rat and guinea pig; type I neurons, in the minority, migrate into the outgrowth and may represent immature, retarded, or abnormal cells; type II neurons, in the majority, do not show migratory activity and appear to correspond to those seen in situ (33, 34). Accessory cells present in these cultures have been described (35); they include satellite cells (which appear to be identical with interstitial cells), small intensely fluorescent cells, Schwann cells, sheath fibroblasts, macrophages, and perineural epithelial cells. Processes of cultured sympathetic neurons are varicose, and they show fluorescence and histochemical and ultrastructural features characteristic of adrenergic nerves growing of regenerating in situ (36). NGF generally increases the size, growth rate, and noradrenaline levels of cultured sympathetic neurons (37).

Studies of dissociated neurons from rat superior cervical ganglion, however, have produced some curiously ambiguous results (38–45). These neurons show enzyme activity for noradrenaline synthesis, have the ability to take up catecholamines, and have typical adrenergic nerve histochemistry and ultrastructure. However, physiological studies of synapses formed between these neurons or with skeletal myotubes revealed excitatory postsynaptic potentials with pharmacological properties of cholinergic nicotinic junctions (41, 43, 44), and iontophoretic application of noradrenaline at these junctions was ineffective (46). Possible explanations for these results will be discussed in the next section. The ciliary ganglion has also been grown in tissue culture for studies of the interaction of cholinergic neurons with smooth muscle (12, 47).

"Attraction" of Autonomic Nerves to Explants of Smooth and Cardiac Muscle

The first report of the influence of explants of autonomic effector organs on the growth of nerves from sympathetic ganglia in culture was by Levi-Montalcini et al. (48). These authors showed that during the first 16 hr in culture the number of nerve fibres originating from the sympathetic ganglion (but not the spinal cord) was consistently higher on the side facing either mouse heart or sarcoma explants. Since then a number of similar experiments have been carried out (17, 18, 49, 50, 51, 52, 65). For example, when sympathetic ganglia are grown at equal distances from explants of potentially densely-innervated muscle (e.g., vas deferens or atrium) and explants of potentially sparsely-innervated muscle (e.g., ureter, uterus, or lung), nerve fibres show preferential growth towards the densely-innervated explants for distances of up to 2 mm (11). In contrast, the direction and amount of nerve growth from spinal cord explants grown together with atrium, vas deferens, or lung was not significantly different from controls (65). This "attraction" of sympathetic nerves is evident soon after the nerve fibres emerge from the ganglion explants, and it was therefore suggested that it might be due to a chemical substance released from the smooth muscle explants (11, 17). Indications that this substance is NGF come from a number of different sources: a) the increased growth of cultured sympathetic or sensory nerves by NGF-producing mouse sarcomas (48, 53); b) the "attraction" of cultured sensory nerves to the tip of capillary tubes containing a solution of NGF, but not to tubes containing saline (50); c) the presence of higher levels of NGF in atrium and vas deferens than in sparsely-innervated tissues (54, 55, 56); d) the increased sympathetic neuron growth, catecholamine fluorescence intensity, and size of nerve cell bodies, when the vas deferens is added to the culture chamber (17); the similarity of this stimulatory effect to that produced when NGF is added to the medium (32, 37).

When irises from 3- to 5-day-old rats are grown 1–3 mm from superior cervical or lumbar sympathetic ganglia, varicose adrenergic fibres become associated with the dilator pupillae, while excitatory cholinergic junctions are formed with the sphincter pupillae (57). This is precisely the pattern of innervation of the iris in vivo, and it therefore raises some interesting questions. For example, Is there a nerve growth factor specific for cholinergic as well as for adrenergic nerves? Do the cholinergic fibres that reach the sphincter pupillae from the sympathetic ganglia arise from a small population of cholinergic neurons in the ganglia? Or are some of the maturing cultured sympathetic neurons (which contain the genetic machinery to produce both acetylcholine and catecholamine) triggered to become cholinergic by "trophic" factors released by sphincter pupillae? Or do they retain a cholinergic nature due to the absence of a "trophic" factor inducing noradrenaline synthesis? Initially all undifferentiated neuroblasts appear to possess an acetylcholine synthesising system (58). Whether a maturing neuron emerges at the end of its differentiation as cholinergic, adrenergic, or of another neuron type appears to be determined by external ("trophic") factors that trigger the expression of the appropriate genetic mechanism (see, for example, 59, 60 61). Presumptive adrenergic neuroblasts taken from the adrenomedullary neural crest area and transplanted into the vagal neural crest area are influenced by splanchnic mesoderm to become fully differentiated cholinergic neurons when they reach the gut (61). It has been shown recently that acetylcholine synthesis in cultured sympathetic neurons is increased 100-fold to 1,000-fold in the presense of several nonneuronal cell types, notably fibroblasts (42, 45). Studies of cultured mouse neuroblastoma cells (62) revealed three types of cells with respect to neurotransmitter synthesis, namely cholinergic, adrenergic, and nonadrenergic non-cholinergic, although all three cell types contained acetylcholinesterase. The authors suggested that the expression of a gene required for the synthesis of one neurotransmitter may restrict the expression of genes for alternate transmitters. In another interesting experimental study, it was claimed that after removal of the superior cervical ganglion and anastomosis of the pre- and postganglionic cervical sympathetic trunks, "the denervated nictitating membranes were reinnervated by cholinergic presynaptic sympathetic fibres that had been modified so that they could release catecholamines in addition to, or instead of, acetylcholine" (63).

Nerves grown from cultured ciliary ganglia penetrated explants of taenia coli or vas deferens 1–2 mm away, and functional excitatory innervation was observed 3–4 days later (47). The muscle responses to nerve stimulation were potentiated by neostigmine and abolished by hyoscine, indicating that the junctions were cholinergic; this was also supported by electron-microscope demonstration of nerve profiles, containing a predominance of small agranular vesicles within 20 nm of muscle cells.

"Recognition" of Isolated Muscle Cells by Autonomic Nerves

When the interactions between sympathetic nerve fibres and single, isolated smooth muscle cells were studied for the first time (16, 17), nerve fibres, upon random contact with a cell, appeared to be able to distinguish between fibroblasts and muscle cells within about an hour. Nerves did not maintain contact with fibroblasts after this time (and nerves never come closer than 30–40 nm), whereas they formed long-lasting, intimate relationships with smooth muscle cells of the potentially densely-innervated vas deferens, which were often maintained up to several weeks. Nerve varicosities in contact with muscle became larger and formed junctions with nerve and muscle separation as little as 10 nm. Once such a relationship was established, long-lasting association with further nerve fibres was inhibited. However, multiple innervation did occur when several nerve fibres reached a muscle cell at about the same time. The junctions that formed between sympathetic nerves and single or small clumps of smooth muscle cells from the vas deferens and sphincter pupillae or between ciliary ganglion nerves and taenia coli and vas deferens became functional 1–3 days after first contact (12). Sympathetic nerve fibres formed long-lasting associations of up to 8 days with single, isolated smooth muscle cells from the densely innervated rabbit ear artery, but not with smooth muscle cells from the sparsely-innervated thoracic aorta (9, 20). It is interesting to note that the nerve-muscle separation in the junctions formed with rabbit ear artery muscle cells was 10–50 nm, i.e., considerably closer than is seen in any blood vessels in vivo (64).

REFERENCES

1. Katz, B.: "The Release of Neural Transmitter Substances." Liverpool: University Press (1969).
2. Hubbard, J. I.: Neuromuscular transmitters – presynaptic factors. In "The Peripheral Nervous System," J. I. Hubbard (Ed.). New York: Plenum Press (1974).
3. Burnstock, G.: In "Smooth Muscle," E. Bullbring, A. F. Brading, A. W. Jones, and T. Tomita (Eds.). London: Edward Arnold (1970).
4. Burnstock, G., and Iwayama, T.: Prog. Brain Res. 34:389 (1971).
5. Shimada, Y., and Kano, M.: Arch. Histol. Jap. 33:95 (1971).
6. Nelson, P. G.: Physiol. Rev. 55:1 (1975).
7. Burnstock, G.: In "Dynamics of Degeneration and Growth in Neurons," K. Fuxe, L. Olson, and Y. Zotterman (Eds.). Oxford and New York: Pergamon Press (1974).
8. Burnstock, G., and Costa, M.: "Adrenergic Neurons: Their Organisation, Function and Development in the Peripheral Nervous System. London: Chapman & Hall (1975).
9. Chamley, J., Campbell, G. R., and Burnstock, G.: In "Functional and Comparative Anatomy of the Artery," C. J. Schwartz (Ed.). New York: Plenum Press (1976).
10. Murrary, M. R.: In "Cells and Tissues in Culture," E. N. Willmer (Ed.). New York: Academic Press, Vol. 2, p. 311 (1965).
11. Chamley, J. H., Goller, I., and Burnstock, G.: Devel. Biol. 31:362 (1973).
12. Purves, R. D., Hill, C. E., Chamley, J., Mark, G. E., Fry, D. M., and Burnstock, G.: Pflüg.Arch. 350:1 (1974).
13. Cook, R. D., and Peterson, E. R.: J. Neurol. Sci. 22:25 (1974).
14. Laqueur, E.: Zbl. Physiol. 28:728 (1914).
15. Lewis, M. R., and Lewis, W. H.: Amer. J. Physiol. 44:67 (1917).
16. Mark, G. E., Chamley, J. H., and Burnstock, G.: Devel. Biol. 32:194 (1973).
17. Chamley, J. H., Campbell, G. R., and Burnstock, G.: Devel. Biol. 33:344 (1973).
18. Chamley, J., Campbell, G. R., and Burnstock, G.: J. Embryol. Exp. Morph. 32:297 (1974).
19. Gröschel-Stewart, U., Chamley, J. H., Campbell, G. R., and Burnstock, G.: Cell Tiss. Res. 165:13 (1975).
20. Chamley, J. H., and Campbell, G. R.: In "Vascular Neuroeffector Mechanisms." Second Int. Symp. on Vascular Neuroeffector Mechanisms, Odense. Bevan, Burnstock, Johansson, Maxwell and Nedergaard (Eds.). Karger: Basel (1976).
21. Purves, R. D., Mark, G., and Burnstock, G.: Pflüg. Arch. 341:325 (1973).
22. Gröschel-Stewart, U., Chamley, J. H., McConnell, J. D., and Burnstock, G.: Histochem. 43:215 (1975).
23. Campbell, G. R., Chamley, J. H., and Burnstock, G.: J. Anat. 117:295 (1974).
24. Chamley, J. H., and Campbell, G. R.: Cytobiol. 11:358 (1975).
25. Yamauchi, A., and Burnstock, G.: J. Anat. (Lond.) 104:1 (1969).
26. Bennett, T., and Cobb, J. L. S.: Z. Zellforsch. 96:173 (1969).
27. Campbell, G. R., Uehara, Y., Malmfors, T., Burnstock, G.: Z. Zellforsch. 117:155 (1971).
28. Fritz, K. E., Jarmolych, J., and Daoud, A. S.: Exp. Molec. Pathol. 12:354 (1970).
29. Chamley, J. H., and Campbell, G. R.: Cell Tiss. Res. 161:497 (1975).
30. Stout, R. W., Bierman, E. L., and Ross, R.: Artery 1:471 (1975).
31. Stout, R. W., Bierman, E. L., and Ross, R.: Circ. Res. 36:319 (1975).
32. Bevan, R. D.: Circ. Res. 37:14 (1975).
33. Chamley, J. H., Mark, G. E., Campbell, G. R., and Burnstock, G.: Z. Zellforsch 135:287 (1972).
34. Perry, R. A., Chamley, J. H., and Robinson, P. M.: J. Anta. (Lond.) 119:506 (1975).
35. Chamley, J., Mark, G. E., and Burnstock, G.: Z. Zellforsch. 135:315 (1972).
36. Burnstock, G., and Bell, C.: In "The Peripheral Nervous System," J. I. Hubbard (Ed.). New York: Plenum Press (1974).

37. Levi-Montalcini, R., and Angeletti, P. U.: Physiol. Rev. 48:534 (1968).
38. Mains, R. E., and Patterson, P. H.: J. Cell Biol. 59:329 (1973).
39. Mains, R. E., and Patterson, P. H.: J. Cell Biol. 59:346 (1973).
40. Mains, R. E., and Patterson, P. H.: J. Cell Biol. 59:361 (1973).
41. O'Lague, P. H., Obata, K., Claude, P., Furshpan, E. J., and Potter, D. D.: Proc. Nat. Acad. Sci. 71:3602 (1974).
42. Patterson, P. H., and Chun, L.: Proc. Nat. Acad. Sci. 71:3607 (1974).
43. Nurse, C. A., and O'Lague, P. H.: Proc. Nat. Acad. Sci. 72:1955 (1975).
44. Burton, H., and Bunge, R.: Brain Res. 97:157 (1975).
45. Patterson, P. H., Reichardt, L. F., and Chun, L. Y.: In "The Synapse" Cold Spring Harbor Symposium Quant. Biol. No. 40 (1976).
46. Obata, K.: Brain Res. 73:71 (1974).
47. Fry, D. M., and Burnstock, G.: Ultrastructure and physiology of the innervation of smooth muscle in tissue culture. In "Electronmicroscopy 1974," Proc. 8th Int. Cong. Electronmic. J. V. Sanders, and D. J. Goodchild (Eds.). Austr. Acad. Sci. (Canberra) Vol. II, 396–397 (1974).
48. Levi-Montalcini, R., Meyer, H., and Hamburger, V.: Cancer Res. 14:49 (1954).
49. Bueker, E. D. Cancer Res. 17:190 (1957).
50. Charlwood, K. A., Lamont, D. M., and Banks, B. E. L.: In "Nerve Growth Factor and Its Antiserum," E. Zaimis (Ed.). London: Athlone Press (1972).
51. Silberstein, S. D., Johnson, D. G., Jacobowitz, D. M., and Kopin, I. J.: Proc. Nat. Acad. Sci. 68:1121 (1971).
52. Johnson, D. G., Silberstein, S. D., Hanbauer, I., and Kopin, I. J.: J. Neurochem. 19:2025 (1972).
53. Bueker, E. D.: Anat. Rec. 102:369 (1948).
54. Bueker, E. D., Schenkein, I., and Bane, J. L.: Cancer Res. 20:1220 (1960).
55. Levi-Montalcini, R., and Angeletti, P. V.: In "Regional Neurochemistry," S. S. Kety and J. Elkes (Eds.) New York: Pergamon Press (1961).
56. Johnson, D. G., Gorden, P., and Kopin, I. J.: J. Neurochem. 18:2355 (1971).
57. Hill, C. E., Purves, R. D., Watanabe, H., and Burnstock, G.: Pflüg. Arch. 361:127 (1976).
58. Filogamo, G., and Marchisio, P. C.: In "Neuorsciences Research," Vol. 4, S. Ehrenpreis and O. Solnitsky (Eds.). New York: Academic Press (1971).
59. Cohen, A. M.: J. Exp. Zool. 179:167 (1972).
60. Norr, S. C.: Develop. Biol. 34:16 (1973).
61. Le Douarin, N. M., Renaud, D., Teillet, M. A., and Le Douarin, G. H.: Proc. Nat. Acad. Sci. 72:728 (1975).
62. Amano, T., Richelson, E., and Nirenberg, M.: Proc. Nat. Acad. Sci. 69:258 (1972).
63. Ceccarelli, B., Clementi, F., and Mantegazza, P.: J. Physiol. 220:211 (1972).
64. Burnstock, G.: In "Methods in Pharmacology," Vol. III, E. E. Daniel, and D. M. Paton (Eds.). New York: Appleton-Century-Crofts (1975).
65. Chamley, J. H., and Dowel, J.: J. Exptl. Cell Res. 90:1 (1975).

Cellular Neurobiology 139—146

Studies on Cell Recognition in the Developing Brain

David I. Gottlieb, Ronald Merrell, Kenneth Rock, Daniel Littman, Roger Santala, and Luis Glaser

Department of Biological Chemistry, Division of Biology and Biomedical Sciences, Washington University, St. Louis, Missouri 63110

Several lines of evidence demonstrate cell-cell receptors on the surface of developing brain cells. Plasma membrane vesicles with regional and temporal binding specificities can be prepared. Active factors that block cell aggregation can be extracted from these membranes and partially purified. Quantitative studies of cell-cell adhesion demonstrate a gradient of adhesive specificity along the dorsoventral axis of the developing retina.

Key words: cell surface, neuronal specificity, gradients

INTRODUCTION

One of the most striking features of the vertebrate central nervous system is the precise spatial arrangement of neuronal cell bodies and processes. Neuronal somata are not scattered randomly, but instead are grouped into laminae or nuclei which are highly characteristic of a particular region of the brain. The spatial arrangement of axons is also highly ordered. Axons run in defined tracts and terminate on restricted populations of target neurons. Populations of axons have the added property of forming ordered two-dimensional arrays, of which the retinotopic projection of the optic nerve is a well-studied example. The molecular basis of these kinds of pattern formation in the nervous system is not known, but it is reasonable to speculate that surface cell-cell receptors might play an important role; consequently several authors have proposed mechanisms involving complementary receptors and ligands on "appropriate" pairs of plasma membranes (1, 2).

Recently, Roth, Roseman, and their co-workers have provided direct evidence for cell-cell receptors on the surface of embryonic cells by showing that single cells derived by dissociating embryonic tissues bind preferentially to aggregates or monolayers of homologous cells (3, 4). These demonstrations of cell-cell receptors raise two related questions: first, "What is the molecular nature of the receptors and ligands involved?" and second, "What role do they play in normal development?" As regards cell-cell receptors in the developing brain, we would like to know if they contribute to the formation of biologically important patterns such as nuclei, laminae, or topographical maps. In this report, we will review our recent efforts to elucidate the structure and function of cell-cell receptors in the developing chick brain.

MATERIALS AND METHODS

Details of the procedures used in these studies are described in the original papers from our laboratory (5—9).

RESULTS

Specific Binding of Plasma Membrane Vesicles to Embryonic Brain Cells

As a first step in trying to isolate cell-cell receptors and ligands from embryonic nervous tissue, we prepared plasma membrane vesicles from 8-day chick neural retina and cerebellum (5). Retina plasma membrane vesicles were shown to bind specifically to retina cells by two methods; direct measurement of binding using radioactive membranes (Fig. 1) and the ability of the vesicles to inhibit the aggregation of homologous cells more effectively than the aggregation of heterologous cells. Cerebellar plasma membranes bound specifically to cerebellar cells when measured in the aggregation inhibition assay. Control experiments indicated that membrane vesicles were not internalized, that they did not irreversibly alter the cell surface, that trypsinized membranes did not bind, and that binding was partially inhibited at 4°C.

A subsequent study, using as an assay the inhibition of cell aggregation by membranes, has shown that membrane inhibition specificities change dramatically during development (Fig. 2) (6). Membrane vesicles from the 8-day retina were more effective in inhibiting the aggregation of 8-day retinal cells than the aggregation of 7 or 9-day retinal cells. On the other hand, membranes from 7- and 9-day retina bind most strongly to cells from 7- and 9-day retina respectively. One additional region was investigated using plasma membranes, the optic tectum (6). As in the case of retinal cells, tectal cell surface specificity also changed dramatically on days 7, 8, and 9 of development. Membranes prepared from the tectum were effective at blocking tectal cell aggregation but not retinal cell aggregation. However, retinal membranes could block both retinal and tectal aggregation. This asymmetry might be explained by the selective loss of an adhesive

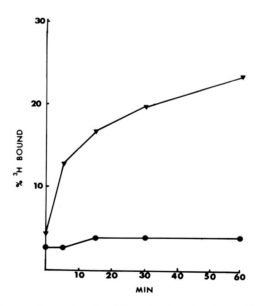

Fig. 1. Binding of radioactive membranes to cells. Cells are incubated at 37°C with [³H] glucosamine-labeled retinal plasma membranes. Membranes bound to cells are determined by differential centrifugation ▲——▲, retinal cells; ●——●, cerebellar cells. (Source: Ref. 5.)

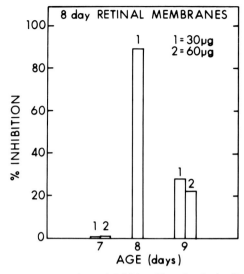

Fig. 2. Effect of retinal cell age on membrane inhibition. Neural retinal cells were obtained from 7-, 8- and 9-day embryos. The cells were allowed to aggregate for 30 min under standard conditions either alone or with the indicated concentration of 8-day retinal membranes. The data show the percentage of inhibition of aggregation by the addition of membranes. In the absence of membranes 80–90% of cells aggregate in 30 min. (Source: Ref. 6.)

component during preparation of the membranes. However, a recent study using an aggregate-collecting assay has shown that tectal aggregates will pick up retinal and tectal cells but that retinal aggregates pick up only retinal cells (10). In light of the numerous important developmental events taking place in the retina and tectum between days 7 and 9, it is perhaps not surprising to find such dramatic changes in surface specificity. However, at present we do not know if the changes are related to the appearance of new cell types or to the maturation of the surface of preexisting cells.

Extraction of an Active Component Involved in Cell Recognition

Having shown that plasma membrane fractions carried specific adhesive components, we proceeded to extract an active binding component from these membranes (7). Acetone powders of plasma membranes were extracted with 3 mM LIS (lithiumdiiodosalicylate). These extracts could reversibly block cell aggregation and exhibited the same regional and temporal specificity as the membranes they were prepared from (Fig. 3). The active component in the LIS extract passed through Amicon PM10 filters but was retained by UM2 filters, indicating that the molecular weight of the factor was roughly between 2,000 and 20,000 daltons; the PM10 filtrate was purified about 200-fold over the starting material on a protein basis and has been further purified by chromatography on DEAE Sephadex. The blocking activity was highly trypsin-sensitive, suggesting that it is either a protein itself or is somehow associated with a protein. Two observations suggest that the factor acts by reversibly blocking adhesive sites rather than modifying them enzymatically. The first is that blocking activity is fully and rapidly reversed by trypsinization of the cells, and the second is that blocking activity can be absorbed from solution by cells of the appropriate type.

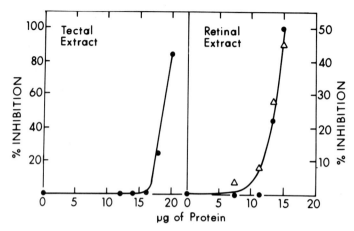

Fig. 3. Inhibition of cell aggregation as a function of LIS extract concentration. Cell aggregation was measured under standard assay conditions with concentrations of extract as indicated. △——△, retinal cells; ●——●, tectal cells. (Source: Ref. 7.)

Studies on the Specificity of Cell-Cell Adhesion Using Intact Cells From the Developing Chick Brain

One of the major goals of our recent work has been to understand the functional role of cell-cell receptors in the formation of nervous tissues. We have approached this problem by trying to determine if there is any relationship between patterns of cell-to-cell adhesive specificity and developmentally important patterns such as gradients of synaptic specificity.

Our experiments measure the rate at which suspensions of labeled cells bind to cell monolayers. The assay we use is a modification of the monolayer adhesion assay of Walther et al. (4), which allows stable monolayers to be formed within one hour of sacrificing embryos (8). Using this assay we were able to demonstrate differences in adhesive specificity between cells from two major brain regions, the tectum and the telencephalon. Radioactively labeled cells were prepared from each of these regions and assayed for their ability to bind to homologous and heterologous monolayers. The results, shown in Fig. 4, were surprising: The most rapid binding occurred between heterologous cells. Tectal cells bound most rapidly to monolayers of telencephalic cells while telencephalic cells bound most rapidly to tectal monolayers. As far as we know, this is the first case of cells that adhere specifically to heterologous cells, and it is therefore worth considering three points. The first is that we are measuring the binding of single cells to confluent monolayers. It is conceivable that the cells on the monolayer block recognition sites on each other's surface and that the adhesive sites left free to interact with single cells in the overlying suspension are a distinct and perhaps quantitatively minor subclass. Second, while the rate of homologous binding is only about one-half that of the rate of heterologous binding, it is still considerably more rapid than binding to a variety of nonneural cell types, including fibroblasts and several established cell lines. Finally, the binding rates we see must be influenced by both the number and affinity of adhesive sites, but we cannot assess the relative contribution these make to the overall binding rate. In spite of these ambiguities, the data clearly show the existence of region-specific adhesive determinants.

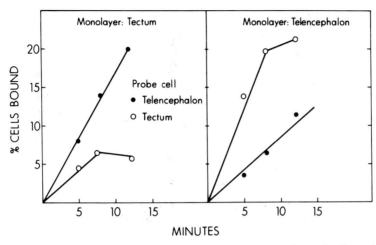

Fig. 4. Binding of tectal and telencephalic probe cells to monolayers. Left panel: telencephalon probe cells show best binding to tectal monolayers. Right panel: tectal probe cells show best binding to telencephalon monolayers.

The retinotopic projection to the optic tectum is the most extensively analyzed example of pattern formation in the nervous system. Sperry's chemoaffinity hypothesis attempts to account for the experimental findings by postulating cell surface determinants on retinal ganglion cells that encode positional information. Roth and his colleagues (see this volume, pp. 73–79) have shown that the binding of retinal cells to the surface of the optic tectum mimicked retinotectal connections in certain respects. Our monolayer adhesion assay proved suitable to show more refined topographic differences in retinal cell adhesive specificity. Nine- or 12-day embryonic retinae were divided into dorsal and ventral halves, and radioactive cell suspensions and monolayers were prepared from each half. Binding assays clearly showed that dorsal cells bound more quickly to ventral cell mono-layers than dorsal cell monolayers. Ventral radioactive cells, on the other hand, bound more quickly to dorsal cell monolayers than ventral cell monolayers (Fig. 5). The binding affinities followed a dorsoventral gradient. To show this, the retina was divided into six horizontal strips of equal width; monolayers were prepared from all six strips and probe cells from the most dorsal and most ventral strips were tested against the set of six mono-layers. Radioactive probe cells from the most dorsal strip had low affinity for monolayers of the three most dorsal strips but a progressively increasing affinity for cells more ventrally displaced from the retinal equator. Cells from the most ventral strip showed the opposite behavior; that is, a low affinity for the three most ventral strips and an increasing affinity for cells dorsal to the equator. The graded nature of adhesive specificity along the dorsoventral axis was further documented and shown to be statistically significant in an additional series of experiments (Fig. 6). These experiments emphasize that probe cells from the extreme dorsal part of the retina cannot distinguish between cells from the two most dorsal strips but can distinguish between cells of the two most ventral strips. Cells from the most ventral strip showed the reciprocal behavior. It is worth noting that previously published models of morphogenetic gradients in the retina predict a key feature of our results, namely, that cells from opposite poles of the gradient should show the highest adhesive affinities (2, 11, and Roth, this volume).

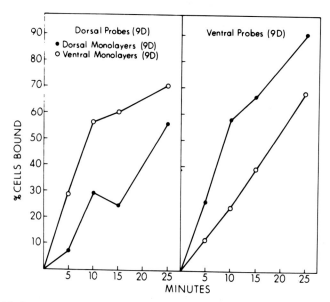

Fig. 5. Cell-cell binding characteristics of dorsal and ventral 9-day neural retinal cells. The left panel shows that cells obtained from the dorsal neural retina adhere more rapidly to a monolayer prepared from ventral neural retinal cells. The right panel shows that ventral probe cells have the opposite behavior. (Source: Ref. 9.)

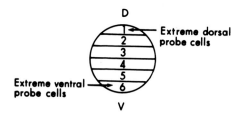

Probe Cell	No. of Experiments	Ratio of Adherence to Monolayer	
		1/2	5/6
Extreme dorsal (area 1)	6	–	0.77 ± .07[1]
Extreme ventral (area 6)	5	–	1.006 ± .06
Extreme dorsal (area 1)	4	1.01 ± .10	–
Extreme ventral (area 6)	4	1.35 ± .22[1]	–

[1]Significantly different from unity at the 0.01 level of confidence.

Fig. 6. Summary of cell-to-monolayer binding experiments showing graded cell adhesive affinities along the dorso-ventral axis of the retina. Probe cells from area 1 bind preferentially to monolayers from area 6 as compared to monolayers from area 5. They do not distinugish between monolayers from areas 1 and 2. Probe cells from area 6 show the converse behavior. (Modified from Ref. 9.)

Our studies on retinal cell binding thus show a striking correlation between a developmentally critical pattern and cell-cell adhesion. However, it would be premature to claim that the determinants responsible for the gradient in adhesive affinity are involved in synaptogenesis. For one thing, we are looking at the interaction of cell somata, while synaptic specificity must involve the surfaces of axons and dendrites. In addition, only a small fraction of retinal cells are retinal ganglion cells, the cells which actually project to the tectum. Thus we have been able to establish that cell surface adhesive sites encode positional information but we do not yet know the role of the determinants in neural development.

Studies of Adhesion of Clonal Neuronal Cells to Embryonic Brain Cells

Many of the difficulties we have encountered in trying to purify the factors responsible for specific cell recognition in the nervous system could be overcome if one could find clonal neural lines that were able to recognize normal neurons. These cells could be grown in large quantities and, perhaps more importantly, they could be labeled to high specific activities with radioactive precursors. In light of these considerations we have used the monolayer adhesion method to search for neuroblastoma lines that would bind specifically to embryonic brain cells. The most promising results to date have been obtained with a neuronal line from the central nervous system of the rat provided by Dr. D. Shubert, (of the Salk Institute), B103. These cells bind very rapidly to monolayers of rat or chick embryonic brain cells, but bind very slowly to monolayers of embryonic fibroblasts, liver cells, or a variety of established lines (Fig. 7). Although in this sense they appear to be specific for brain, we have not been able to demonstrate interregional specific binding of B103 cells. Plasma membranes prepared from B103 cells mimic the binding properties of the cells (Fig. 8). They bind very quickly to embryonic brain cells but only slowly to embryonic liver. The binding is extremely trypsin sensitive. Efforts are underway to extract the factors responsible for binding.

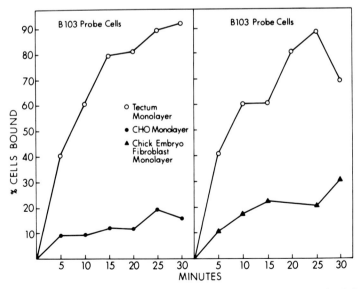

Fig. 7. Cell-to-cell binding behavior of B103 cells. B103 cells bind rapidly to tectal cells but slowly to CHO cells (left panel) and chick embryo fibroblasts (right panel).

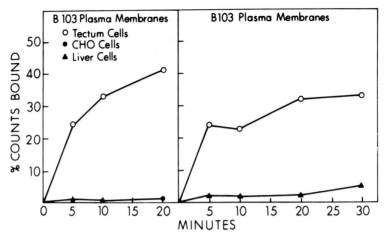

Fig. 8. Plasma membranes prepared from B103 cells bind preferentially to tectal cells when contrasted to CHO cells (left panel) or embryonic liver cells (right panel).

SUMMARY

The studies reviewed in this report have been directed at two closely related goals. The first is to extract, purify, and characterize cell-cell receptors from the developing central nervous system. Our conclusions to date are that cell surface receptors occur on the surface of developing brain cells, and that by functional criteria there are at least seven types of receptor. An active component of cell-cell recognition can be solubilized and partially purified, but limitations in the amount of available starting material have prevented us from purifying this component to homogeneity. Our experiments indicate that clonal neuronal lines may provide a more abundant and convenient source of receptors.

Finally, we have shown a topographic correspondence between the pattern of retinal cell adhesion and a developmentally important gradient of specificity.

REFERENCES

1. Sperry, R. W.: Proc. Nat. Acad. Sci. USA 50:703–710 (1963).
2. Marchese, R. B., Barbera, A. J., and Roth, A.: In "A Molecular Approach to Retino-Tectal Specificity in Cell Patterning. A Ciba Symposium," Amsterdam: Elsevier, Vol. 29, (1975). pp. 315–327.
3. Roth, S., McGuire, E. J., and Roseman, S.: J. Cell Biol. 51:525–535 (1971).
4. Walther, B ᵀT., Ohman, R., and Roseman, S.: Proc. Nat. Acad. Sci. USA 70:1569–1573 (1973).
5. Merrell, R., and Glaser, L.: Proc. Nat. Acad. Sci. USA 70:2794–2798 (1973).
6. Gottlieb, D. I., Merrell, R., and Glaser, L.: Proc. Nat. Acad. Sci. USA 71:1800–1802 (1974).
7. Merrell, R., Gottlieb, D. I., and Glaser, L.: J. Biol. Chem. 250:5655–5659 (1975).
8. Gottlieb, D. I., and Glaser, L.: Biochem. Biophys. Res. Commun. 63:815–821 (1975).
9. Gottlieb, D. I., Rock, K., and Glaser, L.: Proc. Nat. Acad. Sci. USA 73:410–414 (1976).
10. McGuire, E. J., and Burdick, C. L.: J. Cell Biol. 68:80–89 (1976).
11. Barondes, S. H.: In "The Neurosciences: Second Study Program," (Schmitt, F. O., ed.). New York: Rockefeller University Press, 1970, pp. 747–760.

Ca and Na Spikes in Egg Cell Membrane

Susumu Hagiwara and Shunichi Miyazaki

Department of Physiology and the Brain Research Institute, University of California at Los Angeles, Los Angeles, California 90024

Na, Ca and K channels of the cell membrane are distinguished by different kinetics of their currents, by their different ion selectivities, and by their different sensitivities to different pharmacological agents. These channels are already found in unfertilized egg cells in many animals. Elimination of existing channels and creation of new channels occur during the process of differentiation.

Key words: Na channel, Ca channel, ion selectivity, egg cell

INTRODUCTION

According to the Na theory developed by Hodgkin and Huxley (1952) the action potential is produced by a permeability increase of the membrane to Na ions, bringing the membrane potential towards the Na equilibrium potential E_{Na}. This permeability increase is then followed by a K permeability increase which brings the membrane potential rapidly back to E_K which is close to the resting potential. In the last 20 years a considerable body of experimental results has accumulated to show that this principle is applicable to a number of different excitable tissues. Shortly after the Na theory was established, Fatt and Katz (1953) found that this general principle has to be modified slightly in some excitable tissue such as crustacean muscle fibers. In those tissues the action potential is produced by an initial permeability increase for Ca ions instead of Na ions, followed by the K permeability increase. Such action potentials are referred to as Ca spikes and the membrane mechanism responsible for the Ca permeability increase as the Ca channel. The classical action potential, by contrast, should then be called the Na spike (Hagiwara, 1973, 1975).

Hoyle and Smyth (1963) described a giant muscle fiber system in the barnacle Balanus nubilus. The muscle fibers are up to 2 mm diameter and are very convenient for applying various complicated electrophysiological techniques. Our earlier work on the Ca spike was performed mainly with this preparation. The top two records of Fig. 1 show Ca spikes of the same barnacle muscle fiber obtained before and after replacing the external Na ions with impermeant Tris ions. Under this condition any Na spike should disappear; however, the action potential remains virtually unchanged. A slight increase of the resting potential suggests that the resting Na permeability is not negligible. In contrast, changes in the external Ca concentration results in changes in the action potential, which increased in amplitude as the Ca concentration was gradually increased from 20 mM to 338 mM as seen in the middle five records. At the bottom of the figure the membrane potential at the peak of the spike is plotted against the logarithm of the Ca concentration. When the

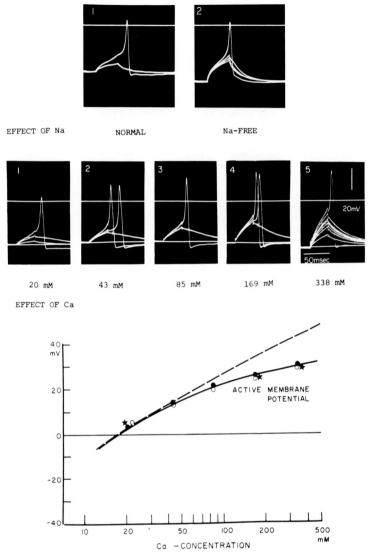

Fig. 1. Action potentials of a barnacle muscle fiber. Top, effect of removal of external Na. Middle, effect of the external Ca concentration. The lower traces are the recorded intracellular potentials; the horizontal line is the reference potential level. Bottom, relationship between the membrane potential at the peak of the action potential and the external Ca concentration. Different symbols represent data obtained from different fibers. The broken line indicates the Nernst slope of a Ca electrode. (Hagiwara and Naka, 1964).

Ca concentration is close to its normal value (20 mM in the barnacle saline), the rate of increase is 29 mV for a tenfold increase in the concentration. This slope would be expected from the Nernst equation for a Ca electrode and is illustrated by a broken line (Hagiwara and Naka, 1964). As the concentration increases the rate becomes smaller; in other words, the relation tends to saturate. A similar saturation phenomenon, which is not usually seen for the Na spike, is often found for Ca spikes in a variety of preparations.

The properties of the Na, Ca, and K channels responsible for the Na and Ca spikes differ in several aspects. In fact, these differences provide the basis for the belief that they correspond to different molecular structures of the membrane. The term channel does not necessarily mean that its structure in the membrane is actually channel-like. The Na, Ca, and K channels are distinguished in the following three major aspects.

KINETICS OF Na, Ca, AND K CURRENTS

A depolarization causes an increase of the Na conductance which is always followed by an inactivation even during a maintained depolarization. In other words, the Na conductance follows m^3h kinetics in the Na theory (Hodgkin and Huxley, 1952). In contrast, the K conductance shows no inactivation and it follows n^4 kinetics. Figure 2A shows membrane currents obtained during voltage clamp of a barnacle muscle fiber. In this preparation the inward current is carried by Ca ions (Hagiwara, Hayashi, and Takahashi, 1969; Hagiwara, Fukuda, and Eaton, 1974). The K current was reduced by adding tetra-ethylammonium (TEA) to the external solution. The number preceding each pair of traces indicates the membrane potential during the voltage clamp. In each record, current traces were obtained before and after replacement of the external Ca. The difference between the paired traces roughly represents the inward Ca current. These records show that the Ca permeability increase is not very fast compared with the increase in the K permeability. Therefore, at relatively positive membrane potentials the K current has already become significant by the time the Ca current reaches its peak value. In Fig. 2B the peak amplitude of the net inward current is plotted against the membrane potential with filled circles while the peak amplitude of the actual inward Ca current obtained as a difference between the two paired traces is plotted with open circles. They deviate significantly as the membrane potential becomes more positive.

Two points emerge from these results. First, the activation of the Ca channel is always faster than that of the K channel; but it seems to be slower when compared with that of the Na channel. This is always the case when the membrane of the same cell includes both Ca and Na channels. The second point is that the inactivation of the Ca current is not very clear or is at least very slow. Therefore, the kinetics of the Ca channel may represent an intermediate position between those of the Na and K channels.

PHARMACOLOGY

Different channels show different sensitivities to various pharmacological agents. The most remarkable one is tetrodotoxin (TTX) (Narahashi, Moore, and Scott, 1964), which blocks the Na channel at 10–15 nM concentration. However, no effect is seen in the Ca or K channels, even when the concentration is raised by a factor of 1,000 (Hagiwara and Nakajima, 1966). Tetraethylammonium blocks only the K channel. D-600 blocks the Ca channel but not the Na and K channels at relatively low concentration. Polyvalent cations such as La, Co, Mn, Ni, and Mg block the Ca channel at relatively low concentration by competitively occupying the Ca site of the Ca channel. The order of effectiveness of blocking is La > Co > Mn > Ni ≫ Mg. For example, the concentration necessary to reduce the maximum Ca current of a barnacle muscle fiber to one half, when the external Ca concentration is 40 mM, is only 330 μM for La. In order to obtain the same effect 5–15 mM is necessary for Co, Mn, and Ni, and 150 mM for Mg (Hagiwara and Takahashi, 1967a).

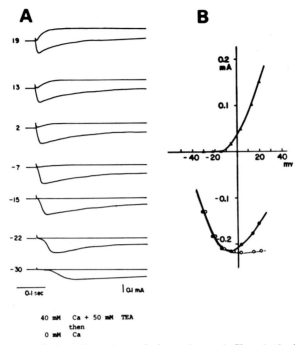

Fig. 2. Membrane current during voltage clamp of a barnacle muscle fiber. A, the fiber was first in a solution containing 40 mM Ca, 100 mM Mg, and 50 mM TEA and then all of the CaCl$_2$ was removed from the solution by replacement with an isomolar amount of NaCl. Paired traces were obtained with (bottom trace) and without Ca (top trace) at the same membrane potential. The number preceding each current record is the membrane potential during the voltage pulse (mV). B, the peak amplitude of the inward current in the bottom trace (filled circles), the maximum amplitude of the outward current in the top trace (filled triangles), and the maximum difference between currents of the paired traces (open circles) are plotted against the membrane potential. (Hagiwara, Fukuda, and Eaton, 1974.)

ION SELECTIVITIES

The most important difference between the channels is in their ion selectivity. It is obvious that the Na channel is permeable to Na ions and the K channel is permeable to K ions. The permeability of either channel to other alkali cations is not zero. Figure 3 shows the selectivity of the Na and K channels in terms of permeability ratios determined from the zero current potential. The X axis is the crystal diameter of the ion. For the Na channel P_{Na} was taken as unity and for the K channel P_K was taken as unity. Continuous lines show the data obtained with frog Ranvier node (Hille, 1972, 1973). Broken lines show the data obtained with a squid giant axon (Chandler and Meves, 1965; Hagiwara, Eaton, Stuart, and Rosenthal, 1972). The Na channel is permeable to Li but not much to K, Rb, Cs. Tl and NH$_4$ are not alkali cations but their ionic diameters are similar, and are moderately permeant in the Na channel. For the K channel, Tl is more permeant than K. An important conclusion one can deduce from the data is that the selectivities of both the Na and K channels are similar for the frog and squid axon. This suggests that the Na or K channels have unique molecular structures regardless of the species of animal.

The Ca permeability of the Na channel of the squid axon is not zero but P_{Ca}/P_{Na} estimated by Baker, Hodgkin, and Ridgway (1971) is less than 1:100. In other words, the permeability to divalent cations is very small. On the other hand, the Ca channel is

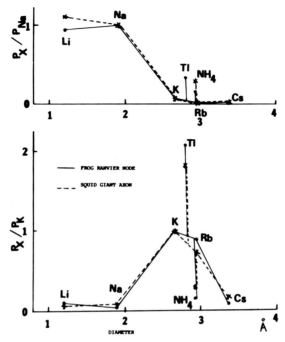

Fig. 3. Ionic selectivity of the Na and K channels in terms of permeability ratios among monovalent cations. Detailed explanation is in the text.

permeable to divalent cations while permeabilities to monovalent cations are negligible. Table I lists divalent cations together with their crystal diameter. It is very difficult to determine the reversal potential for the current of the Ca channel accurately since the internal Ca ion concentration is extremely low. One can therefore compare only the maximum membrane current. The sequence determined by the membrane current differs not only among different preparations but also within the same preparation if other conditions are different (Hagiwara, Fukuda, and Eaton, 1974). It is, however, always true that large cations such as Ca, Sr, and Ba are significantly permeant, whereas small cations such as Mg, Ni, and Co are impermeant. One of the intermediate-sized cations, Mn, shows small but significant permeability in the Ca channel. Figure 4 shows currents of the Ca channel of the membrane in a starfish egg cell obtained in 50 mM $CaCl_2$, $MnCl_2$, $CoCl_2$ and $NiCl_2$, respectively. NaCl in the external artificial sea water had been replaced with sucrose. Mn shows a small but significant inward current, whereas there is no sign of an inward current for Co and Ni.

CHANNELS IN THE EGG CELL MEMBRANE OF A TUNICATE

Both Na and Ca spikes are found in a variety of tissues of vertebrates as well as invertebrates. Na spikes are seen in the axons of annelids such as earthworm, leech, myxicola; mollusks such as squid; and arthropods, protochordates, and vertebrates. Ca spikes are also found in other tissues, in all of those animals. Although Ca spikes are found in Paramecia, so far there is no evidence of a Na spike in Protozoa. It seems interesting to ask how the Na and Ca channels appear either during evolution or during development. Of course, experiments of evolution are difficult, but one can carry out experiments during developmental differentiation. Recently, egg cell membranes have been

TABLE I. The Permeability of the Ca Channel

Ion species	Ionic diameter	Permeability
Mg	1.30	−
Ni	1.40	−
Co	1.44	−
Mn	1.60	+
Ca	1.98	++
Sr	2.26	++
Ba	2.70	++

Ionic diameters are from Electrolyte Solutions by R. A. Robinson and R. H. Stokes. London: Butterworth, 1959.

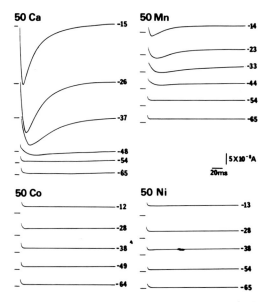

Fig. 4. Comparison of inward membrane currents of a starfish egg cell in Ca, Mn, Co, and Ni media. Membrane potential was clamped from the holding potential of −75 mV to the potential listed for each current recording (mV). The external solution contained 50 mM of either Ca, Mn, Co, or Ni, and no Na. The osmolarity was adjusted by adding sucrose.

found to be electrically excitable in some animals. Both mature unfertilized eggs and fertilized eggs of a tunicate, Halocynthia, show action potentials (Miyazaki, Takahashi and Tsuda, 1972, 1974). In Fig. 5A, the middle record shows a regenerative response in a saline containing 100 mM Ca and 315 mM Na (Miyazaki et al., 1972). There are two steps in the rising phase of the response; step 1 occurs at −45 mV and step 2 at 0 mV (see arrows). Step 1 disappears when Na is removed from the external saline (Fig. 5A). The potential change initiated at step 2 is enhanced when the external Ca concentration is increased (Fig. 5B). Thus the action potential of the tunicate egg cell is considered to have both Na- and Ca-dependent components that show different membrane potential dependencies.

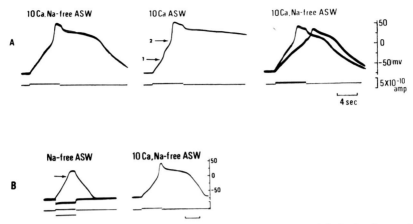

Fig. 5. A, regenerative responses of the tunicate unfertilized egg at 100 mM Ca in the absence (right and left traces) and the presence (middle trace) of Na ions. Ten Ca indicates that the Ca concentration is 10 times that of normal sea water (10 mM). Ten Ca ASW contains 100 mM Ca and 315 mM Na. Note 2 inflections in the rising phase of the response (arrows 1 and 2) in 10 Ca ASW. B, the potential change initiated at step 2 is augmented by the increase of the Ca concentration. Tunicate embryo at 2-cell stage. (Miyazaki, Takahashi, and Tsuda, 1972).

Properties of the membrane currents of the Na and Ca channels of the tunicate egg have been analyzed by using the voltage clamp technique (Okamoto, Takahashi, and Yoshii 1976a, b). Figure 6 shows membrane currents under voltage clamp. Depolarizing steps from a holding membrane potential of -90 mV induce transient inward currents and the results indicate that the current shows an activation and inactivation just as the Na inward current does in various adult excitable tissues (Hodgkin and Huxley, 1952). The time course of the inward current becomes faster as the membrane potential becomes more positive. At a membrane potential of $+15.5$ mV, a step(arrow in Fig. 6A) appears during the decay of the inward current suggesting that another slow component of the in-ward current emerges at this membrane potential. Slow, small components of the inward current is isolated from the major component by holding the membrane potential at -15 mV (Fig. 6B). The major component is inactivated entirely at -15 mV. Thus, Okamoto, Takahashi, and Yoshii (1976a) recorded two types of inward currents by select-ing holding potentials of either -90 mV or -15 mV. Figures 7A and C are current-voltage relations at the peaks of the major component obtained with -90 mV and those of the minor component at -15 mV respectively. The major component becomes significant at -55 mV and maximum amplitude is reached at -25 mV. The amplitude of the maximum inward current is linearly related to the external Na concentration (Fig. 7B). On the other hand, the minor component appears at -10 mV and the relation between the amplitude of the inward current and the external Ca concentration shows a saturation (Fig. 7D). The minor component remains unaltered upon removal of the Na ions from the external saline. Thus, the action potential of the tunicate egg cell membrane is shown to have two inward current mechanisms with different membrane potential dependencies.

Okamoto et al. (1976a) compared the property of the major component with that of the Na channel in adult excitable tissues. As already mentioned, the Na conductance of the squid axon shows m^3h kinetics (Hodgkin and Huxley, 1952). The current of the major components shows m^2h kinetics and the kinetic parameters depend on the mem-brane potential in a way similar to those obtained for the squid axon membrane. The

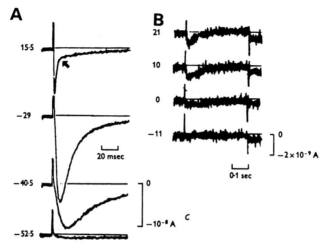

Fig. 6. Inward currents of the tunicate egg cell membrane during voltage clamp obtained under different holding potentials: −90 mV in A and −15 mV in B. Note current and time scales are different in A and B. An arrow in A indicates a step suggesting minor component of the inward current which is demonstrated in B. (Okamoto, Takahashi, and Yoshii, 1976a).

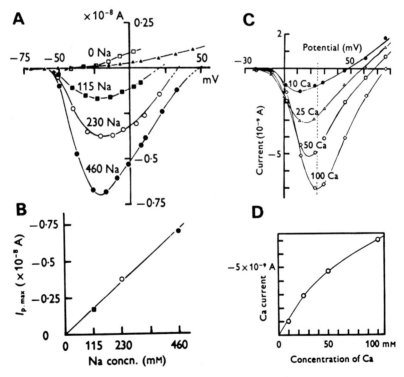

Fig. 7. A and C, current-voltage relations at the peak of the inward current of the tunicate egg cell membrane at various Na or Ca concentrations. Holding potential is −90 mV in A and −15 mV in B, C, and D. Relations between inward currents and Na or Ca concentrations: in B, current was measured at its maximum amplitude; in D, the current was plotted at membrane potential of +25 mV (dotted line in C). (Okamoto, Takahashi, and Yoshii, 1976 a, b.)

permeability ratios among alkali cations are $P_{Li} \geqslant P_{Na}(1.0) > P_k(0.088) > P_{Rb}(0.045) > P_{Cs}(0.027)$. These ratios are very similar to those obtained in adult excitable tissues (Fig. 3A). Therefore, the channel can be considered as Na channel from the criteria of its kinetics and ion selectivity. One of the pharmacological criteria, that is, the TTX sensitivity, is lacking for this channel of the tunicate egg. TTX-resistant Na channels have also been reported in embryonic chicken heart muscle (Sperelakis and Lehmkuhl, 1965; Shigenobu and Sperelakis, 1971), in myotubes formed by fusion of rat myoblasts in tissue culture (Kidokoro, 1973, 1975), in denervated rat skeletal muscle (Redfern, Lund and Thesleff 1970; and in puffer fish tissues (Hagiwara and Takahashi, 1967b; Kidokoro, Grinnell, and Eaton, 1974).

The properties of the minor component of the inward current in the tunicate egg membrane are very similar to those of the current of the usual Ca channels in adult tissues such as crustacean muscle fibers. Sr and Ba can also carry the current (Okamoto et al., 1976b). The inward current is blocked by La and Co very effectively and by Mg less effectively. The tunicate egg cell offers an excellent opportunity to anlyze the kinetics of the current of the Ca channel since there are no significant membrane invaginations that may disturb the space clamp and since the outward K current is very small. Okamoto et al. (1976b) suggests *mh* kinetics for the Ca current and the analysis indicates a definite inactivation for the current of the Ca channel.

Baker, Hodgkin, and Ridgway (1971) showed that a small amount of Ca ions also go through the Na channel. This is found to be the case in the Na channel of the tunicate egg. It is interesting to note that the selectivity among Ca, Sr, and Ba in the Na channel seems to be different from that in the Ca channel. The permeability of Sr and of Ba is substantially smaller than that of Ca in the Na channel of the tunicate egg.

CHANNELS IN THE EGG CELL MEMBRANE IN ECHINODERMS

All-or-none action potentials have been demonstrated in the eggs of the starfishes, Asterina pectinifera (Miyazaki, Ohmori, and Sasaki, 1975) and Patiria miniata (Shen and Steinhardt, 1976). The action potential is both Ca- and Na-dependent with threshold membrane potential ranging from −60 to −50 mV. Two different inward current mechanisms are demonstrated in a giant egg (about 1 mm diameter) of a starfish, Mediaster aequalis, using voltage clamp technique (Hagiwara, Ozawa, and Sand, 1975). Figure 8A illustrates the current-voltage relations at the peak of the inward current. Curve I was obtained in normal sea water. Two peaks and two regions of negative slope indicate that the membrane has two kinds of channels differing in membrane potential dependence. Channel I is activated at −50 to −56 mV and channel II at −7 to −6 mV. Curve II was recorded after the removal of external Na, and curve III is the difference between curves I and II. The thick, continuous curve in Fig. 8A represents the peak inward current through channel II obtained after the current of channel I had been inactivated by holding the membrane potential at −45 mV. Open and filled circles were obtained before and after Na removal, respectively. This indicates that channel II is not permeable to Na ions. Data indicated the properties of channel II resemble in every respect those of the ordinary Ca channel (Hagiwara et al., 1975).

Channel I is both Na- and Ca-dependent as shown by inward current vs Na or Ca concentration relationships (Fig. 8B and C). However, its properties differ from those of the typical Ca or Na channels. 1) Ca carries more current than Na in channel I and this is very different from the property of the Na channel. 2) The Na component of the inward current as represented by curve III of Fig. 8A is linearly proportional to the external Na

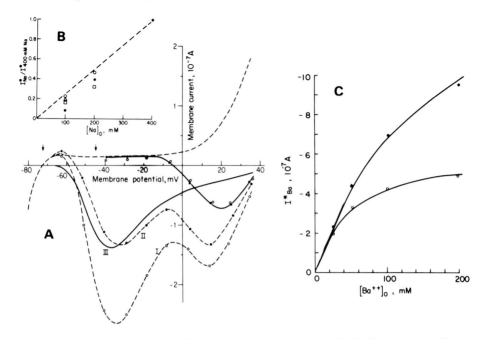

Fig. 8. A, current-voltage relations in the egg cell membrane of the starfish Mediaster aequalis. See text for explanations of each curve. B, relative amplitude of the peak Na current through channel I at varying Na concentration normalized to the value at 400 mM. C, relations between the peak inward current and the Ba concentration. Filled and open circles are for inward currents of channel I at −20 mV and of channel II at +25 mV, respectively. (Hagiwara, Ozawa, and Sand, 1975).

concentration (Fig. 8B), but it is dependent also on the external Ca concentration. The Na current is not detected when the external Ca concentration is less than 5 mM. 3) No selectivity is found among Li, Na, Rb, and Cs, and this is not the case in the ordinary Na channel. 4) Currents of channel I increase with increasing concentration of either Ca, Ba, or Sr (Fig. 8C), and Co^{++} blocks the inward current carried by divalent cations. The current of channel I is completely blocked by 7.3 mM procaine, which does not block the usual Ca channels at this concentration. Thus, channel I differs from the Na and Ca channels both so far reported.

Action potentials have been observed in egg cells of other echinoderms, sea urchins, Strongylocentrotus purpuratus (Jaffe, 1976) and Lytechinus variegatus (Jaffe, unpublished) and sea cucumber, Cucumaria miniata (Hagiwara, Ozawa, and Miyazaki, unpublished). Thus, most echinodern egg cells seem to show action potentials.

EGG CELLS OF OTHER ANIMALS

Action potentials are found in unfertilized mammalian eggs. Takahashi, Okamoto, and Yamashita (personal communication) recorded Ca spikes in rat oocytes and then analyzed them with voltage clamp technique. They could not detect any component of a Na spike. Recently, we examined unfertilized eggs as well as fertilized eggs up to the stage of syncytial blastoderm in Drosophila melanogaster (Miyazaki and Hagiwara, 1976). The Drosophila egg membrane shows no sign of excitability even when the external Ca concentration is raised 10 times.

BIOLOGICAL INTERESTS OF EGG CELL ACTION POTENTIALS

It is interesting to examine how the Na or Ca channel appears during development. The tunicate embryo is a typical mosaic one and blastomeres destined to be muscle cells are determined at the early gastrula stage. The presumptive muscle cells remain large until the striated muscle stage of a tadpole type of larva. Therefore, the preparation offers an opportunity to trace the electrical properties of the membrane throughout the development from egg cell to differentiated muscle cells. The differentiated muscle fiber shows a pure Ca spike (Miyazaki et al., 1972). Since both Na and Ca channels were observed in embryonic cells at all stages, it seems reasonable to postulate that both Na and Ca channels already exist at the very early stage and that differentiation of excitable tissues is characterized by selective elimination of one of the channel types. Is this idea applicable to other kinds of embryos? Unfortunately, there are very few embryos that enable us to trace electrical properties from the egg cell to the differentiated stages. Kidokoro (1973, 1975) found a Na- and Ca-dependent action potential in rat clonal myotubes. Since differentiated muscle of the rat shows pure Na spikes, this work may support the above idea. The Na channel is lacking in rat oocytes and no excitability is found in the gg of Drosophila. Since adult tissues of rat as well as Drosophila have both Na and Ca channels they have to be created during the developmental differentiation. Spitzer and Baccaglini (1976) have shown that the Rohon Beard cell of Xenopus tadpole has a Ca-dependent action potential at an early stage, the action potential becoming both Ca- and Na-dependent at a later stage. Eventually, the Ca channel is eliminated and only the Na channel remains at an even later stage. This suggests that both elimination and creation of channels may occur during differentiation.

ACKNOWLEDGMENTS

The authors wish to express their thanks to Dr. R. Kado for his advice during the preparation of the manuscript. The work was aided by USPHS Grant NS 09012 to Dr. S. Hagiwara.

REFERENCES

Baker, P. F., Hodgkin, A. L., and Ridgway, E. B. (1971). Depolarization and calcium entry in squid giant axons. J. Physiol. 218:709–755.

Chandler, W. K., and Meves, H. (1965). Voltage clamp experiments on internally perfused giant axons. J. Physiol. 180:788–820.

Fatt, P., and Katz, B. (1953). The electrical properties of crustacean muscle fibers. J. Physiol. 120:171–204.

Hagiwara, S. (1973). Ca spike. In: "Advances in Biophysics," Vol. 4, M. Kotani, ed., Tokyo: University of Tokyo Press, pp. 71–102.

Hagiwara, S. (1975). Ca-dependent action potential. In "Membranes," Series of Advances Vol. 3, G. Eisenman, ed., pp. 359–381, Marcel Dekker Inc., New York.

Hagiwara, S., Eaton, D. C., Stuart, A. E., and Rosenthal, N. P. (1972). Cation selectivity of the resting membrane of squid axon. J. Memb. Biol. 9:373–384.

Hagiwara, S., Fukuda, J., and Eaton, D. C. (1974). Membrane currents carried by Ca, Sr and Ba in barnacle muscle fiber during voltage clamp. J. Gen. Physiol. 63:564–578.

Hagiwara, S., Hayashi, H., and Takahashi, K. (1969). Calcium and potassium currents of the membrane of a barnacle muscle fibre in relation to the calcium spike. J. Physiol. 205:115–129.

Hagiwara, S., and Naka, K. (1964). The initiation of spike potential in barnacle muscle fibers under low internal Ca^{++}. J. Gen. Physiol. 48:141–162.

Hagiwara, S., and Nakajima, S. (1966). Differences in Na and Ca spikes as examined by application of tetrodotoxin, procaine and manganese ions. J. Gen. Physiol. 49:793–806.

Hagiwara, S., Ozawa, S., and Sand, O. (1975). Voltage clamp analysis of two inward current mechanisms in the egg cell membrane of a starfish. J. Gen. Physiol. 65:617–644.

Hagiwara, S., and Takahashi, K. (1967a). Surface density of calcium ions and Ca spikes in the barnacle muscle fiber membrane. J. Gen. Physiol. 50:583–601.

Hagiwara, S., and Takahashi, K. (1967b). Resting and spike potentials of skeletal muscle fiber of salt water elasmobranch and teleost fish. J. Physiol. 190:499–518.

Hille, B. (1972). The permeability of the sodium channel to metal cations in myelinated nerve. J. Gen. Physiol. 59:637–658.

Hille, B. (1973). Potassium channels in myelinated nerve. Selective permeability to small cations. J. Gen. Physiol. 61:669–686.

Hodgkin, A. L., and Huxley, A. F. (1952). A quantitative description of membrane currents and its application to conduction and excitation in nerve. J. Physiol. 117:500–544.

Hoyle, G., and Smyth, T., Jr. (1963). Neuromuscular physiology of giant muscle fibres of a barnacle, Balanus nubilus Darwin. Comp. Biochem. Physiol. 10:291–314.

Jaffe, L. A. (1976). Fast block to polyspermy in sea urchin eggs is electrically mediated. Nature 261:68–71.

Kidokoro, Y. (1973). Development of action potentials in a clonal rat skeletal muscle cell line. Nature New Biol. 241:158–159.

Kidokoro, Y. (1975). Sodium and calcium components of the action potential in a developing skeletal muscle cell line. J. Physiol. 244:145–159.

Kidokoro, Y., Grinnell, A. D., and Eaton, D. C. (1974). Tetrodotoxin sensitivity of muscle action potentials in puffer fishes and related fishes. J. Comp. Physiol. 89:59–72.

Miyazaki, S., and Hagiwara, S. (1976). Electrical properties of the Drosophila egg membrane. Develop. Biol. 53:91–100.

Miyazaki, S., Ohmori, H., and Sasaki, S. (1975). Action potential and non-linear current-voltage relation in starfish oocytes. J. Physiol. 246:37–54.

Miyazaki, S., Takahashi, K., and Tsuda, K. (1972). Calcium and sodium contributions to regenerative responses in the embryonic excitable cell membrane. Science 176:1441–1443.

Miyazaki, S., Takahashi, K., and Tsuda, K. (1974). Electrical excitability in the egg cell membrane of the tunicate. J. Physiol. 238:37–54.

Narahashi, T., Moore, J. W., and Scott, W. R. (1964). Tetrodotoxin blockage of sodium conductance increase in lobster giant axons. J. Gen. Physiol. 47:965–974.

Okamoto, H., Takahashi, K., and Yoshii, M. (1976a). Membrane currents of the tunicate egg under the voltage-clamp condition. J. Physiol. 254:607–638.

Okamoto, H., Takahashi, K., and Yoshii, M. (1976b). Two components of the calcium current in the egg cell membrane of the tunicate. J. Physiol. 255:527–561.

Redfern, P., Lund, H., and Thesleff, S. (1970). Tetrodotoxin resistant action potentials in denervated rat skeletal muscle. Eur. J. Pharmacol. 11:263–265.

Shen, S., and Steinhardt, R. A. (1976). An electrophysiological study of the membrane properties of the immature and mature oocyte of the batstar, Patiria miniata. Develop. Biol. 48:148–162.

Shigenobu, K., and Sperelakis, N. (1971). Development of sensitivity to tetrodotoxin of chick embryonic hearts with age. J. Molec. Cell. Cardiol. 3:271–286.

Sperelakis, N., and Lehmkuhl, D. (1965). Insensitivity of cultured chick heart cells to autonomic agents and tetrodotoxin. Am. J. Physiol. 209:693–698.

Spitzer, N. C., and Baccaglini, P. I. (1976). Development of action potential in embryonic amphibian neurones in vivo. Brain Research 107:610–616.

Lectin Activity in Embryonic Chick Muscle: Developmental Regulation and Preliminary Purification

T. P. Nowak and S. H. Barondes

Department of Psychiatry, University of California, San Diego, School of Medicine, La Jolla, California 92093

Soluble extracts of embryonic chick pectoral muscle contain lectin activity. This activity is assayed by agglutination of trypsin-treated, glutaraldehyde-fixed rabbit erythrocytes, and is blocked by specific saccharides such as thiodigalactoside and lactose. Lectin activity of the muscle extracts increased at least 1 order of magnitude between 8 and 16 days of chick embryo development, as the pectoral muscle differentiated. Preliminary purification was achieved by affinity chromatography on Sepharose 4B derivatized with either asialo-bovine glycoprotein, or p-aminophenyl β-D-thiogalactopyranoside as the ligand.

Key words: embryonic chick pectoral muscle, agglutination, thiodigalactoside, affinity chromatography, developmentally regulated lectins

INTRODUCTION

Developmentally regulated lectins (multivalent, carbohydrate-binding proteins assayed as cell agglutinins) have been identified in cellular slime molds as they differentiate to a cohesive form. These lectins are detectable on the surface of cohesive cells and appear to mediate species-specific cell recognition in slime molds by interaction with species-specific cell surface oligosaccharides (reviewed in 1 and 2).

Recently, Teichberg et al. (3) reported that a number of tissues, including electric organ of Electrophorus and skeletal muscle, contain lectin activity. This raised the possibility that lectins from these tissues have some functional similarity to those in slime molds. In the present report we describe results of two types of studies designed to determine the nature and biological function of lectin activity from embryonic chick pectoral muscle. We found that: 1) lectin activity of chick pectoral muscle extracts is developmentally regulated, increasing at least 1 order of magnitude between 8 and 16 days of chick embryo development as the pectoral muscle differentiates; and 2) the lectin activity can be purified by affinity chromatography on derivatized Sepharose 4B with either asialo-bovine glycoprotein or p-aminophenyl β-D-thiogalactopyranoside as the ligand.

MATERIALS AND METHODS

Fertilized White Leghorn chicken eggs were incubated under standard conditions (4). At any given day of development, embryo morphology agreed fairly closely with that described by Hamburger and Hamilton (4). Retarded or defective embryos were discarded. Agglutinins from embryonic pectoral muscle were extracted with 9 vol of 0.1 M NaCl,

© 1977 Alan R. Liss, Inc., 150 Fifth Avenue, New York, NY 10011

2 mM EDTA, 2 mM dithiothreitol titrated to pH 9.1 with NaOH (this mixture is hereafter called DES) containing 0.3 M lactose. The yield of agglutinin was lower if extracts were prepared in DES without lactose. The extracts were sedimented at 100,000 $\times$ g for 1 hr and the supernatant was dialyzed exhaustively against DES for assay of agglutination activity.

Rabbit erythrocytes for agglutination assays were prepared from 50 ml of fresh rabbit blood (collected in Alsever's medium) that had been washed 4 times with 5 vol of 0.15 M NaCl. A 4% erythrocyte suspension (by vol) in 0.1 M Na phosphate, pH 7.4, 0.05 M NaCl containing 1 mg/ml of crystallized trypsin (Calbiochem, Grade A) was incubated at 37°C for 1 hr. The trypsin-treated cells were then washed 4 times with 5 vol of 0.15 M NaCl and fixed in 5 vol 0.075 M NaK phosphate, pH 7.2, 0.075 M NaCl (hereafter called PBS) containing 1% glutaraldehyde for 1 hr at room temperature. Glutaraldehyde fixation was terminated by addition of 5 vol of 0.1 M glycine in PBS at 4°. The fixed erythrocytes were centrifuged, then washed twice in 5 vol of 0.1 M glycine in PBS and then twice in PBS. The cells were then stored as a 10% suspension in PBS. Fresh rabbit erythrocytes were not agglutinated by the extracts. After trypsinization, the cells were agglutinable but could not be kept for long periods of time. With glutaraldehyde fixation the cells could be maintained as stable reagents which could be used for periods of up to 1 month without significant loss in activity. However, there was considerable variation in the agglutinability of different batches of glutaraldehyde-treated trypsinized rabbit erythrocytes. Therefore, in each of the developmental studies shown, all the extracts were assayed against an identical preparation of fixed erythrocytes.

Agglutination assays were done in microtiter V plates (Cooke Engineering) using serial 2-fold dilutions of the extract in DES. Each well contained 0.025 ml of a 4% suspension of glutaraldehyde-fixed, trypsin-treated rabbit erythrocytes in PBS, 0.025 ml of a dilution of the dialyzed extract, 0.025 ml of 0.15 M NaCl and 0.025 ml of 1% bovine serum albumin in 0.15 NaCl. The fixed erythrocytes were added last after which the plates were shaken vigorously for 1 min. Agglutination was determined after 90 min. Unagglutinated erythrocytes formed a clear dot on the bottom of the well whereas agglutinated erythrocytes formed a diffuse mat on the bottom of the well. The transition from an agglutinate to a dot was distinct; i.e. from the end point dilution of extract that still agglutinated the cells, to the next dilution of extract. For sugar inhibition studies, the sugar in question was dissolved at the appropriate concentration in 0.15 M NaCl and added in place of the 0.15 M NaCl. The sugars used were obtained from commercial sources at the highest available level of purity. Protein was estimated by the method of Lowry et al., after dialysis of the extracts against 0.15 M NaCl.

Bovine $\alpha 1$ acid glycoprotein (hereafter called bovine glycoprotein), obtained from Miles, was desialated in 0.1 N H_2SO_4 for 1 hr at 80°. The acid was then neutralized and the glycoprotein was dialyzed against 0.1 M $NaHCO_3$ pH 9.1. The protein was coupled to Sepharose 4B that had been activated with cyanogen bromide (5) (5 mg glycoprotein per ml of Sepharose). p-amino phenyl β-D-thiogalactopyranoside (hereafter called APTG) was coupled to Sepharose 4B by the procedure of Steers et al. (6), using hexanediamine and succinic anyhydride as spacers and 1-ethyl-3-(3-dimethylaminopropyl) carbodiimide hydrochloride as the coupling agent. Affinity chromatography of crude muscle extracts on columns of these 2 types of derivatized Sepharose was performed by reacting the extract with the column, washing, then eluting with lactose as described in Fig. 2.

RESULTS

Developmentally Regulated Lectin in Pectoral Muscle Extracts

Extracts of embryonic chick muscle contained an agglutinin of glutaraldehyde-fixed, trypsin-treated rabbit erythrocytes. The agglutinin was not dialyzable and agglutination activity was completely destroyed by boiling for 10 min.

Agglutination activity of embryonic chick muscle extracts with titers as high as 1:2,048 was completely inhibited by addition of 0.15 M lactose to the agglutination assays. A number of other saccharides also inhibited the agglutination reaction (Table I). The spectrum of saccharides that were relatively potent inhibitors of agglutination activity of extracts from this tissue is quite similar to that observed by Teichberg et al. (3) with extracts from electric organ of Electrophorus. The finding that agglutination activity is inhibited by specific saccharides indicates that the agglutination reaction may be based on binding of a divalent or multivalent carbohydrate-binding protein (lectin) to complementary oligosaccharides on the surface of the test erythrocytes.

Agglutination activity of extracts from embryonic chick pectoral muscle showed a striking increase with maturation of the muscle up to about 16 days of development in ovo (Figs. 1A, 1B). Agglutination activity declined thereafter (Fig. 1A). Experiments with 2 different sets of extracts using 2 different preparations of glutaraldehyde-fixed, trypsin-treated rabbit erythrocytes are shown in Figs. 1A and 1B. In both experiments there was a marked increase in the specific activity of the agglutinin between 8 and 16 days of embryonic life. The major change occurred between days 10 and 12 (Fig. 1B). The results are expressed as the reciprocal of the titer divided by the milligrams protein per ml of the dialyzed extract; but similar curves were obtained when activity was expressed per gram (wet weight) of the muscle tissue used for extraction. With the erythrocyte preparation used for the experiments in Fig. 1A, the specific activity of the extracts from 16-day-old embryos was about 3,500, almost 2 orders of magnitude higher than the specific activity of extracts from the 8-day-old embryos concurrently prepared and concurrently assayed. With another preparation of erythrocytes and with another set of extracts, concurrently prepared, specific activity at 16 days of embryonic life was only about 300, about 1 order

TABLE I. Effect of Saccharides on Agglutination Activity of Extracts From 16-Day Chick Embryo Pectoral Muscle (6) (Reprinted with permission)

Saccharide	Concentration that inhibits 50% (mM)
thiodigalactoside (D-galactosyl-β-thiogalactoside)	0.19
lactose	0.19
α-methyl-D-galactoside	9.4
β-methyl-D-galactoside	37.5
D-galactose	37.5
melibiose	37.5
N-acetyl-D-galactosamine	75
L-fucose	75
D-fucose, D-trehalose, L-rhamnose, D-glucose, α-methyl-D-glucoside, β-methyl-D-glucoside N-acetyl-D-glucosamine, 3-0-methyl-D-glucoside, D-mannose, α-methyl-D-mannoside	>75

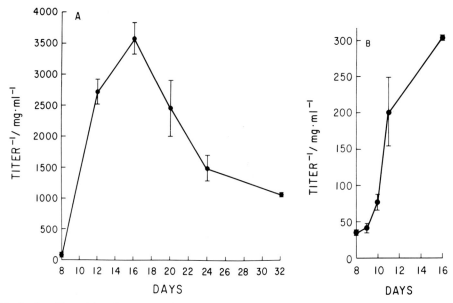

Fig. 1. Specific activity of agglutinin in extracts of pectoral muscle of chick embryos or chicks whose incubation had been begun at day 0. Each point is the mean (± SEM) of separate determinations made with 3 different extracts. About 16 embryos were used for each 8 day extract and smaller numbers giving approximately the same total weight of pectoral muscle were used for later time points. All extracts in (A) were prepared and assayed concurrently. A different batch of glutaraldehyde-fixed, trypsinized rabbit erythrocytes and a different set of extracts was used for the experiment in (B). These extracts were also prepared and assayed concurrently (7). Reprinted with permission.

of magnitude higher than the specific activity of extracts from 8-day-old embryos concurrently prepared and assayed (Fig. 1B). The differences between Fig. 1A and Fig. 1B are due to the erythrocytes, since we have assayed an extract from 16-day-old chick embryos using the erythrocytes used in Figs. 1A and 1B and found specific activities of around 3,500 with the former and around 300 with the latter. The difference in agglutinability of the erythrocytes may be due to special characteristics of the erythrocytes from the specific rabbit used in each case, or to slight variations in the trypsinization or the glutaraldehyde fixation conditions that are presently under investigation. Any of these variables could change the nature and the state of aggregation or aggregability of the saccharides on the erythrocyte cell surface with which the agglutinins presumably interact. In all these experiments agglutination could be completely blocked by lactose.

Preliminary Purification

Attempts to purify the lectin activity by affinity chromatography with columns of derivatized Sepharose have been fairly successful. When either asialo-bovine glycoprotein or APTG was coupled with Sepharose 4B, lectin activity bound to the column and could be eluted with lactose (Fig. 2). With both columns purification was more than 100 fold. However, the adsorptive capacity of both columns was fairly limited, although the APTG column as prepared bound about 10 times as much lectin activity per ml of derivatized Sepharose as the asialo-bovine glycoprotein column. With the APTG column shown in Fig. 2, only about 50% of the lectin activity was bound. Whereas marked reduction of the amount of lectin activity applied to the column reduces the percentage that is not adsorbed,

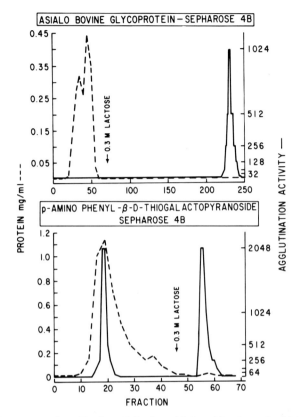

Fig. 2. Affinity chromatography of lectin activity from 16-day-old embryonic chick muscle. Sepharose 4B was derivatized with the indicated reagents, as described in the Materials and Method section and equilibrated with DES. A 500 ml column derivatized with asialo-bovine glycoprotein and a 35 ml column derivatized with APTG were used in these experiments. Extract containing 225 or 125 mg protein, respectively, was applied to the columns. Fraction volumes were 10 ml and 2 ml, respectively. Elution with 0.3 M lactose in DES was begun where indicated. Agglutination activity of fractions containing lactose was determined after dialysis.

our impression is that total adsorption is not possible with the APTG column. This raises the possibility of heterogeneity of the lectin activity in the extract.

Thus far, neither affinity column has provided sufficient material to permit characterization of the product. Further work is in progress.

DISCUSSION

The results indicate that embryonic chick pectoral muscle contains a developmentally regulated agglutinin that can be assayed with appropriate preparations of rabbit erythrocytes. Like the similar agglutinin from electric organ of Electrophorus, the agglutinin from embryonic chick muscle is inhibited by a specific group of saccharides and may therefore be classified as a lectin. The cell type in embryonic chick muscle that synthesizes this lectin is not presently known with certainty. We have previously shown that extracts of L-6 myoblasts contain a similar agglutinin (7). Since this is a clonal myogenic cell line, it seems likely that myoblasts in the chick pectoral muscles are synthesizing the agglutinin assayed in the present studies. However, it remains possible that the lectin activity is also present in fibroblasts and other cell types present in the embryonic chick pectoral muscle; and cellular localization of the lectin activity requires further study. It is also presently unclear how many lectins are actually present in the extract. Indeed, recent preliminary experiments (Mir and Barondes, unpublished observations) suggest that more than one lectin-like activity can be identified in these extracts. This finding may prove an important complication in attempts at purifying lectin activity from these extracts. Preliminary results with the APTG column suggest that the lectin activity that does not bind to the column is discriminable from the activity which does bind.

The biological function of the lectin activity observed here is not clear. Gartner and Podleski (8) have reported that fusion of L-6 myoblasts in culture can be inhibited by saccharides which react with this lectin activity but not by other saccharides. This raised the possibility that the lectin mediates cell fusion. However, Den et al. (9), using primary chick muscle cultures, failed to demonstrate inhibition of fusion by specific saccharides. Therefore, the possible role of the lectin activity in cell fusion remains to be determined.

Clarification of the biological role of the lectin activity is dependent on appropriate purification with which we have had some preliminary success. In principle, antibodies to purified lectin should permit determination of both cellular localization and its biological function, by analogy with similar studies with slime molds in which developmentally regulated lectins apparently mediate specific cell cohesion (1, 2). Affinity chromatography with an APTG column shows promise not only in lectin purification, but also in discriminating different lectin activities in the extract.

NOTE ADDED IN PROOF

We recently found that a column prepared from Sepharose 4B derivatized with p-aminophenyl lactoside has a high adsorptive for chick muscle lectin activity, and provides the best affinity chromatography material thus far tested for its satisfactory purification.

REFERENCES

1. Barondes, S. H., and Rosen, S. D., in "Neuronal Recognition." S. H. Barondes (Ed.). New York: Plenum Press, p. 331 (1976).
2. Barondes, S. H., in "The Nervous System." D. B. Tower (Ed.). vol. I. New York: Raven Press, p. 129 (1975).
3. Teichberg, V. I., Silman, I., Beutsch, D. D., and Resheff, G., Proc. Nat. Acad. Sci. 72:1383 (1975).
4. Hamburger, V., and Hamilton, H. L., J. Morphol. 88:49 (1951).
5. March, S. C., Parikh, I., and Cuatrecasas, P., Anal. Biochem. 60:149 (1974).
6. Steers, E., Jr., Cuatrecases, P., and Pollard, H. B., J. Biol. Chem. 246:196 (1971).
7. Nowak, T. P., Haywood, P. L., and Barondes, S. H., Biochem. Biophys. Res. Comm. 68:650 (1976).
8. Gartner, T. K., and Podleski, T. R., Biochem. Biophys. Res. Comm. 67:972 (1975).
9. Den, H., Malinzak, D. A., and Rosenberg, A., Biochem. Biophys. Res. Comm. 69:621 (1976).

Nerve and Glial-Specific Antigens on Cloned Neural Cell Lines

William B. Stallcup

Developmental Biology Laboratory, Salk Institute for Biological Studies, San Diego, California 92112

Antisera have been prepared which recognize specific surface antigens on a group of cloned cell lines from the rat central nervous system. Six cell lines judged to be neuronal express a common antigen N1. Four of these neurons also have the antigen N2, and 2 of them have a third antigen N3. Glial cells lack all of these antigens, but express either or both of 2 antigens G1 and G2 which are not found on the nerve cells. Muscle cells, like nerve cells, are excitable, yet the 2 muscle cell lines examined express none of the nerve-specific antigens; they do express the glial antigen G1. Two as yet unclassified cell lines judged to be excitable by the sodium uptake assay also lack the neuronal antigens but express the.second glial antigen G2. In addition there are at least 6 antigens or determinants which are shared in various combinations by nerve, muscle, glial, and fibroblastic cell lines.

Cell-specific surface components such as these could be involved in recognition patterns between various cells. Furthermore, these antigens may prove to be useful markers in mapping the lineage of cells in the developing nervous system. This is shown by absorption experiments which demonstrate the presence of the antigens in normal rat brain. N3 is present in the 10 day fetal brain, but disappears before birth. In contrast G2 appears only at the end of the second fetal week and persists into adulthood. Thus these 2 antigens appear to be present on different cell populations in the developing brain.

Key words: surface antigens, cloned cell lines, central nervous system, nerve cells, muscle cells, mapping the lineage of cells

INTRODUCTION

The successful use of antisera against cell-surface components to identify and manipulate various cell types in the immune system has inspired recent efforts to extend this immunological approach to the nervous system. Antisera against specific cell-surface markers would provide us with the means of mapping the lineage and fate of the many cell types in the nervous system. Moreover, we might be able to use these antisera to identify molecules that are involved in cell-cell recognition and pattern formation. Promising studies on antigens in normal brain [1—4], on a variety of brain-specific proteins and enzymes [5—13], and on the surface components of a growing number of neuroblastoma and glioma cell lines [14—21] have indicated that this immunological approach may indeed be a valuable one.

Abbreviations: γG = gamma globulin, BSS = balanced salt solution, NEU = nitrosoethylurea, (N) = neuronal, (G) = glial, (E) = excitable, (F) = fibroblast, (M) = muscle.

The establishment of a series of independently derived and cloned cell lines from the rat central nervous system [22] would appear to offer an excellent starting point for the production of a collection of antisera with a variety of specificities. Studies of morphology, transmitter synthesis, enzymatic make-up, and electrical properties show that this family of cells includes a range of cell types, including nerve, glial, and muscle cells. We have tried to demonstrate that antisera can be raised which are specific for these various classes of cells.

METHODS

Cell Lines

All cell lines were derived from the central nervous system of the BDIX rat (22), except as detailed in Table VI. They were cultured in Dulbecco's Modified Eagle's medium supplemented with 10% fetal calf serum.

By means of electrophysiology [22,34] and sodium uptake studies [23,24], these cells were previously classified as being excitable or nonexcitable. Throughout this article they are identified as being glial (G), neuronal (N), muscle (M), fibroblast (F), or excitable in the sodium uptake assay but not in electrophysiology (E). These electrical properties are also summarized in Table VI.

Antisera

For immunization, cell lines C6B(G) and B9(G) were chosen as examples of glial cells, while B35(N) and B103(N) were used as neuronal cells. Antisera were raised in New Zealand White rabbits by intradermal injection of whole cells in complete Freund's adjuvant on days 0 and 14 followed by intravenous injections of cell suspensions on days 28, 35, and 42. Per injection, 10^7 cells were given. In the case of B35(N) the adjuvant injections were omitted and were replaced by intravenous injections of cell suspensions. Rabbits were bled on days 31, 39, 45, and 48 and the resulting sera pooled and stored at $-20°$C. Gamma globulin fractions were prepared by first passing the serum through DEAE-Sephadex A50 equilibrated in PBS, followed by 2 precipitations of the eluate with 33% saturated ammonium sulfate.

Absorption of these gamma globulin fractions was carried out at room temperature by suspending 1 vol of packed washed cells in from 5 to 10 vol of the serum. After 30 min, the cells were removed by centrifugation, and the process was repeated until the desired level of specificity was attained.

Cytotoxic assays were performed in Falcon Microtest wells. One volume of trypsinized cell suspension was incubated at $37°$C with 1 vol of 30% guinea pig complement (Grand Island Biological Co.) and 1 vol of antiserum at the desired dilution. Lysed cells were detected after 1 hr by a conventional trypan blue exclusion test.

For radioimmune binding assays, goat antibody against rabbit gamma globulin (Cal Biochem) was absorbed with various rat cell lines to reduce background binding, and was then iodinated with ^{125}I (New England Nuclear) using a Chloramine T procedure (25). Cells were grown to confluency in monolayer cultures in Linbro 16 mm wells; 4 wells of each cell type were used, and pains were taken to assure that approximately the same degree of confluency was attained by each cell type at the time of assay. The growth medium was removed and replaced by 0.2 ml of BSS containing 2% fetal calf serum and the rabbit antiserum. Three different dosages of this antiserum were used plus 1 of normal rabbit serum for background; hence the 4 wells. After 30 min at room temperature these solutions were removed and the monolayers were carefully washed 3 times with the BSS + 2% fetal calf medium. The cells were then covered with 0.2 ml of the same medium containing 0.1 mg of the ^{125}I-labelled goat antiserum, allowed to incubate 30 min at room temperature, and washed 3 times with BSS. Finally, 1 ml of BSS was added to each well, and the cells were scraped off with a rubber policeman and centrifuged in small glass tubes. After the supernatants were removed, these tubes were counted in a gamma counter. Protein determinations [26] were also made on the cell pellets so that corrections could be made for variation in cell number. The final treatment of the data then consisted of subtracting the counts bound to cells incubated with the normal serum from the counts bound to corresponding cells incubated with the immune serum.

Absorption With Normal Tissue

In order to demonstrate the presence of antigens on normal brain tissue, we used a quantitative absorption technique much like that employed by Schachner et al [4]. The tissue was finely minced in BSS containing 1% fetal calf serum to retard proteolytic degradation and was then homogenized in the cold in a Dounce homogenizer fitted with a teflon pestle. This homogenate was centrifuged at 2,000 rpm for 5 min. The pellet was washed twice in the BSS fetal calf serum solution and resuspended in the same medium. One aliquot of this suspension was taken for protein determination, and several other aliquots of varying size were placed in small tubes and centrifuged. These latter pellets were resuspended in known amounts of the antiserum to be tested, and the absorptions carried out at room temperature. After 30 min the tissue was removed by centrifugation and the antisera were tested for reactivity with a cell line known to be positive for the antigen in question. The reactivity was compared to that of unabsorbed antiserum. For controls, the antiserum was also absorbed with a cell line known to be negative for the antigen. Thus, such factors as nonspecific absorption and dilution could be taken into account.

RESULTS

Our attempts to characterize the antisera by means of a cytotoxic assay were initially successful. All of the antisera had titers of about 1:200 for any of the cell lines, and after absorption with BDIX rat liver still retained titers of 1:20 or greater. As shown in Table I, however, upon absorption with various neural cell lines, the sera rapidly lost their cytoxicity. For example, after the 2 anti-glial sera anti-C6B(G) and anti-B9(G) were absorbed with B35(N), they still killed several types of glial cells at a 1:3 dilution; however, any attempts at further absorption [such as with B65(N)] removed the cytotoxic activity of the sera. Conversely, the anti-neuronal sera anti-B103(N) and anti-B35(N) could be absorbed with B9(G) but further absorption with C6B(G) left them inactive. It is well known that the complement-mediated cytotoxic activity of an antiserum can decrease sharply as the antiserum becomes more monospecific, particularly if the surface antigen it recognizes is present at low density.

In any case, since even these preliminary results looked promising in terms of distinguishing neuronal and glial cell lines, we sought a more sensitive system to increase the usefulness of the antisera. The radioimmune binding assay, using ^{125}I-labelled goat antibody to recognize rabbit gamma-globulin bound to the cells, appeared to be such a method. Use of the goat serum as the labelled component allowed us to prepare a single

TABLE I. Cytotoxic Activity of Antisera

Cell line	Anti-C6B(G) absorbed with B35(N)	Anti-B9(G) absorbed with B35(N)	Anti-B35(N) absorbed with B9(G)	Anti-B103(N) absorbed with B9(G)
C6B(G)	80%	75%	25%	30%
B9(G)	> 90%	> 90%	< 5%	< 5%
B49(G)	75%	75%	25%	40%
B90(G)	> 90%	80%	10%	10%
B65(N)	25%	35%	> 90%	> 90%
B35(N)	< 5%	< 5%	> 90%	> 90%
B50(N)	< 5%	< 5%	> 90%	> 90%
B103(N)	< 5%	< 5%	> 90%	> 90%
B104(N)	< 5%	< 5%	> 90%	> 90%

Values represent cytotoxic killing efficiency of the various antisera compared to controls without antiserum. See Methods section for details.

radioactive reagent for use with all the various sera. This assay also had the advantage of allowing us to examine cells in monolayer cultures, something we were unable to do effectively with the cytotoxic assay. Not only were we able to avoid the use of trypsin, but we could detect any antigens expressed by morphologically "differentiated" adherent cells.

A considerable amount of data is required to analyze the reactions of 4 separate antisera with this large group of cells. Summaries of the results obtained with each serum are presented in Tables II through V, and a complete summary of all the antigens is given in Table VI. We believe that it will be sufficient to present a small sample of the actual raw data for the anti-C6B(G) serum and show how this data is carried through to the final presentation in Tables II and VI. The principles of this analysis apply to all of the data presented.

Figure 1 illustrates the results of repeated absorption of the anti-C6B(G) anti-serum with the B103(N) cell line. After a single absorption, the antiserum retains a significant amount of reactivity with B103(N) cells. After 3 absorptions the binding to B103(N) has dropped to a low level, while binding to C6B(G) remains high. Three more absorptions with B103(N) do little if anything to alter this picture. Both the low reactivity toward B103(N) and the high binding to C6B(G) appear to have reached plateau levels. Thus we feel assured that C6B(G) expresses surface antigens not found on B103(N). This principle forms the basis for all of the absorptions presented in this paper. Absorptions with a given cell line are carried out until plateau levels of binding are attained for the key cell lines involved. Sometimes this results in complete loss of activity [for example if anti-C6B(G) is absorbed with B90(G), in which case we know that C6B(G) and B90(G) have identical surface antigens as defined by the anti-C6B(G) antiserum].

The small but persistent background binding to "unreactive" cells [for example, B103(N) in the case just discussed] limits our ability to detect small amounts of antigen. Cell lines having less than about 10% as much of a given antigen as the strongly reactive cell lines will be classified as unreactive. Thus, although our data show quantitative differences in antigen expression among the various cell lines, we are not able to draw conclusions of the all-or-none level. It should also be pointed out that detailed studies of the

TABLE II. Absorption of Anti-C6B(G)

Cells used for absorption	Unabsorbed antiserum → Serum 1 B103(N)	Serum 2 B65(N)	Serum 3 B65(N), B23(F)
Reactivities lost	S1	S1, S3	S1, S3, F1
Reactivities retained	S3, F1, G1	F1, G1	G1
Reactivity of cell lines (cpm per 10^5 cells)			
C6B(G)	7,000	4,000	2,700
B90(G)	8,500	4,100	2,300
B19(G)		7,900	2,900
B27(G)		2,200	1,600
B49(G)	6,050	5,400	4,225
B15(G)	3,650	3,700	3,050
B111(G)		7,500	5,875
RN2(G)	3,800	3,950	2,850
L6(M)	7,200	4,100	3,175
B44(M)	10,400	2,225	1,750
B28(G)	6,700	2,150	250
B92(G)	7,110	3,100	325
G26(G)	5,330	2,200	275
B23(F)	5,070	2,300	310
3T3(F)	3,200	1,525	225
B9(G)	6,400	320	325
B65(N)	4,700	450	330
B104(N)	3,150	400	300
B35(N)	3,020	380	290
B11(N)	2,900	350	310
B103(N)	400	360	290
B50(N)	510	420	315
B82(E)	450	460	325
B108(E)	325	330	275

This is essentially a flow sheet for the absorption of the C6B(G) antiserum. The data is derived from experiments described in the text and illustrated in Figs. 1 and 2. The chart shows that Serum 1 is derived from the unabsorbed antiserum through absorption with B103(N) cells (Figs. 1 and 2a), while Serum 2 is derived from unabsorbed antiserum through absorption with B65(N) cells (Fig. 2b). Serum 3 is then derived from Serum 2 by additional absorptions with B23(F) cells. The line labeled "cells used for absorption" presents the sum total of cell lines used to obtain a particular serum. For example, Serum 3 has been absorbed with both B65(N) and B23(F). The "Reactivities lost" category shows the sum of specificities which are lost in making a given serum. B103(N) absorbs out anti-S1 activity, while B65(N) absorbs out both anti-S1 and anti-S3 activities. Finally, in going from Serum 2 to Serum 3, B23(F) absorbs out anti-F1 activity, so that serum 3 lacks anti-S1, anti-S3, and anti-F1 activities. Likewise, the "Reactivities retained" list gives the specificities retained by the antiserum at each step. The "Reactivity of Cell Lines" is expressed in counts per min bound per 10^5 cells, these values having been derived as explained in the text. Values which seem to be significantly above background are given in boldface type to facilitate visual grouping of the cell lines. These reactive cell lines are indicated as being + in Table VI. Different batches of iodinated goat anti-rabbit gamma globulin were used in compiling Tables II–V, and differences in specific radioactivity of this reagent account for many of the differences in both background and significant binding seen in these Tables.

TABLE III. Absorption of Anti-B9(G)

	Unabsorbed antiserum			
	Serum 1	Serum 2	Serum 3	Serum 4
Cells used for absorption	B103(N)	B65(N)	B65(N) B90(G)	B65(N) B108(E)
Reactivities lost	S1	S1, S2	S1, S2, G1	S1, S2, G2
Reactivities retained	S2, G1, G2	G1, G2	G2	G1
Reactivity of cell lines (cpm per 10^5 cells)				
B9(G)	53,000	28,200	18,400	2,200
B108(E)	23,100	22,500	18,150	2,010
B82(E)	12,350		14,900	2,570
B92(G)	24,500		10,550	2,335
B28(G)	49,000		17,200	1,980
G26(G)			9,875	2,050
B49(G)	27,500	27,000	6,000	15,100
B19(G)	39,000		5,600	26,300
B27(G)	14,000		10,720	25,800
C6B(G)	37,200	20,250	2,950	24,100
B15(G)	35,600		2,290	25,000
B90(G)	34,700	21,900	2,100	20,750
B111(G)			2,210	21,830
RN2(G)	23,000	14,100	2,360	16,300
L6(M)	51,000		2,575	25,400
B44(M)	27,000	15,330	2,645	26,100
B23(F)	13,200	1,700	1,900	1,850
B65(N)	50,500	2,060	2,340	2,050
B11(N)	12,900	2,200	2,180	2,175
B103(N)	2,100	2,050	1,975	2,250
B104(N)	2,355	2,280	2,300	2,010
B50(N)	2,700	2,530	2,070	2,130
B35(N)	2,720	2,600	2,350	2,020
3T3(F)	2,250	2,550	2,200	1,950

Legend as in Table II.

dependence of antigen expression on culture conditions, growth time, etc., have yet to be made. Such factors could conceivably alter antigen levels on any of the cell lines tested.

The absorbed C6B(G) antiserum derived from Fig. 1 is now used to collect data on a number of cell lines as shown in Fig. 2. In order to reduce this information to more manageable form, the plateau binding value for each cell line is chosen to represent the reactivity of the antiserum toward these cell lines. These values are listed in the comprehensive data sheet for the anti-C6B(G) serum, namely Table II. Values significantly higher than background binding are listed in boldface type, and these cell lines are represented as being positive (+) for a particular antigen in Table VI, the comprehensive summary of all the antigens.

The sequential absorption of anti-C6B(G) defines 4 antigens: S1, S3, F1, and G1. Obviously, the order in which the absorptions are performed is very important. Different sequences can reveal different relationships between the cells, and therefore many combinations were tried. Only a few are presented here. In Table II for example, if we use B65(N) for the first absorption of anti-C6B(G), we find that this absorbed antiserum still contains anti-G1 and anti-F1 activity, but has lost activity towards a large group of cell lines expressing S1 and S3. However, if we initially absorb with B103(N) which removes only anti-S1 activity, we find that this large group can be divided into those cells which have only S1, and those which have both S1 and S3. Obviously, there may be other reactivities which remain to be revealed by using the appropriate absorption. The anti-F1 activity is revealed after absorptions with B23(F). This F1 antigen is so designated because of its presence on the 3T3(F) mouse fibroblast. It is also expressed by 3 (and possibly more) of the glial cell lines. This finding substantiates a previous report that C6B(G) shares an antigen or antigens with fibroblasts (19).

The anti-B9(G) antiserum (Table III) contains both anti-G1 and anti-G2 activities. These are separated by absorption with either a $G1^+G2^-$ cell line such as B90(G) or a $G1^-G2^+$ cell line such as B108 (E). This double reactivity seems paradoxical in view of

TABLE IV. Absorption of Anti-B103(N)

Cells used for absorption	Unabsorbed antiserum Serum 1 B90(G)	Serum 2 B90(G) B49(G)	Serum 3 B90(G), B49(G) B92(G)	Serum 4 B90 (G), B49(G) B65(N)
Reactivities lost	S1	S1, S6	S1, S6, S4	S1, S6, S4, N1
Reactivities retained	S4, S6 N1, N2	S4, N1, N2	N1, N2	N2
Reactivities of cell lines	(cpm per 10^5 cells)			
B103(N)	120,000	29,000	17,300	11,700
B104(N)	90,000	15,000	15,100	8,900
B35(N)	95,000	16,000	16,750	12,050
B50(N)			14,050	9,225
B65(N)	120,000	8,700	9,000	2,410
B11(N)	87,000	15,500	13,800	2,100
B92(G)	60,000	14,000	2,100	2,180
B82(E)	92,000	9,600	1,850	1,980
B49(G)	60,000	3,000	2,125	2,200
B15(G)	63,000	2,275	2,070	2,190
B19(G)		2,300	2,310	2,100
B27(G)		2,320	2,100	2,000
B28(G)		2,100	2,300	2,125
B111(G)		2,175	2,300	2,270
B108(E)		2,500	2,150	2,120
L6(M)		2,550	2,375	2,200
B44(M)		2,340	2,080	2,190
B90(G)	9,500	2,900	2,400	2,150
C6B(G)	9,000	2,750	2,260	2,275
B9(G)	7,200	2,200	2,050	2,000
RN2(G)	8,100	2,375	2,100	2,130
3T3(F)	8,000	2,190	2,100	2,025
B23(F)		2,400	2,350	2,135

Legend as in Table II.

TABLE V. Absorption of Anti-B35 (N)

	Serum 1	Serum 2	Serum 3	Serum 4	Serum 5
Cells used for absorption	B90(G) B49(G)	B90(G), B49(G) B82(E)	B90(G), B49(G) B65(N)	B90(G),B49(G) B82(E), B65(N)	B90(G), B49(G) B82(E) B103(N)
Reactivities lost	S1, S6	S1, S6, S5	S1, S6, N1, N3	S1, S6, S5, N1, N3	S1, S6, S5 N1, N2
Reactivities retained	S5, N1, N2, N3	N1, N2, N3	S5,N2	N2	N3
Reactivities of cell lines	(cpm per 10^5 cells)				
B35(N)	60,000	24,600	41,000	18,100	9,500
B50(N)	32,000	18,000	30,000	16,500	2,340
B103(N)	29,000	19,000	19,000	12,700	1,900
B104(N)	35,100	21,000	20,000	10,900	2,275
B65(N)	36,000	15,000	2,900	2,225	7,600
B11(N)	27,000	12,000	2,250	2,300	2,150
B82(E)	29,800	3,000	17,000	2,430	2,190
B23(F)	47,000	3,200	21,000	2,200	2,250
B15(G)	18,000	2,900	17,900	1,900	2,000
B49(G)	4,300	2,450	2,700	2,325	2,280
B19(G)		2,165	2,300	2,275	2,250
B27(G)		2,335	2,400	2,100	1,950
B28(G)	2,700	2,470	2,300	2,100	2,210
B111(G)		2,550	2,460	2,190	2,200
B108(E)	3,900	2,900	2,850	2,325	2,320
L6(M)		2,800	2,345	2,400	2,240
B44(M)	4,150	2,775	2,500	2,425	2,100
B92(G)	4,000	2,930	2,345	2,350	2,350
B90(G)	3,450	2,400	2,400	2,270	2,110
C6B(G)	3,950	2,700	2,580	2,430	2,250
B9(G)	3,325	2,550	2,525	2,200	1,930
RN2(G)	3,400	2,200	2,300	2,280	1,775
3T3(F)	3,250	2,600	2,410	2,000	2,030

The top of the table indicates the Unabsorbed antiserum is applied successively to Serum 1 through Serum 5.

Legend as in Table II.

the fact that B9(G) appears to express only G2. There are two possible explanations for this. First, B9(G) may have expressed G1 at the time of immunization and subsequently lost this antigen. This possibility is not borne out by our tests of early-passage B9(G) cells. Second, B9(G) may express G1 in quantities insufficient for detection by our assay (i.e., below the 10% level). This small amount of G1 might nevertheless be sufficient to produce an antibody response, especially if G1 is a strong immunogen. In addition, anti-B9(G) has an anti-S2 activity which reacts with B65(N) but apparently differs from anti-S3 (Table II), since it does not react with B35(N) or B104(N).

The anti-B103(N) and anti-B35(N) neuronal antisera both recognize the neuronal antigens N1 and N2. Anti-B35(N) also recognizes a third antigen, N3. Additionally, anti-B103(N) possesses anti-S4 activity, anti-B35(N) has anti-S5 activity, and both contain anti-

S6 (Table IV and Table V). Once again it is likely that different sequences of absorption will reveal other antigens. It is interesting to note that the excitable muscle cell lines L6(M) and B44(M) do not have the neuronal antigens. Likewise, the excitable cell lines B108(E) and B82(E) do not express them, and on this basis we might classify them as muscle cells, although there is no other evidence to support this.

We used a quantitative absorption procedure (see Methods) to detect these antigens on normal brain tissue. In these initial experiments we used whole brain taken from adult BDIX rats (3 months old) and from embryos of various ages. Figure 3A shows the result of these absorptions in the case of the G2 antigen. The absorbed antisera were tested for reactivity with B9 cells which are known to be positive for G2. Absorptions with the normal tissue are compared to control absorptions with B50 (negative for G2) and B9 (positive for G2). This comparison shows that most of the tissues are positive for G2, the lone exception being 10 day fetal brain. In contrast, Fig. 3B shows that the N3 antigen is present only in the 10 and 15 day fetal brains. These absorptions are compared to absorptions with B35 (positive for N3) and B103 (negative for N3). B35 is the test cell in the case of N3 antisera. The timetable shown in Fig. 4 illustrates the difference between N3 and G2 more directly. Whereas N3 is present very early in development and becomes undetectable before birth, G2 appears at the end of the second fetal week and persists into adulthood.

TABLE VI. Summary of Antigens

Cell line	Origin and reference	Excitability		Antigenic determinants										
		Elec.	Na+	N1	N2	N3	G1	G2	F1	S2	S3	S4	S5	S6
B35(N)	BDIX rat (22)	+	+	+	+	+	−	−	−	−	+		+	+
B50(N)	BDIX rat (22)	+	+	+	+	−	−	−	−	−	−			
B103(N)	BDIX rat (22)	+	+	+	+	−	−	−	−	−	−	+		+
B104(N)	BDIX rat (22)	+	+	+	+	−	−	−	−	−	+			
B11(N)	BDIX rat (22)	+	+	+	−	−	−	−	−	+	+			−
B65(N)	BDIX rat (22)	+	−	+	−	+	−	−	−	+	+	+	−	
B82(E)	BDIX rat (22)	−	+	−	−	−	−	+	−		−	+	+	
B108(E)	BDIX rat (22)	−	+	−	−	−	−	+	−		−	−	−	
B28(G)	BDIX rat (22)			−	−	−	−	+	+			−	−	
B92(G)	BDIX rat (22)	−		−	−	−	−	+	+	+		+	−	
B9(G)	BDIX rat (22)			−	−	−	−	+	−	+	+	−	−	−
G26(G)	C57BL/6 mouse (32)	−		−	−	−	−	+	+					
B49(G)	BDIX rat (22)	−		−	−	−	−	+	+			−	−	+
B19(G)	BDIX rat (22)	−		−	−	−	−	+	+			−	−	
B27(G)	BDIX rat (22)	−		−	−	−	−	+	+			−	−	
B15(G)	BDIX rat (22)	−		−	−	−	−	+	−			−	+	+
B111(G)	BDIX rat (22)			−	−	−	−	+	−			−	−	
B90(G)	BDIX rat (22)			−	−	−	−	+	−			−	−	−
C6B(G)	Wistar rat (29)			−	−	−	−	+	−	+	+	−	−	−
RN2(G)	BDIX rat (31)			−	−	−	−	+	−			−	−	
L6(M)	Wistar rat (30)	+	+	−	−	−	−	+	−			−	−	
B44(M)	BDIX rat (22)	+	+	−	−	−	−	+	−			−	−	
B23(F)	BDIX rat (22)	−		−	−	−	−	−	+	+		−	+	
3T3(F)	BALB/c mouse (33)	−		−	−	−	−	−	+					

A blank space indicates that the cell line was not tested, or that the absorption necessary for a definitive decision has not been performed. Electrophysiological data (Elec.) was taken from Refs. 22 and 34, while sodium flux data (Na⁺) is from Refs. 23 and 24. Immunological data is compiled from Tables II through V of this paper.

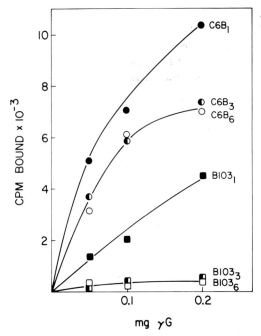

Fig. 1. Absorption of anti-C6B(G) with B103(N). Anti-C6B(G) gamma globulin was absorbed with B103(N) cells and the binding assays were performed as described in the Methods.section. The reactivity of the antiserum toward C6B(G) and B103(N) cells is shown after 1, 3, and 6 absorptions. The subscripts in the figure refer to the number of absorptions. The counts per min show the level of binding to 10^5 cells.

● $C6B_1$ = binding to C6B(G) after 1 absorption
◐ $C6B_3$ = binding to C6B(G) after 3 absorptions
○ $C6B_6$ = binding to C6B(G) after 6 absorptions
■ $B103_1$ = binding to B103(N) after 1 absorption
◧ $B103_3$ = binding to B103(N) after 3 absorptions
□ $B103_6$ = binding to B103(N) after 6 absorptions

The relative insensitivity of this absorption technique means that we cannot establish the absolute absence of antigen in any case. The presence of very few reactive cells would be indistinguishable from the case in which no reactive cells were present. Thus while the qualitative aspects of these data are correct, the accurate detection of very small amounts of antigen will require more sensitive assays.

DISCUSSION

We can make the following summary of our results. 1) Six neuronal cell lines [B11(N), B35(N), B50(N), B65(N), B103(N), and B104(N)] express a common antigen N1. The correlation between this antigen and a positive electrophysiological response is striking. In addition there is an N2 antigen expressed by B35(N), B50(N), B103(N), and B104(N), and an N3 antigen found only on B35(N) and B65 (N). None of these neuronal antigens are expressed by the muscle cell lines L6(M) and B44(M) or by B82(E) and B108(E), the other 2 cell lines previously found to give positive sodium uptake results [24]. 2) There are 2 glial-specific antigens, G1 and G2, and cells may express either or both of these. G1 and G2 are not found on fibroblasts such as 3T3(F), but oddly enough G1 is expressed by the muscle cells L6(M) and B44(M), while G2 is expressed by the excitable cells B82(E) and B108(E). 3) In addition to G1 and G2, there is a third antigen, F1, which is not expressed on any of the neuronal cell lines. This antigen is expressed by several glial lines and also by the 3T3(F) mouse fibroblast (hence the designation F1). An otherwise unclassified cell line B23(F) also expresses this antigen, and on this basis has been tentatively classified as a fibroblast. 4) There are several antigens designated S1 through S6 which are shared by various combinations of nerve, muscle, and glial cells. S1 is probably a relatively uninteresting antigen or antigens common to all cells tested, but the others occur less universally and may prove to be interesting cell markers.

We were rather surprised to find that all 6 neuronal cell lines could be characterized by a single antigen N1, and that only 2 antigens, G1 and G2, were necessary to classify the large list of glial cells. One interpretation of these findings might be that the myriad of diverse cell types in the adult brain arise from a very small number of embryonic precursor cell types, stem cells which pass their N1, G1, and G2 markers on to their differentiating progeny. Alternatively, the method used to induce these neoplastic cell lines (transplacental treatment of 2 week fetuses with nitrosoethylurea [22,27,28]), may selectively transform only particular classes of cells in the embryonic brain. The fact that these NEU-induced tumors arise in many parts of the nervous system, including the cerebellum, the hippocampus, the cerebral hemispheres, and the cranial nerves does not necessarily rule out this latter alternative.

There are a few cell lines on our list which do not fit comfortably into the classes defined by the existing antisera. The nonexcitable cell line B23(F), which expresses F1 but not G1 or G2, may be a fibroblast, but also could represent a new class of glial cell.

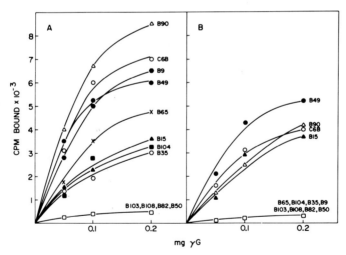

Fig. 2. Reactivity of anti-C6B(G). These antisera were derived as detailed in the text and in Fig. 1. As in Fig. 1 the cpm bound are normalized to 10^5 cells. These results are also presented in Table II.
A. Following absorption with B65(N)
    △ B90(G) ○ C6B(G) ● B9(G) ● B49(G) X B65(N) ▲ B15(G) ■ B104(N)◯B35(N) ▫ B103(N)
    B108(E), B82(E), B50(N)
B. Following absorption with B65(N)
    △ B90(G) ○ C6B(G) ● B49(G) ▲ B15(G) □ B35(N), B104(N), B65(N), B9(G), B103(N),
    B108(E), B82(E), B50(N)

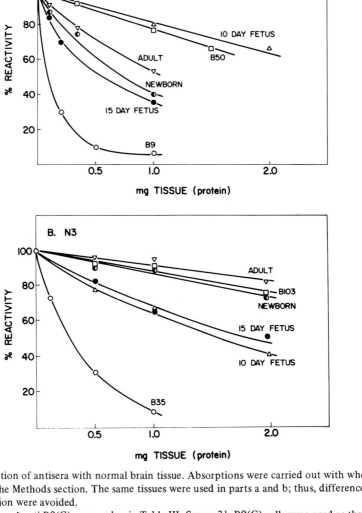

Fig. 3. Absorption of antisera with normal brain tissue. Absorptions were carried out with whole brain as detailed in the Methods section. The same tissues were used in parts a and b; thus, differences in tissue preparation were avoided.

A. Anti-G2 serum [anti-B9(G) prepared as in Table III, Serum 3]. B9(G) cells were used as the test cells to evaluate the reactivities of all absorbed antisera. Control absorptions were done using B9(G) as a G2+ cell and B50(N) as a G2⁻ cell. The 100% level is that given by unabsorbed G2 antiserum.

B. Anti-N3 serum [anti-B35(N) prepared as in Table V, Serum 5]. B35(N) cells were used to evaluate the reactivities of all absorbed antisera. Control absorptions were done using B35(N) as an N3+ cell and B103(N) as an N3⁻ cell. The 100% level is that given by unabsorbed N3 antiserum.

○ Positive cell line   □ Negative cell line   ▽ Adult   ◉ Newborn   ● 15 day fetus   △ 10 day fetus

It is therefore a good candidate to use in making a new antiserum. Somewhat surprisingly, the muscle cells L6(M) and B44(M), and the excitable cells B82(E) and B108(E), do not express any of the neuronal antigens, yet do express the glial antigens G1 and G2, respectively. These cell lines should be used for immunization to check for muscle-specific antigens and to determine whether B82(E) and B108(E) are muscle cells or a new class of neuronal

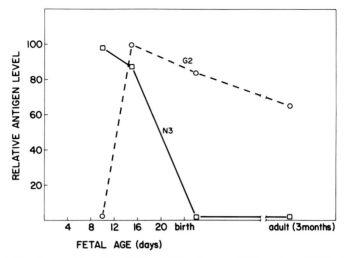

Fig. 4. Developmental profile of G2 and N3 antigens. ○ G2 antigen □ N3 antigen

cells. It may prove significant that B82(E) and B108(E) are judged excitable in the sodium uptake assay but not electrophysiologically.

The shared antigens (S), and the restricted neuronal antigens N2 and N3, serve to subdivide the large classes into smaller groups. In many cases, as shown in Table VI, cell lines appear to be unique in terms of the combination of antigens they express. Examples are the neuronal cells B35(N), B104(N), B11(N) and B65 (N); and B49(G), B92(G), and B15(G) among the glial cells. In some cases the existing data do not distinguish between cell lines, as in the case of the 2 neuronal cells B103(N) and B50(N), and in numerous cases among the glial cells. It seems likely, however, that further absorption of existing antisera, and the production of new antisera, will enable us to distinguish each cell line from all others.

The results of the absorption experiments using normal tissue show that at least 2 of the antigens, N3 and G2, are present in normal rat brain. More important, these 2 antigens appear at different times during development. N3 is present in the early fetus and disappears before birth, while G2 does not appear until the second fetal week and then persists into adulthood. This reinforces our contention that these antigens are indeed expressed by different populations of cells in the brain, a concept that was initially based on the work with the cloned cell lines. This makes us optimistic that antigens such as these will be useful in mapping cell types in the nervous system.

ACKNOWLEDGMENTS

The author is particularly indebted to Drs. Melvin Cohn, David Schubert, Steve Heinemann, and Yoshiaki Kidokoro of the Salk Institute for their advice and for providing most of the cell lines used in this study.

This work was supported by a Basil O'Connor Starter Grant to William B. Stallcup from the National Foundation-March of Dimes, and by National Institutes of Health grants AI-05875 and AI-00430 to Dr. Melvin Cohn.

Figures 1 and 2 and Tables I through VI are reproduced by courtesy of Experimental Cell Research, Academic Press Inc., New York.

REFERENCES

1. Toh, B. H., and Cauchi, M. N., Nature 250:597 (1974).
2. Bock, E., Mellerup, E. T., and Rafaelson, O. J., J. Neurochem. 18:2435 (1971).
3. Raiteri, M., Bertollini, A., and LaBella, R., Nature (New Biol.) 238:242 (1972).
4. Schachner, M., Wortham, K. A., Carter, L. D., and Chaffee, J. K., Dev. Biol. 44:313 (1975).
5. Berg, O., and Bergstrand, H., Neurobiol. 4:191 (1974).
6. Bignami, A., and Dahl, D., Nature 252:55 (1974).
7. Singh, V. K., and McGeer, P. L., Brain Res. 82:356 (1974).
8. Rossier, J., Bauman, A., and Benda, P., FEBS Lett. 36:43 (1973).
9. Eng, L. F., Uyeda, C. T., Chao, L. P., and Wolfgram, F., Nature 250:243 (1974).
10. Saito, K., Barber, R., Wu, J. Y., Matsuda, T., Roberts, E., and Vaughn, J. E., Proc. Nat. Acad. Sci. USA 71:269 (1974).
11. Hokfelt, T., Efendic, S., Johansson, O., Luft, R., and Arimura, A., Brain Res. 80:165 (1974).
12. Van Nieuw Amerongen, A., Roukema, P. A., and Van Rossum, A. L., Brain Res. 81:1 (1974).
13. Haglid, K., Hamberger, A., Hansson, H. A., Hyden, H., Persson, L., and Ronnback, L., Nature 251:532 (1974).
14. Schachner, M., Nature (New Biol.) 243:117 (1974).
15. Schachner, M., Proc. Nat. Acad. Sci. USA 71:1795 (1974).
16. Schachner, M., and Carnow, T. B., Brain Res. 88:394 (1975).
17. Akeson, R., and Herschman, H., Nature 249:620 (1974).
18. Martin, S. E., Nature 249:71 (1974).
19. Day, E. D., and Bigner, D. D., Cancer Res. 33:2362 (1973).
20. Coakham, H., Nature 250:328 (1974).
21. Fields, K. L., Gosling, C., Megson, M., and Stern, P. L., Proc. Nat. Acad. Sci. USA 72:1296 (1975).
22. Schubert, D., Heinemann, S., Carlisle, W., Tarikas, H., Kimes, G., Patrick, J., Steinbach, J. H., Culp, W., and Brandt, B. L., Nature 249:224 (1974).
23. Stallcup, W. B., and Cohn, M., Exp. Cell Res. 98:277 (1976).
24. Stallcup, W. B., and Cohn, M., Exp. Cell. Res. 98:285 (1976).
25. Greenwood, F. C., Hunter, W. M., and Glober, T. S., Biochem. J. 89:114 (1963).
26. Lowry, O. H., Rosebrough, N. J., Farr, A. L., and Randall, R. G., J. Biol. Chem. 193:265 (1951).
27. Druckrey, H., Preussmann, R., and Ivankovic, S., Ann. N.Y. Acad. Sci. 163:676 (1969).
28. Wechsler, W., Kleihues, P., Matsumoto, S., Zulch, K. J., Ivankovic, S., Preussmann, R., and Druckrey, H., Ann. N.Y. Acad. Sci. 159:360 (1969).
29. Benda, P., Lightbody, J., Sato, G., Levine, L., and Sweet, W., Science 161:370 (1968).
30. Richler, C., and Yaffe, D., Develop. Biol. 23:1 (1970).
31. Pfeiffer, S. E., and Wechsler, W., Proc. Nat. Acad. Sci. USA 69:2885 (1972).
32. Zimmerman, H. M., Amer. J. Pathol. 31:1 (1955).
33. Armelin, H. A., Proc. Nat. Acad. Sci. USA 70:2702 (1973).
34. Kidokoro, Y., Heinemann, S., Schubert, D., Brandt, B. L., and Klier, F. G. in "Cold Spring Harbor Symposium," Vol. XL, p. 373 (1976).

Biochemical Studies of the Common and Restricted Antigens, Two Neural Cell Surface Antigens

Kay L. Fields

Medical Research Council Neuroimmunology Project, Department of Zoology, University College, London, England

Two cell surface antigens on rat neural tumor cells are defined by antisera from mice immunized with a rat glioma cell line, 33B. The Common antigen is on rat brain and embryo, and is strongly expressed on the surface of all, or most, rat glioma and neuroblastoma cell lines and tumors. The other Restricted antigen is not present at detectable levels on normal rat tissues, but is on 33B, and on 11 other rat neural tumors or cell lines developed from such tumors, though many other tumors are negative. These 2 antigens are on cell membrane preparations from cells and tumors, and have been further characterized using a quantitative antigen assay. Both antigens are heat labile, and can be destroyed by digestion with proteolytic enzymes. The Common antigen is 10 times more sensitive than the restricted antigen to pronase digestion. Furthermore, spacially separate sites for the 2 antigens are indicated by blocking experiments with pepsin digested antisera. Attempts to purify these antigens further have been frustrated by loss of antigenic activity upon detergent-induced release from the membrane.

The tissue and tumor distributions of recently described mouse and rat surface antigens are reviewed. Many of these antigens are present on both brain and kidney, but not on other tissues, though several are shared with embryonic cells or sperm. Several new antigens have been described which may be neuronal specific.

Key words: neural antigens, cell surface markers, neuronal and glial tumors

INTRODUCTION

Considerable progress has been made recently in defining cell surface antigens useful for neurobiologists, in most cases using cell lines derived from nervous system tumors. Previous work had concentrated on purified cytoplasmic protein antigens such as S-100 and 14-3-2 (1,2), or on surface antigens which were not shown to be brain specific (3). The only purified surface components for which antisera are available are the nicotinic acetylcholine receptor, which can be purified and detected using neurotoxins, and the theta alloantigen, which is purified using immunoadsorbents. In the absence of purified brain specific proteins, most new surface antigens must be defined starting with antisera which are multispecific, and have been raised against complex mixtures of many antigens. Adequate adsorption of the antisera with nonneural tissues, and careful analysis of the antigen distribution on the remaining normal tissues, has been the usual procedure for producing relatively specific reagents. Once an antigen is defined, and reproducible sera available, then purification of the antigen using immunological methods may be practical.

In one approach normal neural tissue homogenates have been used as immunogens and the resulting antisera tested for activity against cell surface antigens, using as target cells either normal neural cell suspensions, which are difficult to prepare or, more commonly, tumor cell lines of neuronal or glial origin. The assumption that neural tumor cells will continue to express brain specific antigens rests largely on the experience of immunologists defining surface antigens in animal and human lymphocytic tumors (4,5). A second approach, which also assumes that tumor cell lines express differentiation antigens, is to immunize directly with the tumor or cell line material, hoping thereby to eliminate the heterogeneity of cell types expected in unfractionated brain material.

In this paper I describe the biochemical characterization of 2 cell surface antigens, the Common and Restricted rat antigens, which have been shown to be relatively specific to the nervous system or nervous system tumors (6). Their properties are compared with other brain specific cell surface antigens recently described.

Both antigens are defined by mouse antisera against a rat glioma, 33B. The Common antigen is present on normal adult brain, and is also on adult kidney to a lesser extent, while other adult tissues are negative. However, the antigen is diffusely distributed in 12–19 day rat embryos in amounts roughly equal to brain homogenates. During early development it is a widespread antigen, which after birth persists in the nervous system. With very few exceptions, neural tumors are highly positive, having about tenfold more antigen than normal brain. Nonneural tumors, or fibroblastic cell lines, are low or negative.

In contrast, the Restricted antigen has not been detected on any normal tissues, and is present on fewer tumors. The glioma cell line 33B, which was used for immunizing and as the target cell, the in vivo tumor 33B, 5 other transplanting neural tumors, and 5 other neural cells lines, are definitely positive for this antigen. Positive cell lines do not have uniform differentiated characteristics; 33B and 2 of the Salk Institute cell lines are probably gliomas, RN22 is from a neurinoma, and 2 electrically active, neuronal cell lines (7) are positive. Brain, embryo, or other tissues do not have the antigen: either it is not present on fetal or adult animals, or too few cells express it for them to be detected. Thus, it is operationally a tumor specific antigen, even though it differs from most such antigens in that it is not associated with a defined cell type or with viral transformation; moreover, it is not specific for an individual tumor.

The experiments described below concern the biochemical nature of the 2 rat antigens and their relationship to each other on the cell surface.

METHODS

Antisera

A serum specific for the Common antigen was raised as previously described (6) but in A/Strong mice. After 6 injections of 33B cells, ascites fluid was obtained which was absorbed with rat liver, spleen, and thymus. Unlike the original sera (6), this antiserum contained no trace of anti-Restricted antibody. Sera from C3H mice had both activities and were made specific for the Restricted antigen by adsorption with liver, spleen and thymus, and 21A tumor cells. Both antigens were then detected on 33B cells in cytotoxicity tests. Anti-Ag-B2 alloantiserum was the gift of Dr. J. Howard.

Quantitative Antigen Measurements

Ten μl aliquots of antisera at a dilution which gave 30–80% of maximum kill were incubated for 30 min with serial dilutions of antigen (10 μl) (whole cells, tissue homogenates, or membrane preparations). Then 2×10^4 Na$_2$ ^{51}CrO$_4$ labelled 33B cells were added (20 μl) and incubation continued for 30 min at 37°C. The cells were washed by centrifugation with 250 μl of cold PBS or Dulbecco's modified Eagle's medium with 10% fetal calf serum, and then resuspended in 20 μl of rabbit complement diluted 1:5. After 60 min at 37°C, release of ^{51}Cr from the cells was measured after dilution and centrifugation. The amount of antigen required to give 50% inhibition of antibody- and complement-specific chromium release was determined for each antigen sample and could be compared on a per cell, per packed volume, or per mg protein basis as appropriate. The usual level of sensitivity was 50% inhibition by 10^4 33B (antigen rich) cells, or by 200 ng protein of a membrane preparation from 33B tumors. For brain homogenates an extra centrifugation was necessary after the first incubation, and the supernatant (20 μl of diluted, adsorbed antiserum) was then transferred to a second tube, followed by the addition of labelled 33B target cells. If this was not done, nonspecific inhibition was found with mouse or rat brain homogenates.

Membrane Preparations

Cells or tumor material in PBS were washed and disrupted with an Ultraturrax homogenizer (60 sec). The lysate was spun at 1,500 g for 20 min, and both supernatant and resuspended pellet were further fractionated on a sucrose step gradient. The lysate was made 1.66 M in sucrose and overlayered with 0.46 M and 1.0 M sucrose, underlayered with 2.3 M sucrose, and then spun for 90 min at 75,000 (R$_{av}$) g in a swinging bucket rotor. Visible bands were collected, diluted with buffer, and concentrated by centrifugation at 100,000 g for 60 min. The pellets were resuspended by gentle sonication in storage buffer (2 vol of 1 mM EDTA in 0.05 M potassium phosphate buffer, pH 6.8 to 1 vol glycerol) and kept at −15°C. The major fraction of antigen-containing membranes from in vivo tumors usually contained 4–10 mg/ml protein, and had an inhibition titer of 1/80–1/600.

Enzyme Digestion

Whole cells were digested in PBS with pronase (BDH Ltd.), trypsin, pepsin, chymotrypsin, papain, collagenase, hyaluronidase, or neuraminidase (all from Sigma Chemical Co.). The cells were then washed and tested either for sensitivity to cytotoxic antisera, or for their ability to adsorb antibody. Digestion and destruction of antigen from membrane preparations is further described in the legend to Fig. 3.

Pepsin Digested Antisera

Crude, unadsorbed A/Strong anti-33B ascites fluid or normal ascites fluid was diluted 1:8 with 0.1 M acetate buffer, pH 4.2, and incubated 20 hr at 37°C with pepsin at 1 mg/ml. Digestion was stopped by adding enough 1M Tris to bring the pH to 7, PBS, and fetal calf serum (10%). The cytotoxic titer of the digested antiserum was reduced from 5,000 to < 10. We then tested whether preincubation of target cells with the digested serum protected the cells from lysis by a limiting dilution of specific anti-Common or anti-Restricted sera.

RESULTS

The quantitative assay for the Common and Restricted antigens is shown in Fig. 1. Cell lines could easily be titrated for antigen over a one-hundred-fold range. It is shown that 33B cells have both antigens, 21A cells have only the Common antigen, and B28 cells have neither one (< 1%). The same method could be used for tissue homogenates, provided that particulate matter was removed at an intermediate stage of the test; otherwise, brain homogenates showed nonspecific inhibition. As shown in Table I, brain and embryo showed 5–10% of the antigen content of 33B. Rat kidney had too little antigen to be distinguished from liver, spleen, or thymus (presumed negative controls) by this method, leading to the rather unexpected conclusion that repeated adsorptions are a more sensitive method for detecting these antigens. It was difficult to maintain the assays at equal sensitivity for both antigens. In particular, the titer of the anti-Restricted antibody would fall, presumably due to fluctuations in the amount of

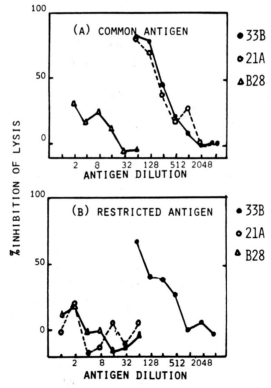

Fig. 1. Inhibition of specific antisera by cell lines differing in antigen content. Cells were grown in vitro, harvested with EDTA, and frozen with cryoprotectants. They were thawed, washed, and dilutions of a 50% suspension (roughly 200 × 10⁶ cells/ml) were tested for their ability to inhibit lysis in a cytotoxicity test. The antibody was specific for (A) the Common, or (B) the Restricted antigen.

TABLE I. Antigens on Tissue and Tumor Homogenates

Rat tissue	Common antigen		Restricted antigen	
	Inhibition titer		Inhibition titer	
33B in vitro cells	512	(100)	128	(100)
33B in vivo tumor	512	100	64	50
Embryo	64	12	< 1	< 1
Brain	32	6	< 1	< 1
Liver	4	1	< 1	< 1
Spleen and thymus	2	< 1	< 1	< 1

The inhibition titer is the dilution of a 50% tissue or cell suspension which gave 50% inhibition of lysis in a test which included removal of particulate material.

Restricted antigen on the target cell surface, and more antiserum had to be used to get sufficient lysis. As a consequence, more antigen was then necessary for inhibiton.

For the purification, separation, or characterization of the 2 antigens we wanted a stable, bulk preparation. It was difficult to obtain single cells without enzymatic digestion because 33B cells grew as a fibrous mat with many processes in culture. Therefore, a simple procedure for the preparation of membranes from in vivo tumor tissue or in vitro cells was developed, as shown in Fig. 2. It differs from procedures for fibroblasts or other tissue culture cells (8) only in that after homogenization the majority of antigen was found in the low speed pellet, not in the supernatant. Recovery of antigen from the supernatant was poor. When the low speed pellet material was banded in sucrose, the largest amount of antigen was recovered at the 0.46/1.0 M sucrose interface. The highest specific activity was always found in that fraction, and this was true for both antigens. This sucrose concentration is where plasma membrane markers usually band (8, 9). Recovery in that fraction was 25–50% of the starting antigenic units, which is comparable to that reported for other membrane antigens (10). Most preparations have been stable for many months. The specificity of inhibition by membrane fractions was very good. As shown in Table II, membranes prepared from 21A cells did not contain the Restricted antigen to any significant extent.

The finding that both antigens were concentrated on similar membrane material said little about their biochemical similarity. However, in Table III it is shown that both the Restricted and the Common antigens were sensitive to heat inactivation, substantial loss occurring at temperatures as low as 52°C, with less than 5% remaining after 10 min at 80°C. Such sensitivity would be expected of many protein antigens, but not carbohydrates or glycolipids.

In agreement with the results of heat inactivation, it could be shown that enzymatic digestion of viable cells with large amounts of trypsin, chymotrypsin, pepsin, or pronase reduced their ability to absorb anti-Common or anti-Restricted antisera (data not shown). In addition, the antigens really could be destroyed by pronase digestion of membrane preparations (Fig. 3). Small amounts of pronase increased the total amount of antigen; larger amounts destroyed it. The Common antigen is five- to tenfold more sensitive than the Restricted antigen to pronase digestion. Other experiments showed that digestion with pronase or trypsin led first to the release of antigenic material from the membranes, and then to its destruction. Most proteases destroyed or released the antigen, but neuraminidase had no effect. Trypsin action was largely blocked by soybean trypsin inhibitor.

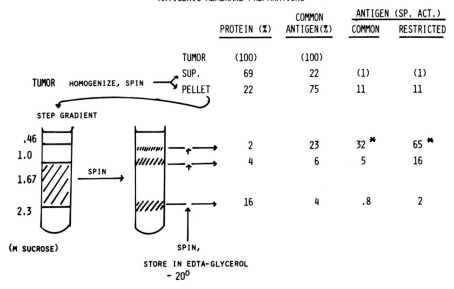

ANTIGENIC MEMBRANE PREPARATIONS

	PROTEIN (%)	COMMON ANTIGEN(%)	ANTIGEN (SP. ACT.) COMMON	ANTIGEN (SP. ACT.) RESTRICTED
TUMOR	(100)	(100)		
SUP.	69	22	(1)	(1)
PELLET	22	75	11	11
	2	23	32 *	65 *
	4	6	5	16
	16	4	.8	2

Fig. 2. An outline of the preparation of high specific activity antigen. Material from the Pellet–0.46/1.0M sucrose band (*) was used for further experiments.

TABLE II. Antigenic Specificity of Membrane Preparations

Antigen source	Protein (mg/ml)	Common antigen Inhibition titer	Common antigen Sp. act	Restricted antigen Inhibition titer	Restricted antigen Sp. act
33B in vivo tumor (Pellet–0.46/1.0)	10	676	65	610	58
21A in vitro cells (Pellet–0.46/1.7)	14	314	21	< 2	< 0.2

The antigen fractions were from the preparation outlined in Fig. 2.

TABLE III. Heat Lability of Antigens

Incubation temperature (°C)	Remaining antigen (%) Common	Remaining antigen (%) Restricted
0	100	100
52	36	20
65	25	≤ 10
80	4	4

Aliquots of membranes from the highest specific activity fraction from 33B tumor were incubated for 10 min at the indicated temperature, and then assayed for antigen content.

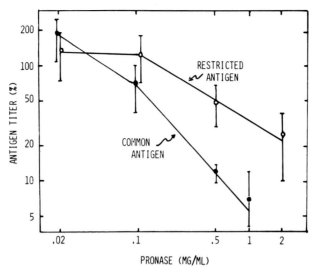

Fig. 3. Destruction of antigens by pronase. Equal volumes of 33B tumor membrane preparations (2 mg/ml) and pronase, at the indicated concentrations, were combined and incubated 30 min at 37°C. Fetal calf serum (1.5 vol) was added and the remaining antigen determined by the quantitative antigen assay. Antigen titers are expressed as the % of the control antigen sample, incubated without added pronase. Data are the average of 3 experiments ± SEM.

In order to decide whether the 2 antigens are on the same molecule, it would be helpful to be able to solubilize them with nondenaturing detergents. Several detergents (Lubrol PX, Triton X100, deoxycholate, and others) were added to membrane preparations at 0°, then excess bovine serum albumin was added [which protected the target cells from detergent lysis, a technique used successfully with histocompatibility antigens (11)] . The samples were centrifuged and assayed for antigen in the supernatant and pellet. We found that if antigen was lost from the pelletable membranes, it did not appear in the supernatant but was destroyed. Whether this was due to an interaction of the antigenic determinants with detergents, or to proteolysis, was unclear, but our inability to solubilize the antigens has precluded their purification.

An indirect method of asking whether the Common and Restricted antigens are physically associated on the cell surface is with blocking antibody (12). When crude serum containing anti-Common (and other more general specificities) was pepsin digested until no longer cytotoxic, it still blocked cytotoxicity of the specific anti-Common antiserum (Fig. 4). On the same test cells, it did not block the specific anti-Restricted antiserum at all. Pepsin alone, or pepsin digested nonimmune sera, had no blocking activity. These results make it unlikely that the Common and Restricted antigenic determinants are on the same cell surface protein. So far, though 33B cells could be killed with allogeneic anti-AgB2, there was no blocking by pepsin digested serum. Therefore, we have no evidence for an association of the Common antigen with rat histocompatibility antigens.

DISCUSSION

Progress in the molecular identification of these 2 antigens is greatly hampered by the difficulties in solubilizing the antigenic activities. However, their location on low

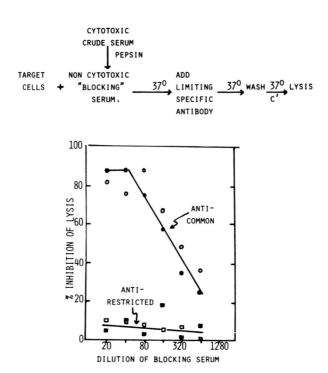

Fig. 4. Blocking of cytotoxic antibody by pepsin treated serum. Target cells were preincubated with serial dilutions of pepsin digested crude anti-33B serum. A limiting amount of cytotoxic antibody specific for the Common antigen (upper curve) or the Restricted antigen (lower curve) was then added, and incubations continued, as for a normal cytotoxic test. Filled symbols are from one experiment, open symbols from a second.

density membranes, their heat lability, and their sensitivity to digestion by proteolytic enzymes establish that they are both cell surface protein antigens. All the quantitative results indicate considerable differences in the 2 antigens, and blocking experiments do not favor a model of separate antigenic sites on the same protein.

These conclusions should be compared to the results for other surface antigens for which similar data are available. Theta antigen (Thy-1) has always been known to be on thymus and the nervous system (13, 14), but is now known to be on peripheral T lymphocytes, epidermal cells, and fibroblasts as well. It has been purified, is a glycoprotein, has a molecular weight of 25,000, is heat labile at 80°C, is sensitive to pronase, and is solubilized by many detergents (15, 16). It increases from a low level at birth to maximal levels in the first 5 weeks of life, and antigen levels vary about fivefold within the nervous system (13, 14). Theta in brain has been studied using most of the approaches available. By fluorescence, theta was demonstrated predominantly in myelinated tracts (17), but myelination deficient mutants had as much theta as normal littermate controls (18). Work with tumor cell lines has not been very decisive. Small amounts of theta were found on in vivo C1300 tumors (19), but might be due to stromal elements. We have been unable to detect theta on our rat glioma 33B, or on other rat or mouse gliomas (Stern and Fields, unpublished). Using a mouse anti-rat thymocyte serum, we were unable to detect any substantial amount of rat theta antigen on the neuronal cell lines. Other cell lines may be positive (20). Using normal mouse brain cultures, theta has been seen on a minority of neuronal cells, but not on other glial type cells (21).

Unfortunately, despite all these approaches, it is really not yet clear whether theta is preferentially expressed by neurons or glia. Since it develops late in brain tissue, the key to its expression may be to increase the "differentiation" of the various cell types. In contrast, the Common rat antigen is well expressed on tumors. Its expression on embryo and brain suggests that it may be a characteristic of the maturation of nonneural cell types to shut off synthesis of the Common antigen.

The properties of the rat antigens we have characterized are very different from those of a prominent fibroblast surface protein. The heaviest band of protein detected by lactoperoxidase catalyzed labeling of fibroblasts has a molecular weight of 220–250,000 on gels, and is now called the LETS protein [see (22) for a review]. This protein is probably identical to a fibroblast surface antigen (SFA) found on fibroblasts and on human glia (23). When fibroblasts were disrupted and the lysate sedimented through sucrose, the LETS protein was not found with plasma membranes, but at a much higher density, banding at 45–50% sucrose (24). The LETS protein was thought to be associated with an extracellular matrix layer (24), and was extremely sensitive to cleavage by proteolytic enzymes (22). A rat cell line B28 (7) which was positive by fluorescence for SF antigen (Beverley and Fields, unpublished) was completely negative for both neural antigens. Thus, our rat neural antigens seem unrelated physically or antigenically to the LETS or SFA glycoprotein.

Several other brain specific surface antigens have been described. Their properties have been reviewed before (25), and are summarized in Tables IV and V. Very little is

TABLE IV. Recent Nervous System Cell Surface Antigens

		Normal tissue distribution					Distribution on tumors		
Antigen	Immunization	Brain	Kidney	Liver Thymus Spleen	Embryo	Sperm	Neuroblas- tomas	Gliomas	Tera- tomas
Anti-neuroblastoma C1300									
MBA-1	Rat anti-in vivo tumor	++	+	0	?	?	1+/1	?	?
N18-DS	Rabbit anti- clone N18	++	+	0	?	?	1+/1	0+/1	?
NS-3	Rabbit anti- in vivo tumor	++	+	0	0	0	1+/1	5+/5	2+/2
Anti-gliomas									
NS-1	Mouse anti-G26	+	0	0	0	0	0+/1	3+/4	?
NS-2	Rabbit anti- glioblastoma	+	0	0	0	0	0+/1	5+/5	?
Common	Mouse anti-33B rat glioma	++	+	0	++	0	5+/5	40+/45	?
Restricted	Mouse anti-33B	0	0	0	0	0	2+/5	9+/31	?

TABLE V. More Recent Nervous System Cell Surface Antigens

Antigen	Immunization	Brain	Kidney	Liver Thymus Spleen	Embryo	Sperm	Neuroblastomas	Gliomas	Teratomas
Natural autoantibody									
MBA-2	None (C3H mouse)	++	++	0	+	?	4+/6	0+/6	1+/2
Anti-teratoma									
C (stem cell)	Syngeneic anti-SIKR cell line	+	+	0	+	+	0+/1	0+/2	5+/5
Anti-cerebellum									
CBL	Rabbit anti-healed cells	++	+	0	?	+	2+/2	0+/2	0+/1
CBL-specific	Rabbit anti-healed cells	±	?	0	?	?	?	?	?
NS-4	Rabbit anti-homogenate	++	0	0	+	+	0+/1	2+/4	?
NS-5	Mouse anti-homogenate	++	+	0	+	(+)	0+/1	0+/5	?

known about their chemistry, except that NS-2 is removed with chloroform:methanol extraction, and may be a glycolipid (26).

One group of brain specific antigens is defined by various sera raised against mouse neuroblastoma C1300. All 3 antigens so far described (27, 28, 29) are on brain and kidney, an association which is more common than anyone had anticipated, but is without an explanation. None of the C1300 antigens has been convincingly shown to be neuronal specific. Indeed NS-3 is not, since all 5 gliomas tested for it were positive (29). The N-18 differentiation specific antigen (28) is associated with process formation in C1300 cell lines (30), but gliomas and teratomas have not been tested. N18 cells grown in suspension lack the antigen, a situation similar to that for a C6 antigen (3). Another independent mouse neuroblastoma tumor, a terato-neuroblastoma cell line (31), and rat neuronal cell lines (7) should be tested for this antigen, for it would be very interesting if the antigen were found specifically on neurons. Akeson (32) has shown that C1300 and human neuroblastomas share antigens. Boosting with the same cell type of another species seems a clever way to produce antibodies only against the common, hopefully cell type specific antigen. Antigen MBA-2 of a terato-neuroblastoma cell line defined by naturally occurring antibody is also found on several mouse and human neuroblastomas, but not on mouse or human gliomas (31). It seems unlikely that N18-DS and MBA-2 are the same antigen, since MBA-2 is not on C1300, but it has not been directly tested.

Another teratoma antigen found on brain is the teratoma stem cell antigen, C (33). This antigen is expressed by embryo cells, sperm, and by brain and kidney (33). The immunization, and some of the properties of the antigen, except possibly its expression on brain and kidney, are very like those described for the antigen F9 [recently reviewed (34)]. The distribution of the C antigen (Table IV) is very like that of several other mouse brain antigens.

Indeed, are several antigens, MBA-2, C, and NS-5 (35) all variants of the same antigen? All of them are absent from C1300, present on brain and kidney, and (where tested) absent from gliomas. All are defined by mouse antibodies and, from their known properties, it even seems worthwhile to propose that the 3 antigens are identical. At least, this should be easy to disprove.

Two recent candidates for glial specific antigens are NS-1 and NS-2, defined by sera raised against an oligodendroglioma (36), or a glioblastoma (26), respectively. Neither antigen is shared with kidney. They are distinct antigens as tested by tumor distribution, association with myelin, and blocking tests (26).

Finally, one of the most interesting antigens in this whole field has been defined using normal cell preparations for immunization and for characterization (37). Seeds' rabbit antiserum against dissociated, reaggregated mouse cerebellar cells, after adsorption, revealed an antigen (CBL) again shared by brain and kidney, and present on cerebellar cells and neuroblastoma C1300, but missing from tested gliomas or a teratoma. At this stage it seems different from NS-4 (38). It is most interesting that further adsorption with cortex left antibody reacting with a minority population of neuronal looking cerebellar cells (37). Exactly what population seems an important question. Whatever the answer, this is an encouraging step forward toward neurobiologically interesting antisera. Another positive report, from the view of finding cell type specific antigens, is that of Stallcup (39, and this volume). If the definition of such antigens can be translated into strong antisera specific for single antigens, the remaining problems of localizing antigens in in vitro cultures, and in vivo sections should combine to enable the wide application originally hoped for from the immunological approach.

ACKNOWLEDGMENTS

I am grateful to Mrs. Carole Gosling for her excellent technical assistance, to my colleagues at University College for their comments on the manuscript, and to Dr. Melitta Schachner for stimulating discussion.

REFERENCES

1. Moore, B. W., Cicero, T. J., Perez, V. J., and Cowan, W. M., in "Cellular Aspects of Neural Growth and Differentiation," Pease, D. E., (Ed.). Univ. of California Press, Berkeley and Los Angeles, p. 481 (1971).
2. Herschman, H. R., Grauling, B. P., and Lerner, M. P., in "Tissue Culture of the Nervous System," Sato, G., (Ed.). Plenum Press, New York, p. 187 (1973).
3. Pfeiffer, S. E., Herschman, H. R., Lightbody, J. E., Sato, G., and Levine, L., J. Cell Physiol. 78:145 (1971).
4. Warner, N. L., Harris, A. W., and Gutman, G. A., in "Membrane Receptors of Lymphocytes," Seligmann, M., Preud'homme, J. L., and Kourilsky, F. M. (Eds.). North Holland, Amsterdam, p. 203 (1975).
5. Greaves, M. F., in "Progress in Hematology," Vol. IX, Brown, E. B. (Ed.). Grune and Stratton, New York, p. 255 (1975).
6. Fields, K. L., Gosling, C., Megson, M., and Stern, P. L., Proc. Nat. Acad. Sci. USA 72:1296 (1975).
7. Schubert, D., Heinemann, S., Carlisle, W., Tarikas, H., Kimes, B., Patrick, J., Steinbach, J. H., Culp, W., and Brandt, B. L., Nature 249:224 (1974).
8. DePierre, J. W., and Karnovsky, M. L., J. Cell Biol. 56:275 (1973).

9. Lelievre, L., Biochem. Biophys. Acta 291:662 (1973).
10. Bridgen, J., Snary, D., Crumpton, M. J., Barnstable, C., Goodfellow, P., and Bodmer, W. J., Nature 261:200 (1976).
11. Springer, T. A., Strominger, J. L., and Mann, D., Proc. Nat. Acad. Sci. USA 71:1539 (1974).
12. Boyse, E. A., Old, L. J., and Stockert, E., Proc. Nat. Acad. Sci. USA 60:886 (1968).
13. Reif, A. E., and Allen, J. M., J. Exp. Med. 120:413 (1964).
14. Reif, A. E., and Allen, J. M., Nature 209:523 (1966).
15. Letarte-Muirhead, M., Barclay, N., and Williams, A. F., Biochem. J. 151:685 (1975).
16. Barclay, A. N., Letarte-Muirhead, M., and Williams, A. F., Biochem. J. 151:699 (1975).
17. Moore, M. J., Dikkes, P., Reif, A. E., Romanul, F. C. A., and Sidman, R. L., Brain Research 28:283 (1971).
18. Schachner, M., Brain Research 56:382 (1973).
19. Schachner, M., Nature (New Biol.) 243:117 (1973).
20. Acton, R. T., Addis, J., Carl, G. F., and Bridgers, W. F., cited in reference 16.
21. Mirsky, R., and Thompson, E., Cell 4:95 (1975).
22. Hynes, R. O., Cell 1:147 (1974).
23. Vaheri, A., Ruoslahti, E., Westermark, B., and Pontén, J., J. Exp. Med. 143:64 (1976).
24. Graham, J. M., Hynes, R. O., Davidson, E. A., and Bainton, D. F., Cell 4:353 (1975).
25. Fields, K. L., in "Membranes and Disease," Bolis, L., Hoffman, J. F., and Leaf, A., (Eds.). Raven Press, New York, p. 369 (1976).
26. Schachner, M., and Carnow, T. B., Brain Research 88:394 (1975).
27. Martin, S. E., Nature 249:71 (1974).
28. Akeson, R., and Herschman, H. R., Nature 249:620 (1974).
29. Schachner, M., and Wortham, K. A., Brain Research 99:201 (1975).
30. Akeson, R., and Herschman, H. R., Exp. Cell. Res. 93:492 (1975).
31. Martin, S. E., and Martin, W. J., Cancer Res. 25:2609 (1975).
32. Akeson, R., and Seeger, R., (personal communication).
33. Stern, P. L., Martin, G. R., and Evans, M. J., Cell 6:455 (1975).
34. Bennett, D., Cell 6:441 (1975).
35. Zimmerman, A., and Schachner, M., Brain Research 115:297 (1976).
36. Schachner, M., Proc. Nat. Acad. Sci. USA 71:1795 (1974).
37. Seeds, N. K., Proc. Nat. Acad. Sci. USA 72:4110 (1975).
38. Schachner, M., Wortham, K. A., Carter, L. D., and Chaffee, J. K., Dev. Biol. 44:313 (1975).
39. Stallcup, W. B., and Cohn, M., Exp. Cell Res. 98:285 (1976).

Interaction of the Lipid-Associating Domain of Glycophorin With Phospholipid Bilayers

Alice Y. Romans and Jere P. Segrest

Departments of Pathology and Biochemistry, University of Alabama in Birmingham Medical Center, Birmingham, Alabama 35294

The MN-blood group bearing glycoprotein of the human red cell membrane, glycophorin, has been shown to traverse the membrane in vivo such that the NH_2-terminal portion is exposed to the external, and the COOH-terminal portion exposed to the cytoplasmic, milieu. The intervening 23 residue lipid-associating domain (LAD) of glycophorin has been shown to have a unique overall hydrophobicity.

The LAD of glycophorin can be obtained intact within an aqueous insoluble tryptic peptide, T(is). Under appropriate conditions (the reaction not being spontaneous), T(is) can be associated with phospholipid bilayers. Freeze fracture studies of T(is): phospholipid vesicles suggest that T(is) forms multimeric torus-shaped intramembranous structures 80 Å in diameter with n > 4. The plot of T(is) concentration versus multimer density suggests there is a critical multimer concentration (CMC) for T(is) in phospholipid bilayers (L/P = 200/1).

Various physico-chemical techniques such as pyrene fluorescence spectroscopy, differential scanning calorimetry, and ionic permeability were used to investigate the T(is)-lipid association. Results indicate that this system is an excellent one in which to study the boundary lipid phenomenon. In addition, T(is) association with lipid bilayers is being correlated with the natural state of glycophorin in the red cell membrane.

Key words: biological membrane, cell membranes, MN glycoprotein, glycophorin, phospholipid bilayer, hydrophobic interactions, lipid-associating domain, freeze-fracture electron microscopy, fluorescence, boundary lipids, differential scanning calorimetry, ionic permeability

Biological membranes comprise a complex barrier to many ionic and polar molecules and in so doing play a crucial role in almost all cellular activity. This remarkable function is dependent upon the structure of the cell membrane — the arrangement of its lipid, protein, and carbohydrate-containing, that is, glycolipid and glycoprotein, components. The phospholipid bilayer is the main structural unit in membranes and dominates their general properties (1). Less is known about the role of the protein than lipid components in membrane structure.

Both the electrostatic association of proteins with the polar surfaces of phospholipid bilayers and the hydrophobic interaction between proteins and the hydrocarbon-like interior of the bilayer are combined into a unified theory of membrane structure in the fluid mosaic model of Singer and Nicolson (2). This theory postulates two types of membrane proteins, one of which is electrostatically loosely associated with the membrane while the other is tightly bound to the membrane by hydrophobic interactions and can be removed only by disruption of the membrane structure.

An example of the second type of membrane protein is a glycoprotein, containing the MN blood group activity, that was isolated from the human red cell membrane over ten years ago (3). This MN glycoprotein, also known as glycophorin, comprises 10% of the red cell membrane protein and contains numerous receptor sites on that portion of its structure exposed to the extracellular milieu (4,5).

Glycophorin has been shown to traverse the membrane in vivo (4, 6), such that the NH_2-terminal portion is exposed to the external milieu and the COOH-terminal portion is exposed at the cytoplasmic membrane surface. The intervening 23 residue lipid-associating domain of glycophorin (4,7,8) has been shown by computer analysis to have a unique overall hydrophobicity matched as yet only by that of a 19 residue segment from the B coat protein of filamentous bacteriophages (9), which associates with the bacterial cell membrane during bacteriophage synthesis (10).

The lipid-associating domain is located intact within a tryptic peptide T(is) derived from glycophorin. T(is) is insoluble in aqueous buffers (7, 8). Under appropriate conditions T(is) can be associated with phospholipid bilayers.

Circular dichroism studies indicate that T(is) is about 75% α-helical when associated with egg lecithin in proteoliposomes (11). Proton magnetic resonance studies show that T(is) association with egg lecithin bilayers leads to a broadening of those peaks that have been assigned to the choline, methylene, and terminal methyl groups of the lipid (11). This broadening suggests that T(is) penetrates deeply into the bilayer, with its α-helical length parallel to the direction of the fatty acyl chains of the lipid.

Lipids such as egg lecithin will also form planar bimolecular membranes or black films. The conductance of these black films increases by a factor of 100 when T(is) is incorporated at concentrations as low as one mole T(is) per 350 moles lecithin (12).

The nature of the T(is)-egg lecithin complex was studied by freeze-fracture electron microscopy (13). Freeze-fracture electron micrographs of hydrated egg lecithin multilamellar vesicles reveal smooth fracture faces of the hydrocarbon interior of the bilayer. Incorporation of T(is) in the liposomes results in the appearance of torus-shaped particles 80 Å in diameter, as shown in Fig. 1.

The number of particles increases linearly with the T(is) (13) (Fig. 4c). This suggests a micelle-like phenomenon in which T(is) prefers to associate with itself rather than with surrounding phospholipids at a certain critical T(is) concentration, the critical multimer concentration. It can be calculated that each particle represents a multimer of four or more T(is) molecules.

The relative intensities of pyrene excimer (excited oligomer) and monomer fluorescence have been shown to be a linear function of the microviscosity of the pyrene environment in micelles and lipid vesicles (14, 15). Pyrene fluorescence has been used as a probe to monitor viscosity changes in dimyristoyl phosphatidylcholine bilayers upon incorporation of various concentrations of T(is). Pyrene is a small molecule forced to remain in the hydrocarbon interior of the lipid bilayers because of its low solubility in aqueous solutions. Its small size is thought not to disrupt packing of the fatty acyl chains of the bilayer to a large extent (15).

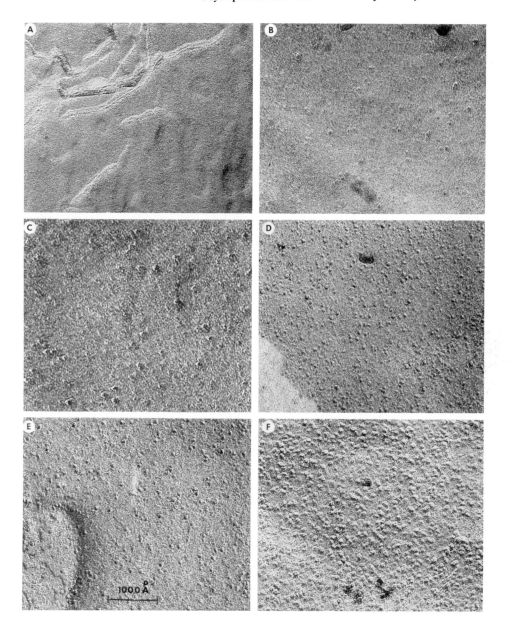

Fig. 1. Freeze-cleavage replicas of T(is)-lecithin complexes at increasing T(is) concentrations.
A) Lecithin; B) 1 mole of T(is) in 40 moles of lecithin; C) 1 mole of T(is) in 30 moles of lecithin;
D) 1 mole of T(is) in 20 moles of lecithin; E) 1 mole of T(is) in 15 moles of lecithin; F) 1 mole of
T(is) in 10 moles of lecithin.

Figure 2 shows the relative intensities of the pyrene excimer ($\simeq$ 470 nm) and
monomer ($\simeq$ 392 nm) fluorescence of dimyristoyl phosphatidylcholine bilayers containing increasing concentrations of T(is) with the pyrene concentration held constant.
Results indicate that the microviscosity of the phospholipid bilayers increases upon
incorporation of T(is).

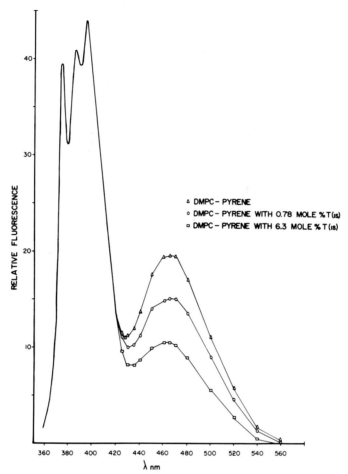

Fig. 2. Relative intensities of pyrene excimer and monomer fluorescence in DMPC bilayers containing increasing concentrations of T(is). Samples contained 0.25 mg DMPC and 0.005 mg pyrene with the T(is) concentrations shown on the graph.

The initial fairly large increases in viscosity as T(is) is added quite likely result from immobilization of lipid due to hydrophobic binding to peptide molecules. Smaller increases in viscosity at higher levels of T(is) incorporation can be explained by the formation of multimers of T(is); that is, T(is) molecules that interact with each other are not available for interacting with and immobilizing boundary lipids. Boundary lipids are those immobilized by proteins and thus unavailable for participating in reactions of the bulk lipid such as cooperative melting.

The temperature and heat content (ΔH) of the phase transitions in lipid bilayers are very sensitive to the packing properties of the membrane components (16). Differential scanning calorimetry experiments were performed to discern the effect of T(is) association upon the thermotropic properties of dimyristoyl phosphatidylcholine bilayers. Representative thermograms are shown in Fig. 3.

The addition of T(is) to the phospholipid bilayers destroys the lipid premelt, lowers the transition temperature slightly ($\simeq 2^\circ$), and lowers the enthalpy of the transition ΔH_t quite markedly. The decrease in enthalpy upon the association of T(is)

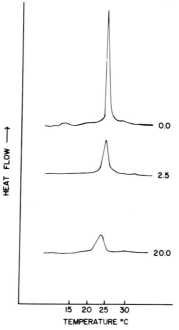

Fig. 3. Differential scanning calorimetry of DMPC bilayers prepared in the presence of T(is). Each mixture contains 2 μmoles DMPC in 1.5 ml of 100 mM NaCl buffer at pH 7.4 plus different amounts of T(is) as indicated by the numbers to the right of each thermogram. These indicate the ratio by weight of T(is) to lipid.

with the lipid bilayers can be best explained by assuming that the lipid bound to the protein is relatively immobilized and thus does not participate in the cooperative melting of the bulk lipid (17). In contrast to the case with the N-2 apoprotein from myelin (17), ΔH for the association of T(is) does not decrease linearly with increasing protein incorporation. Figure 4a is a plot of the enthalpy of transition as a function of increasing T(is) concentration. There is a slope discontinuity at 0.5 mole% T(is) lecithin. These results can be explained by the postulated multimeric association of T(is) molecules. At higher T(is) concentrations, association of the peptide with itself results in less lipid association per unit peptide and, therefore, a nonlinear dependence on concentration, as shown in Fig. 4a.

T(is) increases the flux of $^{22}Na^+$ across egg lecithin bilayers, as shown in Fig. 4b. Similar increases are observed for $^{42}K^+$. The T(is)-induced flux of Na^+ across egg lecithin bilayers is relatively low compared to that caused by known channel-forming peptides such as gramicidin A (18). Studies are currently underway to determine if the T(is) peptide functions as an ion-specific channel, for example, for Ca^{++} across lipid bilayers.

If T(is) multimers form pores to facilitate the flux of ions across bilayers, then one would expect a small positive slope at low concentrations of T(is) and a larger positive slope at higher concentrations of T(is), where multimers are present. This is not found to be the case. Indeed, at low concentration of T(is) the increase in flux is greater than at higher concentrations. This behavior seems to indicate that the ions are leaking through the bilayer at points where deformities in the packing of fatty acid chains occur, namely where T(is) is inserted into the bilayer.

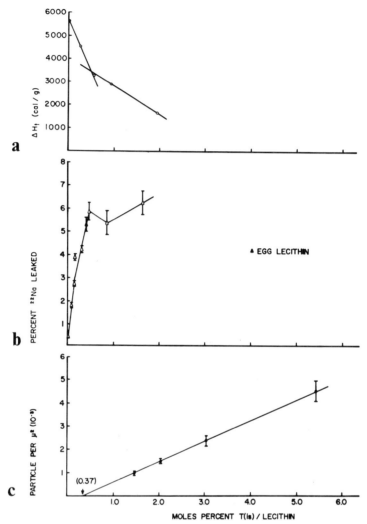

Fig. 4. a) Enthalpy of transition ΔH_t of DMPC bilayers as a function of T(is) concentration. Each sample contains 2 μmoles DMPC and T(is) as indicated. b) Ionic permeability (as measured by ^{22}Na leakage) of egg lecithin bilayers as a function of T(is) concentration. c) Density of particles seen in freeze-cleavage electron microscopy of egg lecithin vesicles as a function of T(is) concentration.

This increase in the cation permeability of phospholipid bilayers is consistent with the perturbation of the bilayer hydrocarbon region by the association of T(is) peptides.

That the plots of ΔH_t, ionic flux, and particle density versus T(is) concentration all show abrupt changes in slope near the same T(is) concentration lends strength to the supposition of multimeric association of T(is) in lipid bilayers. Studies are under way to correlate this multimeric association of T(is) in lipid bilayers with the natural state of glycophorin in the red cell membrane. In addition, the T(is)-lipid model system is an excellent one in which to study the boundary lipid phenomenon.

REFERENCES

1. Davson, H., and Danielli, J. F., in "The Permeability of Natural Membranes," 2nd. ed. London: Cambridge University Press, (1952).
2. Singer, S. J., and Nicolson, G. L., Science 175:720 (1972).
3. Winzler, R. J., in "Red Cell Membranes; Structure and Function," (G. A. Jamieson and T. J. Greenwalt, eds.). Philadelphia: J. B. Lippincott (1969).
4. Segrest, J. P., Kahane, I., Jackson, R. L., and Marchesi, V. T., Arch. Biochem. Biophys. 155:167 (1973).
5. Romans, A. Y., Parrish, D. O., and Segrest, J. P., in "Receptors in Pharmacology," (J. R. Smythies, ed.). New York: Marcel Dekker. (In press.)
6. Bretscher, M. S., Nature New Biology, 236:ii (1972).
7. Segrest, J. P., Jackson, R. L., Marchesi, V. T., Guyer, R. B., and Terry, W., Biochem. Biophys. Res. Commun. 49:961 (1972).
8. Tomita, M., and Marchesi, V. T., Proc. Natl. Acad. Sci. USA 72:2964 (1975).
9. Segrest, J. P., and Feldmann, R. J., J. Mol. Biol. 87:853 (1974).
10. Woolford, J. L., and Webster, R. E., J. Biol. Chem. 250:4333 (1975).
11. Segrest, J. P., in "Mammalian Cell Membranes," (G. A. Jamieson and A. M. Robinson, eds.). London: Butterworth. (In press.)
12. Lea, E. J. A., Rich, G. C., and Segrest, J. P., Biochim. Biophys. Acta 382:41 (1975).
13. Segrest, J. P., Gulik-Krzywicki, T., and Sardet, C., Proc. Natl. Acad. Sci. USA 71:3294 (1974).
14. Pownall, H. J., and Smith, L. C., J. Am. Chem. Soc. 95:3136 (1973).
15. Soutar, A. K., Pownall, H. J., Hu, A. S., and Smith, L. C., Biochemistry 13:2828 (1974).
16. DeKruijff, B., Cullis, P. R., and Radda, G. K., Biochim. Biophys. Acta 406:6 (1975).
17. Papahadjopoulos, D., Moscarello, M., Eylar, E. H., and Isac, T., Biochim. Biophys. Acta 401:317 (1975).
18. Myers, V. B., and Haydon, D. A., Biochim. Biophys. Acta 274:313 (1972).

Adhesion Among Neural Cells of the Chick Embryo

Jean-Paul Thiery, Robert Brackenbury, Urs Rutishauser, and Gerald M. Edelman

The Rockefeller University, New York, New York 10021

Cell-cell binding of both retinal and brain cells of the chick embryo varied as a function of developmental age, brain cells acquiring their binding properties at an earlier time than retinal cells. Brain and retinal cells of the appropriate age bound as well to each other as to themselves. Antibodies prepared against a molecule released by retinal cells in culture were able to inhibit cell-cell binding between homologous and heterologous pairs of retinal and brain cells. These results suggest that the molecular mechanism of cell-cell binding is the same in these 2 tissues. Analysis of cell surface proteins precipitated by these antibodies suggest that one of the molecules involved in adhesion has a molecular weight of 150,000, and may be derived from a larger precursor. The possible mechanisms of cell-cell binding are discussed in terms of the properties of this molecule.

Key words: initial cell-cell binding, brain and retinal cells, cell surface proteins

INTRODUCTION

An analysis of the mechanism of adhesion among vertebrate cells is of central importance in understanding tissue formation during embryogenesis. Although the interaction between cell surfaces has been described in detail at the morphological (1,2) and ultrastructural (3) levels, the molecular mechanism of cell adhesion remains unknown. To solve this problem, a number of workers have attempted to isolate molecules or membrane fragments that can enhance reaggregation of dissociated cells or that demonstrate a tissue-specific affinity for the surface of intact cells (4,5,6). In each case, active molecules or factors have been described, but the relationship of these substances to each other or to the mechanism of cell adhesion has not been established.

In our studies of cell adhesion, we have used a different approach based on 2 major experimental procedures: 1) the quantitative analysis of initial cell-cell binding among individual cells from different neural tissues as a function of embryonic age; and 2) the identification of molecules involved in adhesion according to the ability of antibodies against these molecules to inhibit spontaneous binding among individual cells. These antibodies have also been used to isolate and characterize these molecules as they exist on the cell surface.

METHODS

Preparation of Tissues and Cells

Whole neural retina and brain tissues were obtained from chick embryos of various ages. To prepare single cell suspensions, these tissues were treated with 0.5% trypsin (1–250 Nutritional Biochemicals Corp.) in phosphate-buffered saline, pH 7.4, for 20 min at 37°C. After washing in minimal essential medium (MEM) containing 20 μg/ml of pancreatic DNAse, the cells were dispersed using a Pasteur pipette. The dissociated cells were then allowed to recover from the trypsinization in spinner cultures with calcium- and magnesium-free MEM containing 1% fetal calf serum, or as monolayers with Dulbecco's modified Eagle's medium (DMEM) containing 5% fetal calf serum.

Cell-Cell Binding Assay

This assay is based on the immobilization of cells on culture dishes and a subsequent analysis of the ability of cells in suspension to bind to immobilized cells. A uniform monolayer of cells was obtained by centrifugation of 10^7 cells onto a 35 mm diameter culture dish previously derivatized with wax bean agglutinin (7,8). After washing, anti-wax bean agglutinin antibodies (200 μg/ml) were added to prevent further binding of cells by the lectin. Cells in suspension (2×10^6 cells) in 2 ml DMEM were then added to the monolayer and incubated on a reciprocal shaker at 70 RPM for 30 min at room temperature. The cytoplasm of the cells in suspension had previously been labeled with fluorescein (9) by treatment with fluorescein diacetate (20 μg/ml) for 10 min at room temperature and washing several times in MEM. At the end of the assay the dishes were washed, and the number of suspension cells that had bound to the monolayer was determined by fluorescence microscopy (Fig. 1).

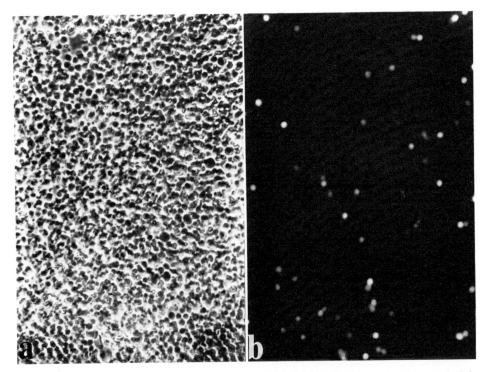

Fig. 1. Cell-cell binding among embryonic neural cells using cells immobilized in a wax bean agglutinin-coated dish. (a) Immobilized cell monolayer as viewed by phase contrast microscopy. (b) Cells containing fluorescein that have bound to the immobilized cells and observed by fluorescence microscopy.

Isolation of Proteins From Cultures of Retinal Cells

Four hundred retinas from 10-day-old embryos were dissociated and the cells cultured as monolayers in DMEM containing 5% fetal calf serum. After 24 hrs, the monolayers were washed extensively with phosphate-buffered saline, pH 7.4 (PBS) and were incubated for an additional 48 hrs in serum-free DMEM containing the protease inhibitor Trasylol. This medium (MCS) was collected and centrifuged to remove debris. After a 30-fold concentration by ultrafiltration through Amicon PM-10 membranes, the MCS was passed through a DEAE cellulose (DE-52, Whatman) column in 0.01 M Tris-0.4 M KCl, pH 7.2, to remove most of the nucleic acids, and then fractionated on a 0.5 × 10 cm column of DE-52 in 0.01 M Tris, pH 7.2, using a linear gradient of KCl from 0.01 M to 0.40 M. Fractions containing the protein called F1 (Fig. 2) were identified by analytical polyacrylamide gel electrophoresis, pooled, and further separated by preparative gel electrophoresis on 1 cm × 10 cm cylindrical gels of 6.5% acrylamide in Tris-glycine buffer. F1 was located by scanning the gel at 280 nm with a Gilford spectrophotometer, and was eluted from the appropriate gel slice by electrophoresis (10). The purity of F1 was assessed by polyacrylamide gel electrophoresis in 0.1% sodium dodecyl sulfate (SDS).

Preparation of Antibodies

Rabbits were immunized at monthly intervals with fractionated MCS proteins in Freund's adjuvant. The immunoglobulin fraction from the antisera was used in all experiments.

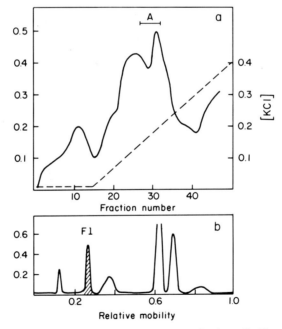

Fig. 2. Isolation of the F1 protein from culture supernatants of retina cells. The vertical axis indicates the absorbance at 280 mμ. (a) Ion-exchange chromatography of monolayer culture supernatant (MCS) on DE-52. F1 is contained in fraction A. (b) Scan of preparative gel electrophoresis of fraction A on polyacrylamide gels in Tris-glycine. F1 was eluted from the region of the gel indicated by the hatched peak.

To determine if a protein purified from MCS is present on the cell surface, cells were incubated with fluorescein-labeled antibody (1 mg/ml, 15 min, 37°C), washed, and examined by fluorescence microscopy.

Immunoprecipitation of NP40 Extracts of ^{125}I-labeled Cell Surface Proteins (11)

Proteins on the surface of cells from monolayer and suspension cultures were labeled with ^{125}I by the lactoperoxidase procedure. The proteins were then extracted with 0.5% NP40, immunoprecipitated by incubation with rabbit antibodies to purified MCS proteins followed by goat-anti-rabbit antibody, solubilized in 2% SDS-2% 2-mercapto-ethanol, and fractionated by electrophoresis on 6.5% polyacrylamide gels in 0.1% SDS (12). The fractionated proteins were detected by measurement of radioactivity in 2 mm gel slices.

RESULTS

Binding Among Retinal and Brain Cells From Embryos of Different Ages

In studying the mechanism of adhesion among embryonic cells, our experiments were first directed towards an evaluation of the specificity of binding among individual retinal and brain cells. Using the cell-cell binding assay described above, it was possible to quantitate both homotypic and heterotypic binding. Freshly trypsinized cells did not bind significantly to each other. If, however, the cells were allowed to resynthesize their cell surface proteins for 6–12 hours in suspension cultures, rapid binding occurred between cells of certain types. We therefore used cells that had been cultured in suspension for 15–20 hrs in all cell-cell binding experiments. The binding among dissociated retinal and brain cells from embryos of various ages is summarized in Table I. High levels of binding were obtained between pairs of 8-day retinal cells, pairs of 6-day brain cells, and between pairs consisting of an 8-day retinal cell and a 6-day brain cell. The number of cell-bound cells in these experiments represented at least 20% of the total number of cells added in the assay, indicating that the assay was not detecting the binding properties of a minor subpopulation of cells. In contrast, 13-day retinal cells and 10-day brain cells bound poorly to themselves and to each other, and only slightly better to 8-day retinal cells and 6-day brain cells.

It therefore appears that cells in both neural tissues have the capacity to resynthesize their cell surface components and to use these components to form cell-cell bonds. The capacity to reaggregate, however, is gradually lost with increasing developmental age, with the loss of binding occurring 3–4 days earlier in the brain than in the retina. It is not as yet known whether the inability of cells from older embryos to reaggregate reflects the failure to express a cell surface molecule directly involved in ligation, or if the cells no longer have some dynamic property or intracellular structure required for cell-cell binding. In any case, it is striking that the loss of this binding capacity for cells from each tissue is temporally correlated with the rate of increase of cell number in that tissue. In fact, the number of cells in a brain or retina reaches a plateau at about the same time that the cells begin to lose their ability to reaggregate (13).

Isolation and Characterization of Proteins From Monolayer Culture Supernatants

In searching for proteins involved in cell adhesion, our strategy was based on the assumption that if a molecule is directly involved in initial cell-cell binding, then antibodies to that molecule should block the binding. This approach required a

TABLE I. Binding Among Retinal and Brain Cells From Embryos of Different Ages

Cell-cell binding between:*		Cell-bound cells†
Cell in monolayer	Cell in suspension	
R_8	R_8	423
B_6	B_6	413
R_8	B_6	390
R_{13}	R_{13}	122
B_{10}	B_{10}	8
R_8	R_{13}	175
R_8	B_{10}	41

*R_8 and R_{13} are cells from retinas of 8- and 13-day-old chick embryos; B_6 and B_{10} are cells from brains of 6- and 10-day-old embryos.

†Expressed as number of cells in suspension that had bound to 1 mm^2 of cell monolayer.

source of cell surface proteins and a fractionation procedure. Direct solubilization of cell surface proteins by detergents was not employed because such treatments eliminate a number of useful fractionation techniques. Instead, we used medium from monolayer cultures (MCS), which contain soluble proteins or fragments that have been shed from the cell surface. Fractionation of MCS by ion-exchange chromatography followed by gel electrophoresis yielded a number of proteins (Fig. 2). Of the antibodies produced against these proteins and labeled with fluorescein, only those directed against the fraction containing protein F1 and its fragments gave detectable staining of retinal or brain cells as assayed by fluorescence microscopy. This protein, isolated from a single band on nondissociating polyacrylamide gels, also migrated as a single component with an apparent molecular weight of 140,000 on gels in 0.1% SDS with 2% 2-mercaptoethanol (Fig. 3A). The native molecular weight of F1 was also found to be 140,000 by gel exclusion chromatography. F1, therefore, appears to be a single polypeptide chain.

If the protease inhibitor Trasylol was omitted from the monolayer cultures, F1 could still be isolated as a single component on nondissociating gels. This protein, however, was found to be internally cleaved in that it dissociated into several smaller fragments either by treatment with SDS (Fig. 3B), or upon prolonged storage in phosphate-buffered saline. The major fragment (F2) had a molecular weight of 55,000 in SDS (Fig. 3B) and could be isolated on nondissociating acrylamide gels. Although this fragment was derived from F1, immunodiffusion studies indicated that anti-F1, which reacts strongly with F1, only reacts weakly with the fragment, and strong antibodies to the fragment react weakly with F1.

Effect of Antibodies to MCS Proteins on Cell-Cell Binding

Of all the proteins purified from MCS, only F1 and its fragments gave rise to antibodies capable of inhibiting cell-cell binding. Whereas antibodies reactive with the fragments caused an almost complete inhibition of both homotypic and heterotypic adhesion among retinal and brain cells (Table II), antibodies to intact F1 caused only a slight decrease even at high concentrations.

Identification of Cell Surface Molecules Containing F1

Cell surface proteins sharing antigenic determinants with F1 or its fragments were identified by SDS polyacrylamide gel electrophoresis of precipitates obtained by

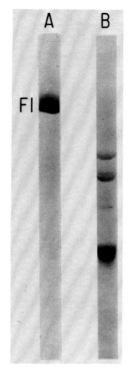

Fig. 3. Polyacrylamide gel electrophoresis in SDS of the F1 protein isolated from cultures, (A) with the protease inhibitor Trasylol, and (B) without Trasylol.

TABLE II. Effect of Antibodies on Binding Among Retinal and Brain Cells

Cell-cell binding between:*		Cell-bound cells	
Cell in monolayer	Cell in suspension	Control	+ Antibody†
R_8	R_8	423	37
B_6	B_6	413	32
R_8	B_6	390	41

*R_8 and B_6 are cells from retinas and brains of 8- and 6-day-old chick embryos, respectively.
†Both the cells in the monolayer and those in suspension were incubated for 15 min at 25°C with antibodies to fragments of F1 (1 mg/ml) prior to cell-cell binding.

combining antibodies to these molecules with an NP40 extract of cells labeled with ^{125}I by lactoperoxidase. When cells from monolayer cultures were used, anti-F1 precipitated a family of molecules with molecular weights (M.W.) ranging from 200,000 to 280,000. However, with cells grown in suspension culture, these components were nearly absent. With antibodies to F1 fragments, quite different results were obtained. These antibodies mainly precipitated a polypeptide of M.W. 150,000 from extracts of suspension and monolayer cells. Antibodies to other MCS proteins or from unimmunized rabbits did not precipitate significant amounts of iodinated protein.

DISCUSSION

The data on initial binding among individual brain and retinal cells suggest that the molecular mechanism of cell adhesion is the same in these 2 tissues. Not only can cells from these 2 tissues bind to each other as well as to themselves, but in all cases binding can be inhibited by antibodies to the same molecule. The binding properties of each cell type, however, did vary with respect to developmental age, indicating that there is a temporal program for cell adhesion that is different for retinal and brain cells.

Immunoprecipitation of cell surface molecules by the antibodies that block cell adhesion has been used for provisional identification of the components that bind the antibodies that prevented cell-cell ligation. The antibodies that completely blocked adhesion precipitated a cell surface protein with a M.W. of 150,000 from NP40 extracts of cells grown in suspension. On the other hand, antibodies to F1, which only weakly blocked adhesion, precipitated large (200,000 to 280,000 M.W.) cell surface proteins from NP40 extracts of monolayer cells, but not from extracts of suspension cells.

Because the antibodies that strongly block adhesion and precipitate the 150,000 M.W. component were made against fragments of F1, the precipitation of higher molecular weight polypeptides by anti-F1 suggests the possibility that the 150,000 M.W. molecule may be derived from or related to a larger precursor. Furthermore, the fact that the antibodies precipitating the 150,000 M.W. species block adhesion completely whereas the anti-F1 antibodies are relatively ineffective in this respect suggest that inhibition of cell ligation occurs through an inactivation of the 150,000 M.W. component by antibody.

These conclusions, of course, rely on the specificity of the antibodies obtained against F1 and its fragments. Inasmuch as the effect of a minor contaminant in the antigens used to produce these antibodies could be magnified in either the inhibition of adhesion or the identification of cell surface molecules, it will be necessary to do further structural and functional experiments to exclude this possibility.

With these reservations in mind, we have formulated a working hypothesis for the mechanism of cell adhesion that assumes that the 150,000 M.W. molecule on the cell surface is directly involved in the formation of cell-cell bonds, which can be inhibited by the binding of antibody specific to that molecule. In addition, there is the possibility that this molecule is derived from a large precursor by proteolytic cleavage. The 150,000 M.W. polypeptide could function by being self-complementary, so that a cell-cell bond would be a symmetrical dimer. Alternatively, this molecule may bind to one or more unrelated molecules. We have found in preliminary experiments that incubation of only 1 of the 2 cells involved in each binding event with monovalent Fab' antibody is sufficient to prevent adhesion. This result is more compatible with mechanisms in which 2 molecules having the same antigenic determinant are involved in the formation of each cell-cell bridge.

Whatever the actual mechanism of cell-cell adhesion, it will be important to explain the temporal specificity of cell adhesion during embryogenesis in terms of molecular events. Our previous studies on the binding of neural cells to nylon fibers coated with the antibodies that block adhesion (13) indicate that a temporal variation occurs in this cell-fiber interaction that parallels the variation seen in direct cell-cell binding (Table I). This raises the possibility that adhesion may in part be modulated by changes in the amount, structure, or dynamic properties of the 150,000 M.W. cell surface protein.

ACKNOWLEDGMENTS

This work was supported by U.S. Public Health Service Grants HD 09635, AI 11378, AI 09273, and AM 04256. J-P.T. is a fellow of the International Agency for Research on Cancer, Lyon, France, and R.B. is a fellow of the Jane Coffin Childs Memorial Fund for Medical Research.

REFERENCES

1. Holtfreter, J., Arch. Entwicklungmench. Organ. 139:110 (1939).
2. Moscona, A. A., J. Cellular Comp. Physiol. 60 Suppl. 1:65 (1962).
3. Trelstad, R. L., Hay, E. D., and Revel, J. P., Dev. Biol. 16:78 (1967).
4. Hausman, R. E., and Moscona, A. A., Proc. Nat. Acad. Sci. USA 72:916 (1975).
5. Merrell, R., Gottlieb, P. I., and Glaser, L., J. Biol. Chem. 250:5655 (1975).
6. Balsamo, J., and Lilien, J., Nature 251:522 (1974).
7. Edelman, G. M., and Rutishauser, U., Methods in Enzymology 34:195 (1974).
8. Sela, B., Lis, H., Sharon, N., and Sachs, L., Biochim. Biophys. Acta 310:273 (1973).
9. Bodmer, W. F., Tripp, M. and Bodmer, J. Application of the fluorochromatic cytotoxicity assay to human leukocyte typing. In "Histocompatibility Testing," E. S. Curtoni, P. L. Mattiuz, and R. M. Tosi (Eds.). p. 341 Munksgaard, Copenhagen (1967).
10. Stephens, R. E., Anal. Biochem. 65:369 (1975)
11. Henning, R., Milner, R. J., Reske, K., Cunningham, B. A., and Edelman, G. M., Proc. Nat. Acad. Sci. USA 73:118 (1976).
12. Laemmli, U. K., Nature 227:680 (1970).
13. Rutishauser, U., Thiery, J-P., Brackenbury, R., Sela, B-A., and Edelman, G. M., Proc. Nat. Acad. Sci. USA 73:577 (1976).

Factors Influencing Degradation of Extrajunctional Acetylcholine Receptors in Skeletal Muscle

C. Gary Reiness, Patrick G. Hogan, Jean M. Marshall, and Zach W. Hall

Department of Neurobiology, Harvard Medical School, Boston, Massachusetts 02115

George E. Griffin and Alfred L. Goldberg

Department of Physiology, Harvard Medical School, Boston, Massachusetts 02115

During development and after both denervation and reinnervation in adult mammalian skeletal muscle, the level of acetylcholine (ACh) receptors in the extrajunctional membrane undergoes wide variation. We have determined the rate of extrajunctional receptor degradation in denervated muscles in organ culture under a variety of conditions by measuring the rate at which α-bungarotoxin bound to the receptors is degraded. Direct electrical stimulation of muscles for several days dramatically reduced the levels of extrajunctional ACh sensitivity, and also reduced the rate of receptor degradation. Since the effect of activity on the rate of receptor degradation is in the opposite direction of the observed change in receptor levels, we conclude that activity must also decrease the rate of receptor synthesis. Receptor degradation was also examined in muscles at various times after denervation. The half-time of degradation increased from approximately 7 hr at 2—5 days after denervation to approximately 14 hr at 10—14 days. Hypophysectomy, which decreases the average rate of protein degradation in muscle, also decreased the rate of extrajunctional receptor degradation, but thyroxine, which restores the normal rate of overall protein breakdown in hypophysectomized animals, did not affect receptor breakdown. Since hypophysectomy did not increase the level of extrajunctional ACh receptors, it must also affect ACh receptor synthesis.

INTRODUCTION

The acetylcholine (ACh) receptor in skeletal muscle of vertebrates is a membrane protein that binds ACh and thereby increases sodium and potassium permeabilities. Because the interaction of ACh with the receptor causes a change in membrane potential, electrophysiological methods have been used to define the physiological role of the protein and many of the characteristics of the permeability changes that it causes (1).

C. Gary Reiness and Zach W. Hall are now at the Department of Physiology, University of California Medical School, San Francisco, California.

Jean M. Marshall was on leave from the Division of Biological and Medical Sciences, Brown University, Providence, R.I.

Recently, the discovery of a group of small protein toxins that bind tightly and specifically to the receptor and can be radiolabelled (2) has made it possible to isolate the ACh receptor and to study its biochemical properties in vitro. Receptor has been highly purified both from muscle (3,4) and from the electric organs of Electrophorus and Torpedo, which provide an exceedingly rich source of the protein (5–7). Although less extensive studies have been made on the structure and properties of the muscle receptor, ACh receptors from all 3 sources appear to be similar. All are large (ca. 4×10^5 daltons), hydrophobic glycoproteins with complex subunit structures.

The ACh receptor in muscle is a particularly interesting surface protein, because 2 distinct populations of the molecule occur in the membrane. One group of receptors is found in the highly enfolded muscle membrane at the motor endplate. The protein occupies the crests of the folds beneath the nerve terminals, where it occurs in very high density (ca. $3 \times 10^4/u^2$) (8–12). It is not clear when in development these receptors first appear, but after formation of the neuromuscular junction, their number is relatively constant and remains so even after denervation (13).

A second population of ACh receptors occurs in the muscle membrane outside the junction, and in contrast to the junctional receptors, undergoes wide changes in density during development, and after denervation and reinnervation in the adult. Both developing and denervated muscle have a high density of extrajunctional receptors, while their density in innervated muscles is low (2, 12, 14–17). One important factor regulating the level of receptors in the extrajunctional muscle membrane is muscle activity; thus, stimulation of denervated muscles reduces the number of extrajunctional receptors (18–20), and the elimination of activity in innervated muscles increases their number (18, 21–23).

The properties of junctional and extrajunctional receptors are generally similar, but subtle differences between them, both in the membrane and purified preparations, can be detected. They can be distinguished by differences in sensitivity to d-tubocurarine (24–26), in the characteristics of the permeability changes they cause (27), in the isoelectric points of the isolated proteins (26), and in their immunological properties (28).

The ability to identify the ACh receptor biochemically makes it possible to study the turnover of the protein in the membrane. Our laboratory, along with others, has examined the degradation of junctional and extrajunctional ACh receptors, using an indirect method in which ^{125}I-α-bungarotoxin is bound to the receptor in the membrane, and the degradation of bound toxin is measured either by following the loss of radioactive toxin from the tissue or by measuring the release of ^{125}I-mono-iodotyrosine from the muscle (29–31). We briefly describe here earlier work on degradation of toxin bound to junctional and extrajunctional receptors (32), along with more recent work on factors that influence degradation of extrajunctional receptors in denervated muscle.

METHODS

The basic design of experiments measuring receptor degradation was to give denervated or normal rats an intrathoracic injection of ^{125}I-α-bungarotoxin to label ACh receptors in the diaphragm. After several hours to allow the removal of free toxin by the circulation, hemidiaphragms were removed, pinned to Sylgard-lined culture dishes, and incubated at 37°C in modified Trowell's medium in an atmosphere of CO_2 and O_2. The loss of bound toxin was measured either by comparing the radioactivity in samples of muscles at 0 and 24 hr, or by measuring the radioactivity appearing in the medium with time. In the latter case, radioactivity remaining in the muscle at the end of the experiment was measured and the results expressed as percentage of the original radioactivity in the tissue. Further details of the methods of culture and measurement of degradation rates are given in (32). Recent studies (G. E. Griffin, unpublished experiments) have shown that muscles cultured according to these procedures remain in net nitrogen balance for at least 3 days.

Procedures for muscle stimulation (33) and for measuring ACh sensitivity (22) and toxin-binding (28) have been described.

Hypophysectomy and treatment with thyroid hormone were carried out as described by Griffin and Goldberg (35).

Animals for the experiments on hormonal influence were male CD rats from Charles River Laboratories, and in all other cases were Sprague-Dawley rats from Gofmoor Farms.

RESULTS AND DISCUSSION

Junctional and Extrajunctional Receptors

In previous experiments from this laboratory (32), we compared the loss of ^{125}I-α-bungarotoxin bound to junctional receptors with that of toxin bound to the extrajunctional receptors that appear after denervation. Normal and denervated rats were injected with radioactive toxin, their hemidiaphragms subsequently cultured for 24 hr, and the amount of radioactive toxin present in the muscle at the beginning and end of the incubation compared. In the case of normal muscle, radioactivity specifically associated with the endplate was measured, while in denervated muscle, only regions of muscle without endplates were examined. A striking difference was observed in the 2 cases. During the 24 hr culture period, only about 20% of the radioactive toxin was lost from junctional receptors, while over 80% of the toxin bound to extrajunctional receptors was lost. When the behavior of toxin bound to receptors at the original endplate in denervated muscle was examined, the rate of loss was similar to that seen in normal muscle. Thus the faster loss of toxin from extrajunctional than from junctional receptors represents a difference between the 2 types of receptor, and cannot be attributed to a change in protein degradation in denervated muscle.

We and others (29, 31) have observed a comparable difference in the loss of toxin bound to junctional and extrajunctional receptors in vivo. In experiments in which the muscles were labelled and allowed to remain in the animal, the half-time of loss from extrajunctional receptors has been estimated to be about 18 hr, while that from junctional receptors is 6–7 days.

Mechanism of Toxin Loss

We have examined the process by which toxin is lost from extrajunctional receptors of denervated muscles in organ culture. As the number of junctional receptors is smaller and the rate of toxin loss slower, we have not investigated the mechanism of loss from junctional receptors.

A number of observations on the loss of toxin from extrajunctional receptors are consistent with the hypothesis that the loss represents intracellular degradation of toxin-receptor complex. First, the radioactivity appears in the medium as ^{125}I-mono-iodotyrosine, indicating that the toxin is degraded. Second, association of the toxin with the receptor appears to be necessary for degradation, since free toxin added to the medium is not broken down to iodotyrosine. Third, toxin degradation is blocked by inhibitors of energy metabolism and is decreased by protein synthesis inhibitors, both of which are characteristics associated with intracellular degradation of proteins in other mammalian tissues (29).

Important support for the idea that toxin degradation represents breakdown of toxin-receptor complex is provided by experiments of Devreotes and Fambrough (30), who have observed a process of toxin degradation similar to that described here in primary muscle cell cultures from chick. They showed that when cycloheximide is included in the medium to inhibit protein synthesis, the rate of decrease in total number of receptors in cells cultured without toxin is identical to the rate of degradation of radioactive toxin bound to receptors in parallel cultures. This correspondence suggests that the presence of toxin does not perturb receptor turnover and that toxin degradation is a valid measure of the normal breakdown of receptors.

Activity

Because muscle activity plays an important role in regulating levels of extrajunctional ACh receptor, we were interested to examine the effect of activity on receptor degradation. In initial experiments we established that stimulation in vitro in our culture system could reduce extrajunctional receptor levels. Muscles were cultured over platinum electrodes embedded in recessed troughs in the Sylgard and stimulated continuously at 2–10 Hz. As had been previously reported by Purves and Sakmann (36), stimulation for several days decreased the extrajunctional sensitivity developed by denervated muscles in culture. Muscles that had been denervated for 5 days and subsequently cultured for 4 days with electrical stimulation contained fibers with lower sensitivities than those from comparable muscles that were cultured without stimulation (Fig. 1A). A similar result was obtained when muscles were cultured with or without stimulation for 4 days directly after denervation and allowed to develop extrajunctional sensitivity in culture (Fig. 1B). No detectable change in ACh sensitivity of muscles denervated for 5 days was seen after 24 hr of stimulation.

The effect of muscle stimulation on degradation of ^{125}I-α-bungarotoxin bound to extrajunctional receptors was then examined. Muscles were labelled and cultured for 24 hr with and without stimulation at 2–10 Hz. In all experiments, degradation of toxin was slower in the stimulated muscles. The half-times of loss for stimulated muscles ranged from 16 to over 30 hr, and for unstimulated muscles from 8 to 14 hr. Tetrodotoxin (10^{-5} g/ml) abolished the effects of stimulation.

The effect of muscle stimulation on toxin degradation was reversible, and the change in rate that occurred when muscle activity was changed was accomplished within several hours of onset or cessation of activity. Figure 2 shows the results of an experiment in which stimulation of different muscles was either stopped or started during the course of an experiment. For reference, one muscle was stimulated continuously, and another left unstimulated. In the 2 cases in which activity was changed, a change in rate of toxin degradation was detectable within 3 hr (Fig. 2).

These results suggest that muscle activity decreases the rate of degradation of the ACh receptor. This may not be specific to the receptor, since in normal muscles, activity has been observed to decrease the average rate of protein degradation (37). In any case, the effect of activity on receptor degradation is in the wrong direction to explain the

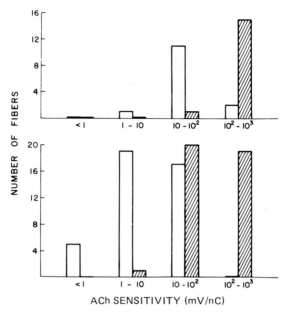

Fig. 1. Effect of electrical stimulation on extrajunctional ACh sensitivity of muscles in culture. In one series of experiments (upper) muscles that had been denervated for 5 days were cultured for 4 days either with continuous stimulation at 10 Hz or with no stimulation. In another series (lower) normal muscles were cultured for 4 days under the same conditions. After the period in culture, extrajunctional sensitivity was determined by iontophoretic application of ACh from micropipettes that contained 2 M acetylcholine bromide and had resistances between 80 and 120 megohms. No attempt was made to select fibers that had been active in culture. ACh sensitivity is expressed in millivolts per nanocoulomb.

decrease in extrajunctional receptor levels that muscle activity causes. These experiments thus provide indirect evidence that activity changes receptor levels by changing the rate of receptor synthesis.

Time After Denervation

After denervation of adult muscle fibers, extrajunctional receptors begin to appear after about 48 hr. Their density increases rapidly for 10–14 days, and then undergoes a slow decline. The rate of receptor degradation as a function of time after denervation was investigated during the period of receptor accumulation. A group of rats were denervated at various times before injection of ^{125}I-α-bungarotoxin and culture of the hemidiaphragms as described above. During the period from 2.5 to 9 days after denervation, the half-time of toxin loss increased; little or no difference was found between 9 and 14 days (Fig. 3). Whether or not the decrease in degradation rate with time after denervation represents a general effect on membrane proteins is not known. The average rate of degradation of total muscle protein is increased after 10 days of denervation (37), but because turnover of extrajunctional receptor in normal muscle cannot be measured, a direct comparison is not possible. Clearly, however, the decrease in rate of receptor degradation that occurs during the first 10 days after denervation must contribute to the continued accumulation of receptor. Whether or not the rate of receptor synthesis continues to increase during this period remains to be determined.

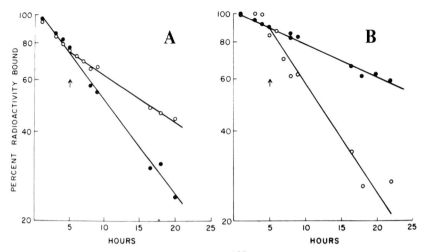

Fig. 2. The effect of muscle activity on degradation of ^{125}I-α-bungarotoxin bound to extrajunctional ACh receptors in denervated muscle. Hemidiaphragms from animals that had been denervated 5 days previously were labelled in vivo by injection of radioactive toxin and were transferred 3 hr later to organ culture. After several changes of medium to reduce the level of unbound toxin in the muscle, release of radioactivity from each muscle was monitored by sampling the medium, and radioactivity remaining in each muscle at the end of the experiment was measured. Each value for the left hemidiaphragms was corrected by subtracting, on a per weight basis, the corresponding value for the right hemidiaphragm from the same animal. The total amount of radioactivity initially associated with extrajunctional receptors was calculated as the sum of the corrected values of radioactivity released into the medium plus that remaining in the muscle. Stimulation was at 2 Hz. The results presented are from 1 experiment, but are presented in 2 figures for clarity. A) One muscle (●) was unstimulated throughout the experiment; and one muscle (○) was stimulated starting at 5 hr. B) One muscle (●) was stimulated continuously; and one muscle (○) was stimulated only for the first 5 hr of the experiment.

Devreotes and Fambrough (30) found no change in the rate of receptor degradation in myotubes in culture over a period of 22 days after fusion.

Hormonal Influence

The overall rate of protein degradation in muscle is determined by a variety of factors, including muscle activity, nutrient supply, and endocrine factors (e.g., insulin). Recently it has been demonstrated that the average rate of protein breakdown in skeletal muscle is decreased following hypophysectomy, but can be restored to normal by administration of replacement doses of thyroid hormone (35). Such doses of the hormone induced net growth of the animals. Larger doses of thyroxine increase degradation of protein in muscle even further. Under these conditions, the rates of proteolysis exceed rates of synthesis. Consequently, net muscle wasting occurs. To see if degradation of the receptor is controlled by the same factors as average muscle protein, we examined the rates of degradation of toxin bound to extrajunctional receptors in denervated hemidiaphragms from normal rats, from hypophysectomized rats, and from hypophysectomized rats treated with thyroxine.

Toxin loss was consistently slower in diaphragms of hypophysectomized animals than in those from normal animals (Fig. 3). Thus the decreased degradation seen 4 weeks after hypophysectomy suggests that the rate of receptor degradation is under hormonal influence. This effect was not reversed, however, even by treatment with large (catabolic)

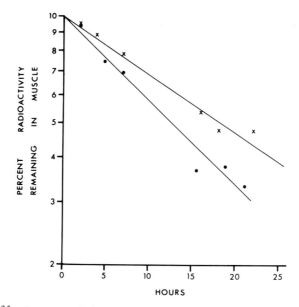

Fig. 3. Loss of ^{125}I-α-bungarotoxin bound to extrajunctional ACh receptors in denervated hemi-diaphragms of normal and hypophysectomized animals. Animals were hypophysectomized, as indicated, 1 month prior to culture. Left hemidiaphragms of 50–60 g. rats were then denervated and 5 days later were injected with ^{125}I-α-bungarotoxin and cultured as described in the legend to Fig. 2. Values from muscles from normal animals (●) and hypophysectomized animals (x) are plotted as indicated. Half-times of toxin loss were determined by least squares analysis of the data. Numbers on ordinate should be multiplied by 10.

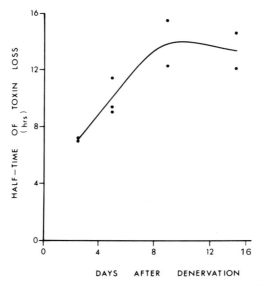

Fig. 4. Half-time of toxin loss from extrajunctional receptors at various times after denervation. Rats (40–50 g) were kept for 14 days and denervated at the indicated times before culture. Experiments were performed as described in the legend to Fig. 1, and half-times derived from least squares analysis of the data.

doses of thyroxine (Table I) in contrast to overall cell proteins. Further work will be required to determine the pituitary hormone (or hormones) that accelerates degradation of extrajunctional receptors. Possibly adrenal corticosteroids may be responsible for such effects, since they selectively promote atrophy of denervated muscles (38).

Even though hypophysectomy reduced the rate of receptor degradation, the level of receptor in both normal and denervated diaphragms was not changed by hypophysectomy (Table II). This result must indicate that hypophysectomy also decreases the rate of synthesis of extrajunctional receptor. Hypophysectomy has long been known to reduce overall protein synthesis in muscle, primarily because of a lack of pituitary growth hormone (39).

TABLE I. Effect of Hormones on Rate of ACh Receptor Degradation

	Half-time of toxin loss (hr)
Normal	13.4 ± 0.9 (6)
Hypophysectomized	19.6 ± 0.8 (4)*
Hypophysectomized and Thyroxine-treated	18.1 ± 1.0 (4)*†

Half-times were obtained as described in the legend to Fig. 3. Hypophysectomized animals were tested 4 weeks following the operation; Thyroxine-treated animals were given 200 ug/day for 6 days prior to testing. Values represent the mean $\pm$ S.E.M., and the number in parentheses indicates the number of muscles tested.

*values different from those of normal animals ($p < 0.02$).
†values not different from those of hypophysectomized animals ($p > 0.10$).

TABLE II. Binding of ^{125}I-α-Bungarotoxin in Innervated and Denervated Hemidiaphragms of Normal and Hypophysectomized Rats

	^{125}I-α-Bungarotoxin bound (fmoles/mg tissue)	
	Normal	Hypophysectomized
Innervated		
Junctional regions	4.6 ± 0.5 (4)	6.9 ± 0.8 (3)
Extrajunctional regions	1.5 ± 0.3 (4)	2.0 ± 0.4 (3)
Denervated		
Junctional regions	16.3 ± 1.6 (4)	15.2 ± 0.8 (3)
Extrajunctional regions	13.9 ± 0.8 (4)	10.8 ± 1.3 (3)

Muscles were incubated with ^{125}I-α-Bungarotoxin, washed, and divided into regions with and without endplates, as described previously (34). They were then weighed and counted in a gamma counter. Values represent the mean $\pm$ S.E.M., and the number in parentheses is the number of muscles examined in each case. In no case are the values from hypophysectomized animals different from those obtained with normal animals ($p > 0.05$).

REFERENCES

1. Rang, H. P., Quart, Rev. Biophysics 7:283 (1975).
2. Lee, C. Y., Tseng, L. F., and Chiu, T. H., Nature 215:1177 (1967).
3. Brockes, J. P., and Hall, Z. W., Biochemistry 14:2092 (1975).
4. Dolly, J. O., and Barnard, E. A., FEBS Lett. 57:267 (1975).

5. Karlin, A., and Cowburn, D. A., Proc. Nat. Acad. Sci. 70:3636 (1973).
6. Meunier, J. C., Sealock, R., Olsen, R., and Changeux, J.-P., Eur. J. Biochem. 45:371 (1974).
7. Raftery, M. A., Vandlen, R. L., Reed, K. L., and Lee, T., Cold Spring Harbor Symp. Quant. Biol. 40:193 (1975).
8. Porter, C. W., Chiu, T. H., Wieckowski, J., and Barnard, E. A., Nature (New Biol.) 241:3 (1973).
9. Porter, C. W., and Barnard, E. A., Exp. Neurol. 48:542 (1975).
10. Fertuck, H. C., and Salpeter, M. M., Proc. Nat. Acad. Sci. 71:1376 (1974).
11. Daniels, M. P., and Vogel, Z., Nature 254:339 (1975).
12. Fertuck, H. C., and Salpeter, M. M., J. Cell Biol. 69:144 (1976).
13. Frank, E., Gautvik, K., and Sommerschild, H., Acta Physiol. Scand. 95:66 (1975).
14. Axelsson, J., and Thesleff, S., J. Physiol. 188:53 (1959).
15. Miledi, R., J. Physiol. 151:1 (1960).
16. Diamond, J., and Miledi, R., J. Physiol. 162:393 (1962).
17. Hartzell, H. C., and Fambrough, D. M., J. Gen. Physiol. 60:248 (1972).
18. Lomo, T., and Rosenthal, J., J. Physiol. 221:493 (1972).
19. Drachman, D. B., and Witzke, F., Science 176:514 (1972).
20. Lomo, T., and Westgaard, R. H., J. Physiol. 252:603–626 (1975).
21. Thesleff, S., J. Physiol. 151:598 (1960).
22. Berg, D. K., and Hall, Z. W., J. Physiol. 244:659 (1975).
23. Chang, C. C., Chuang, S.-T., and Huang, M. C., J. Physiol. 250:161 (1975).
24. Beranek, R., and Vyskocil, F., J. Physiol. 188:53 (1967).
25. Lapa, S. J., Albuquerque, E. X., and Daly, J., Exp. Neurol. 43:375 (1974).
26. Brockes, J. P., and Hall, Z. W., Biochemistry 14:2100 (1975).
27. Katz, B., and Miledi, R., J. Physiol. 224:665 (1972).
28. Almon, R. R., and Appel, S. H., Biochem. Biophys. Acta 393:66 (1975).
29. Berg, D. K., and Hall, Z. W., Science 184:473 (1974).
30. Devreotes, P. N., and Fambrough, D. M., J. Cell Biol. 65:335 (1975).
31. Chang, C. C., and Huang, M. C., Nature 653:643 (1975).
32. Berg, D. K., and Hall, Z. W., J. Physiol. 252:771 (1975).
33. Hogan, P. H., Marshall, J. M., and Hall, Z. W., Nature 261:328 (1976).
34. Berg, D. K., Kelly, R. B., Sargent, P. B., Williamson, P., and Hall, Z. W., Proc. Nat. Acad. Sci. 69:147 (1972).
35. Griffin, G. E., and Goldberg, A. L., Science, in press.
36. Purves, D., and Sakmann, B., J. Physiol. 237:157 (1974).
37. Goldberg, A. L., Jablecki, C., and Li, J. B., Ann. N. Y. Acad. Sci. 228:190 (1974).
38. Goldberg, A., and Goodman, H. M., J. Physiol. 200:667 (1969).
39. Korner, A., Ann. N. Y. Acad. Sci. 148:408 (1968).

Cellular Neurobiology 217—226

The Morphogenesis of Spinal Ganglia From Neural Crest Cells

James A. Weston, John E. Pintar, Michael A. Derby, and David H. Nichols

Department of Biology, University of Oregon, Eugene, Oregon 94703

Neural crest cells migrate extensively in the vertebrate embryo before they differentiat into sensory or autonomic neurons, pigment cells, and various other neuroendocrine and nonneuronal derivatives. Some trunk neural crest cells migrate from their origin at the top of the neural tube ventrally along the lateral wall of the tube. Ultimately, these crest cells coalesce to form spinal ganglia. During their migration, crest cells appear to be surrounded by amorphous extracellular material. This material may be stained with Alcian blue at appropriate pH and ion concentrations, and depleted by specific enzymes that degrade glycosaminoglycans (GAG). The coalescence of crest cells into ganglia is accompanied by a relative decrease in Alcian blue staining material surrounding cells and an increase in close cell-cell association. Crest cells that migrate laterally between the somite and the ectoderm, however, remain dispersed and surrounded by higher levels of extracellular matrix material. Many of these cells differentiate into melanocytes.

When spinal and sympathetic ganglia are explanted in vitro, pigment cells often differentiate in the cultures. The cells that differentiate into melanocytes under these conditions appear to be the precursors of supportive cells within ganglia or nerve bundles. Pigment differentiation occurs when explanted ganglia are cultured under conditions that prevent or fail to maintain close cell association, whereas pigment cells often fail to differentiate when ganglia are cultured so that cell contact is preserved. Results will be presented that help to define both the specific cell interactions involved in regulating neurogenesis and melanogenesis by crest cells, and the environmental factors that affect such interactions.

Key words: neural crest, glycosaminoglycan, spinal ganglia, morphogenesis

INTRODUCTION

Vertebrate spinal and autonomic ganglia are derived from embryonic neural crest cells (1). This unique population of cells is also the developmental antecedent of a large number of other differentiated cell types, including neuroendocrine tissues such as the adrenal medulla and the calcitonin-producing ("C") cells (2), and the glial (Schwann sheath and satellite) cells of the peripheral nervous system. Integumental pigment cells and cells that form skeletal and connective tissue of the head and face (3) are also derivatives of the embryonic neural crest.

David H. Nichols is now at the Department of Zoology, University of Minnesota, Minneapolis, MN 55455.

There is now considerable evidence that crest cells are pluripotent in early migratory stages and, therefore, that the initial migration and subsequent differentiation is, at least partially, regulated by environmental conditions. The most compelling support for this conclusion is provided by the results of heterotopic grafting operations in which crest from one embryonic region is transplanted to another location. For example, Noden (4) has demonstrated that the precise migratory pathways followed by crest cells in the embryo are characteristic of particular axial levels; and that when labeled crest from one axial level of an embryo is grafted heterotopically into an unlabeled host, the pattern of cell migration corresponds to that characteristic of the graft site rather than that of the origin of the grafted crest cells. To some extent, then, the migratory pathways of crest cells may be specified by cues in their immediate environment (see also 1, 3, 5).

Likewise, the differentiation of neural crest cells into particular neuronal derivatives is influenced by local environmental conditions. This was recently shown by LeDouarin and her coworkers (6, 7) by means of heterotopic, interspecific (chick-quail) grafting procedures which utilized differences in nuclear staining properties to distinguish cells of chick or quail origin (8). Crest of the posterior metencephalic (postotic) axial region of avian embryos normally contributes some cells to the cholinergic enteric plexi of the gut, whereas crest from the mid-trunk region normally contributes some of its cells to the adrenergic neurons of the sympathetic chain and the adrenal medulla. When neural tubes from these two axial levels were exchanged in a series of grafting operations, the crest cells from the donors not only migrated but also differentiated as would crest cells normally arising in the host area. In this case, then, it appears that crest cells differentiate in response to environmental cues encountered during migration rather than in response to earlier cues (see also 14).

Crest cell differentiation can also be influenced by environmental cues in vitro. For example, regardless of their normal developmental capabilities or fates, whenever avian or amphibian crest cells are cultured without specific interactions with other embryonic components (9–11), most of the cultured crest cells will make pigment. However, if cranial neural crest is cultured in association with either pharyngeal endoderm (12) or extracellular products produced in vitro by retinal pigment epithelium (13), the cultures produce cartilage, a tissue formed in vivo by head crest. Moreover, sympathetic neurons will differentiate if trunk crest cells from chicken embryos are permitted to associate closely in vitro with somitic mesenchyme (14) that has been "conditioned" by suitable interactions with ventral neural tube tissue (15).

Differentiation of spinal ganglion neurons from cultured crest cells has not yet been demonstrated, although such neurons can be maintained in culture once the initial neurogenic events within spinal ganglia have occurred (16). However, metaplasia in cultures of spinal or sympathetic ganglia provides additional evidence that crest cells may be pluripotent and that local environmental factors continue to play an important role in eliciting the expression of particular crest phenotypes. Peterson and Murray reported, for example, that pigment cells frequently appeared in cultures of embryonic spinal ganglia (17). We have analyzed this phenomenon further and have suggested that the degree of dispersion (or conversely, the extent of association) of crest-derived cells plays a role in determining the differentiative pathway they follow (18–20). Additional information on this system will be presented below. In a similar culture system, Newgreen and Jones (21) have reported that catecholamine-containing sympathetic neurons can differentiate under certain conditions from cultured spinal ganglia, although they would never normally do so in vivo.

Finally, Patterson and his colleagues (22, and this volume) have reported that primary sympathetic neurons from neonatal rat superior cervical ganglia grown in the absence of other (nonneuronal) cell types normally found in the ganglion can synthesize and store the transmitter noradrenalin. In mixed cultures of these neurons and nonneuronal cells, however, the level of acetylcholine increases markedly — again suggesting that metaplasia of crest-derived cells depends on precise environmental interactions. The role of nonneuronal cells in the differentiation of ganglia is clearly complex. They have been reported to enhance neuron survival when dissociated spinal ganglion neurons are cultured in the absence of nerve growth factor (NGF) (23), for example, and additional insights into their own developmental capabilities will be presented below.

In this paper we will address two important questions concerning the early migration of neural crest cells and their contributions to peripheral ganglia. First, we will discuss the relationship between environmental factors (both cellular and extracellular) and cell movement and associations during initial phases of the morphogenesis of crest derivatives. Second, we will report some of our results that indicate how cell associations might affect cellular metaplasia in cultured spinal ganglia.

ROLE OF ENVIRONMENT IN CONTROLLING CREST CELL MIGRATION

The onset and extent of crest cell migration appear to be regulated by changes in the embryonic tissue environment. Thus, Pratt et al. (24) have recently shown that cranial crest cell migration is preceded by the appearance in the embryo of a cell-free space filled with an extracellular matrix rich in hyaluronic acid. Likewise, trunk neural crest cells begin to migrate from their origin at the top of the neural tube in close association with components of extracellular matrix. Initially, migrating crest cells associate closely with basement membranes of the neural tube and the overlying ectoderm (see 25). Subsequently, crest cells enter and are surrounded by a matrix of amorphous extracellular material. The glycosaminoglycan (GAG) components of this extracellular material (ECM) may be characterized qualitatively using both their specific interactions with the cationic dye Alcian blue at various magnesium ion concentrations (27), and its susceptibility to enzymes that selectively degrade GAG components of the matrix. The relative amounts of Alcian blue bound in histological sections may be estimated by microspectrophotometry, using the two-wavelength method (sec 32).

Initiation of Migration

Transverse sections of avian and murine embryos were examined at the stage and axial level where trunk crest cell migration had just begun. In the region of migrating crest cells there is considerable material that binds Alcian blue under conditions that allow all GAG to stain (0.1 M $MgCl_2$; pH 2.6). Microspectrophotometry (32) reveals that approximately 60% of this staining is lost when histological sections are pretreated with Streptomyces hyaluronidase that specifically degrades hyaluronic acid (26). In contrast, the amount of Alcian blue stain in the somitic region of these same embryo sections appears to be about one-third the amount found in the region of the neural crest, and only about 30% of this stain is susceptible to hyaluronidase treatment.

Likewise, when such sections are stained under conditions that are thought to limit reaction of the Alcian blue to sulfated material (0.3 M $MgCl_2$; pH 5.8) (27) microspectrophotometry indicates about twice as much stain in the crest region as in the somite. The

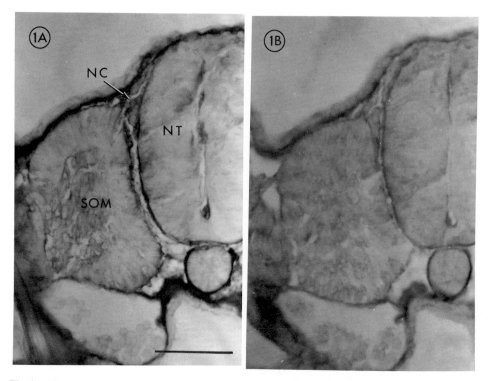

Fig. 1. Adjacent cross-sections through 14th somite of 20 somite paraffin-embedded quail embryo that had been fixed in 4% formaldehyde in 0.12 M Millonig's phosphate with 0.5% CPC and 0.5% PVP and stained for sulfated GAG as described in text. A) Buffer control: note greater Alcian blue stain in area where crest cells are initiating migration, compared to adjacent areas of neural tube and somite; B) Chondroitinase ABC digest: amounts of stain in crest area and adjacent areas still differ, but the same proportion of control values has been degraded in each area. NC = neural crest; NT = neural tube; SOM = somite; bar = 50 μ.

proportion of stain sensitive to Chondroitinase ABC, which degrades chondroitin sulfate and dermatan sulfate, is about the same in the two regions (Fig. 1).

From these results we infer the following: 1) there is more GAG in the region where crest cells begin to migrate than in nearby somite; 2) the proportion of hyaluronidase-sensitive stain (hyaluronic acid) in the region of the neural crest is more than twice that in the somite; and 3) the proportion of Chondroitinase ABC-sensitive stain (chondroitin sulfate and dermatan sulfate) is about the same in the two regions.

Restriction of Migration

Heterochronic grafts, in which crest cells were placed into developmentally older host regions, suggested that the extent of crest cell migration in the region of the somite is progressively restricted, and that this restriction is related to a change in the ability of the somitic region to support crest cell migration (28). It was of considerable interest, therefore, that when transverse sections of older embryos were examined, a different Alcian blue staining pattern was observed, which showed striking correlations with changes in crest cell morphogenetic behavior. Thus, photometric comparisons of Alcian blue staining in the region dorsolateral to the neural tube, and the region between the ectodermal

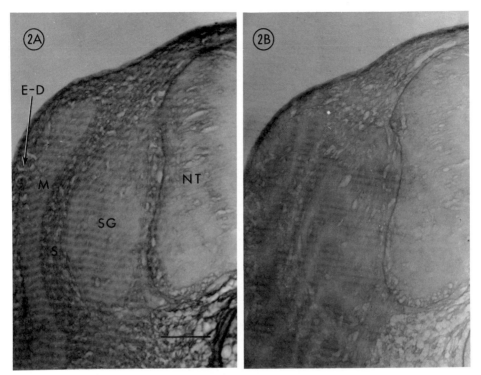

Fig. 2. Adjacent cross-sections through thoracic region (level of 18th ganglia) of Stage 23 quail embryo fixed and stained as in Fig. 1. A) Buffer control: note that there is relatively less stain in the spinal ganglion and other areas of compact cell masses (myotome and neural tube) compared to ectoderm-dermatome and sclerotome regions; B) Chondroitinase ABC digested: microspectrophotometry (see 32) reveals that a high proportion of stainable material in both ectoderm-dermatome and sclerotome regions is enzyme-sensitive. NT = neural tube; SG = sensory ganglion; E-D = ectoderm-dermatome region, M = myotome; S = sclerotome; bar = 50 μ.

epithelium and the dermatome, demonstrated that the extracellular material included both hyaluronic acid and sulfated GAG. Likewise, in somitic mesenchyme, Alcian blue staining matrix components were present, although in reduced amounts compared to the above regions. However, where crest cells had begun to coalesce to form spinal ganglia, significantly less Alcian blue staining was observed compared to the other regions (Fig. 2).

The pattern that emerges seems clear: early crest cell migration proceeds into extracellular spaces containing a variety of materials, including collagen, proteoglycans, and hyaluronic acid. Where crest cells remain dispersed, as appears to be the case for prospective melanoblasts under the ectodermal epithelium, the crest cells are surrounded by Alcian blue staining material. Where crest cells coalesce to form spinal ganglia, however, this close cell association seems to be correlated with a relative decrease of GAG in the extracellular matrix. It is not yet known whether the change in extracellular material actually precedes coalescence of crest cells into ganglia, but it is of some interest that the apparent loss in ability of the somitic region to support crest cell migration revealed by heterochronic grafting of crest (see above and 28), corresponds roughly in stage of development and in embryonic region (Stg. 25; midthoracic level of the chicken embryo) to the decrease in the proportion of hyaluronic acid in axial mesenchyme reported by Toole (29).

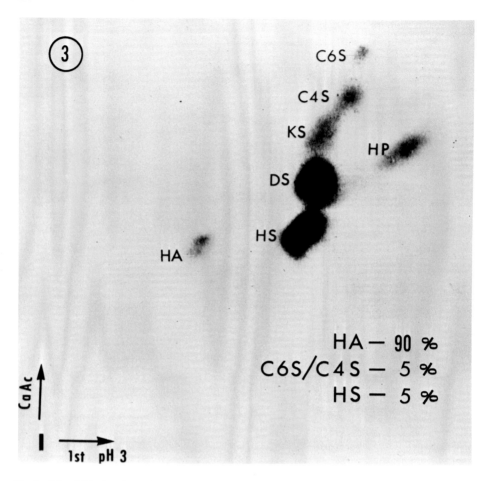

Fig. 3. After 24 hr in culture, isolated trunk crest cells were incubated in the presence of 10 μCi ^{3}H-glucosamine. GAG were isolated from the media after 24 hr and separated by 2 dimensional cellulose acetate electrophoresis (modified from [33]). Percentages were derived from counts co-migrating with authentic standards that were susceptible to enzymes specific for certain classes of GAG. HA = hyaluronic acid; HS = heparan sulfate; DS = dermatan sulfate; KS = keratan sulfate; C4S = chondroitin-4-sulfate; C6S = chondroitin-6-sulfate; HP = heparan.

SYNTHESIS OF GAG

The sources of GAG in the extracellular spaces are not known; nor is it known what mediates the changes in the amounts and proportions of GAG in different axial regions and at different times. However, several lines of evidence suggest that crest cells themselves make at least some of the hyaluronate found in the matrix. Thus, we have found that primary cultures of crest cells from explanted quail neural tubes cultured by standard methods (10, 11) incorporated ^{3}H-glucosamine largely into hyaluronic acid (Fig. 3). A small amount of sulfated GAG may also be made by crest cells in vitro. Similar results, using slightly different methods, have recently been obtained by Greenberg and Pratt (30) for cultured cranial neural crest cells. In contrast, cultures of somitic mesenchyme from the same embryos incorporate a larger percentage (up to 60%) of labelled precursors into chondroitin sulfate and other sulfated GAG, but seem to make hyaluronic acid as well. The pattern of synthesis by these tissues correlates well with observed Alcian blue staining that indicated the composition and relative proportions of GAG in the regions of crest cell migration and the somite.

CELL ASSOCIATION AND GANGLIOGENESIS

Coalescence of crest cells to form spinal ganglia within somitic mesenchyme is clearly accompanied by a local reduction of Alcian blue staining material. Loss of this extracellular material very likely favors cell association, which in turn appears to be involved in neuronal differentiation of crest cells (19, 23).

When it can first be excised from the embryo, the nascent sensory ganglion already contains several different cell types. These include large and small neurons and neuroblasts, as well as supportive (satellite and Schwann sheath) cells and their precursors. In addition, the ganglion is ultimately surrounded by a capsule of meningeal fibroblasts that probably arise from somitic mesenchyme. In light of the cellular metaplasia exhibited by cultured ganglia (see above, and 17, 18), it is of considerable interest to know the source(s) of the adventitious cell types, and the environmental conditions that promote their appearance.

Source of Pigment Cells in Ganglion Cultures

Cultures of 5-day spinal ganglia contain a characteristic population of small, stellate cells with intensely staining nuclei that strikingly resembles cultured crest cells (11, 31). These cells are clearly distinguishable from larger, fibroblastic (meningeal) cells, and from neuronal cells with which they are closely associated. Moreover, they are morphologically similar to the melanosome-containing pigment cells that appear in prolonged cultures of these 5-day ganglia. It seemed possible, therefore, that these small stellate cells were in fact the antecedents of the adventitious pigment cells that appear in cultured spinal ganglia. Since similar small cells with dark-staining nuclei are observed to associate closely with nerve fiber bundles in vivo and in vitro, it was possible to test for their ability to make pigment by culturing peripheral nerve removed from Stage 26 (5-day) chick embryos. Such explants contain the small stellate cells associated with nerve fibers, and some fibroblastic cells from the fiber sheath, but are usually devoid of nerve cell bodies or neuroblasts. In these cultures, the fibers soon degenerate, leaving behind on the substratum a population of the small stellate cells that resemble the cells observed in cultures of spinal ganglia. After several days in suitable culture medium, some of these cells undergo melanogenesis (Table I). These results suggest that at least one source of the pigment cells that appear in cultured spinal ganglia is the population of small stellate cells that normally associate with nerve cell bodies and fibers and that appear to be supportive (satellite or Schwann sheath) cells or their precursors.

Regulation of Melanogenesis in Cultured Ganglia

Close examination of ganglion cultures undergoing mealnogenesis reveals that pigment cells differentiate only in populations of small stellate cells that are not associated with neurons or fibers. To investigate further the relationship between cell association and melanogenesis, several types of experiments were performed. First, a variety of culture conditions were utilized that favored the dissociation of supportive cells from neurons. These conditions included: 1) cultures on plastic substrata of enzymatically

TABLE I. Melanogenesis in Cultured Peripheral Nerve*

Source	Days in culture	Number of cells counted	Number of melanocytes	Percent melanocytes
Spinal nerve (Stg. 26; 5 day)	6	968	164	19
Brachial plexus (Stg. 26; 5 day)	7	1,570	117	7

*From (31).

TABLE II. Melanogenesis in Spinal Ganglia Explanted on Plastic and Fibroblastic Substrata*

Substratum	Number of cells counted	Number of melanocytes	Percent melanocytes
Plastic	1,063	333	31.3
Fibroblasts	2,480	12	0.5

*From (20).

dissociated ganglia in a "permissive" medium containing serum and embryo extract; 2) cultures of intact young ganglia on plastic or collagen substrata in "permissive" media. Under these conditions, numerous small stellate cells were observed that were not associated with neurons or their fibers, and many of these cells formed pigment.

In contrast, when ganglia were cultured on (meningeal) fibroblastic substrata or on agar substrata, both of which favored the maintenance of association between nerve cells or fibers and supportive cells, melanogenesis did not occur even though the cultures were maintained in a "permissive" medium (Table II). Results from cultures of ganglia partially on a substratum of meningeal fibroblasts and partially on plastic were particularly instructive. Under nutritional conditions that are probably identical for all cells (although very short-range cellular effects may alter nutritional microenvironments), pigment appeared only in regions of the ganglion situated on plastic. On plastic substrata, many of the small stellate (supportive) cells seem to have deserted the neurons and fibers in favor of the plastic, whereas most of the supportive cells remained associated with nerves when the alternative substratum was a meningeal cell monolayer.

Finally, when ganglia were cultured in the initial absence of Nerve Growth Factor (NGF) activity, and then transferred to pigment-permissive medium, melanogenesis among the surviving cells, which had many fewer neurons left with which to associate, was enhanced (20).

These results are all compatible with the idea that some of the supportive cells had undergone metaplasia and that association between supportive cells and neurons was inimical to this process. They further suggest that when supportive cells, which normally associate closely with nerve cell bodies or fibers, are given access to alternative substrata in vitro, the choice is not made at random. The preference of supportive cells or their precursors for neurons over meningeal fibroblasts suggests that meninges may normally promote gangliogenesis in vivo by preventing association of supporting cells with each other, more "seductive" substrata, thereby preventing such tissue disruption as occurs on artifical substrata in vitro.

CONCLUSIONS

In general, then, these results further buttress the idea that crest cells are pluri-potent initially, and that some remain so for a considerable period during development. Further, the results suggest how one aspect of cell social behavior — cell association — might affect cell differentiation, and how this, in turn, might be regulated by environ-mental factors: crest cells migrate into embryonic tissue spaces filled with extracellular material composed of collagens, proteoglycans, and glycosaminoglycans. Hyaluronic acid, an important GAG constituent that is plentiful in regions where early crest migration occurs (24), may be produced, in part, by crest cells themselves immediately preceding the onset of migration. The hyaluronate-rich extracellular matrix provides a medium that seems to favor crest cell proliferation and locomotion and tends to keep the cells apart. Later, there is a change in the ability of the somitic region to support crest cell migration that may be correlated with a decrease in the proportion of hyaluronic acid in the extra-cellular matrix. In any case, the coalescence of crest cells into coherent ganglia is seen to be accompanied by a dramatic local reduction in Alcian blue staining material. The cell associations that result from this coalescence favor neuron and supportive cell differentia-tion and survival. Conversely, the disruption of these associations that sometimes occurs when attractive alternative substrata are presented in vitro, leads still-pluripotent crest-derived cells to embark on other differentiative pathways.

REFERENCES

1. Weston, J. A., Adv. Morph. 8:41−114 (1970).
2. LeDouarin, N., and LeLievre, C., C. R. Acad. Sci., Paris, Ser. D. 270:2857−2860 (1970).
3. Johnston, M. C., Bhakdinaronk, A., and Reid, Y. C., in "Fourth Symposium on Oral Sensation and Perception." J. F. Bosma (Ed.). USGPO (1974).
4. Noden, D., Devel. Biol. 42:106−130 (1975).
5. Weston, J. A., Devel. Biol. 6:279−310 (1963).
6. LeDouarin, N., Teillet, M., and LeDouarin, G., P.N.A.S. 72:728−732 (1975).
7. LeDouarin, N., Devel. Biol. 30:217−222 (1973).
8. LeDouarin, N., and Barg, L., C. R. Acad. Sci., Paris, Ser. D. 269:1543−1546 (1969).
9. Dorris, F., W. Roux Arch. f. Entwick-Mech. 138:323−335 (1938).
10. Cohen, A., and Konigsberg, I., Devel. Biol. 46:262−280 (1975).
11. Maxwell, C., Devel. Biol. 49:66−79 (1976).
12. Drews, U., Kocher-Becker, U., and Drews, U., W. Roux Arch. f. Entwick-Mech. 171:17−37 (1972).
13. Newsome, D., Devel. Biol. 49:476−507 (1976).
14. Cohen, A., J. Exp. Zool. 179:167−182 (1972).
15. Norr, S., Devel. Biol. 34:16−38 (1973).
16. Okun, L., J. Neurobiology 3:111−151 (1972).
17. Petersen, F., and Murray, M., Am. J. Anat. 96:319−355 (1955).
18. Cowell, L., and Weston, J. A., Devel. Biol. 22:670−697 (1970).

19. Weston, J. A., in "Cellular Aspects of Growth and Differentiation in Nervous Tissue." D. Pease (Ed.). U.C.L.A. Forum in Medical Sciences 14:1−22 (1971).
20. Nichols, D., Kaplan, R., and Weston, J. A., (in preparation).
21. Newgreen, D., and Jones, R., J. Emb. Exp. Morph. 33:43−56 (1975).
22. Patterson, P., Reichardt, L., and Chun, L., Cold Spring Harbor Symposium on Quant. Biology. 40: 389−398 (1975).
23. Burnham, P., Raiborn, C., and Varon, S., P.N.A.S. 69:3556−3560 (1972).
24. Pratt, R., Larsen, M., and Johnston, M. C., Devel. Biol. 44:298−305 (1975).
25. Cohen, A., and Hay, E., Devel. Biol. 26:578−605 (1971).
26. Pintar, J., Derby, M., and Weston, J., J. Cell Biol. 70:371a (1976).
27. Scott, J., and Dorling, J., Histochemie 5:221−233 (1965).
28. Weston, J., and Butler, S., Devel. Biol. 14:246−266 (1966).
29. Toole, B., Devel. Biol. 29:321−329 (1972).
30. Greenberg, J., and Pratt, R., (submitted; personal communication).
31. Nichols, D., and Weston, J. A., (in preparation).
32. Pollister, A. W., Swift, H., and Rasch, E., in "Physical Techniques in Biological Research," A. W. Pollister (Ed.). V. III (c), pp. 201−251 (1969).
33. Hata, R., and Nagai, Y., Anal. Biochem. 45:62−468 (1972).

Selective Enzymatic Hydrolysis of Nerve Terminal Phospholipids by β-Bungarotoxin: Biochemical and Morphological Studies

Peter N. Strong*, John E. Heuser[+], and Regis B. Kelly *[+]

*Departments of *Biochemistry and Biophysics and [+]Physiology, University of California, San Francisco, California 94143*

β-Bungarotoxin, a presynaptic protein neurotoxin isolated from the venom of the snake Bungarus multicinctus, modifies release of neurotransmitter at the neuromuscular junction. The toxin has a potent phospholipase activity toward both natural membranes and phospholipid liposomes. Studies of ionic requirements and selective chemical modification demonstrate that β-bungarotoxin can only modify synaptic transmission under conditions in which the phospholipase is active. Morphological studies on frog cutaneous pectoris neuromuscular junctions incubated with β-toxin and horseradish peroxidase-conjugated β-toxin support the hypothesis that β-toxin specifically interacts with presynaptic plasma membranes and selectively hydrolyzes nerve terminal phospholipids.

Key words: neurotoxin, phospholipase A$_2$, synaptic transmission, freeze fracture, horseradish peroxidase

INTRODUCTION

A number of animal and bacterial toxins have now been found to block transmitter secretion from motor nerve terminals (1–3). These toxins are being actively studied to gain information on the molecular processes with which they interfere. We have been particularly concerned with one of these neurotoxins, β-bungarotoxin (4–9), since this toxin is calcium-dependent (9). We hoped to use this toxin to discover the molecular events that underlie excitation-secretion coupling, since, in many other secretory tissues (10) as well as at the synapse, secretion is triggered by calcium influx across the plasma membrane (11).

In this paper, we review some previous findings from our laboratory and provide some new biochemical, electrophysiological and anatomical evidence, which, taken together, have led us to hypothesize that the endogenous phospholipase activity of β-bungarotoxin is responsible for its presynaptic toxicity. We also present some ideas and speculative models at the molecular level, to account for our observations that phospholipases in general do not modify neurotransmitter release.

MATERIALS AND METHODS

Reagents

Crude venom from the snake Bungarus multicinctus was obtained from the Ross Allen Reptile Institute, Silver Springs, Florida. Soybean phosphatidylcholine was the gift of Dr. M. Eikermann (Nattermann and Co., Cologne). Purified Vipera russellii phospholipase A_2 was the gift of Dr. J. Salach (Veterans Administration Hospital, San Francisco). Sodium deoxycholate, horseradish peroxidase, N-bromosuccinimide, diaminobenzidine and 4-bromophenacyl bromide were obtained from Sigma; sodium cyanoborohydride was obtained from Apache Chemicals.

Purification of β-Bungarotoxin

The toxin was purified to homogeneity, as previously described (5,12). Purified toxin was stored at $20°C$ in 50% (v/v) ethylene glycol/Tris-HCl (10 mM, pH 7.6) without loss of activity over 6 months.

Phospholipase A Assay

Phospholipase A activities were measured as previously described (12) using a pH-stat (Radiometer) and measuring the linear rates of phospholipid hydrolysis of pH 8.0 and $37°C$.

Electrophysiological Recording

Synaptic events were recorded intracellularly from muscle fibers of the rat diaphragm as previously described (5,9). The data from all cells with resting potentials below -60 mV and with detectable miniature end plate potentials were used without further selection in calculating average values and standard errors. All measurements were made at $22-25°C$.

Chemical Modification Studies

Twenty μl of β-toxin (1.8 mg/ml) was diluted to 1 ml in 100 mM NaCl, 10 mM sodium cacodylate buffer (pH 6.0), and either 5 μl of 4-bromophenacyl bromide (14 mM in acetone, 40 molar excess) or 5 μl of N-bromosuccinimide (1.4 mM in acetone, 4 molar excess) was added. Each reaction was shaken at $37°C$ and, at regular intervals, 20 μl aliquots were removed and assayed for phospholipase activity. The control consisted of incubating the buffered β-toxin solution with 5 μl of acetone at $37°C$. Immediately after the last time point was taken from each reaction, an aliquot (200–900 μl) was injected intraperitoneally into mice and the toxicity of the sample determined, as previously described (5).

Treatment of Erythrocytes With β-Toxin

Fresh human erythrocytes from acid-citrate dextrose treated blood were centrifuged (10 min, 3,000 × g, $0°C$) and washed 4 times in buffer ($0°C$, 150 mM NaCl, 0.25 mM $CaCl_2$, 0.25 mM $MgCl_2$, 0.05 mM Tris-HCl, pH 7.4). One ml of packed erythrocytes were then washed again in calcium-free medium (150 mM NaCl, 1 mM EDTA, 0.05 mM Tris-HCl, pH 7.4) and then incubated with 25 μl β-toxin (4.0 mg/ml, final toxin concentration 100 $\mu g/ml$).

Trapping of β-Toxin Inside Resealed Ghosts

The method is that of Zwaal et al. (13), with slight modifications. Fresh human erythrocytes were washed 4 times in calcium buffer as above. After centrifugation, 10 ml of packed cells were lysed (5 min, 0°C) with 72 ml of 10 mM NaCl, 1 mM EDTA, 0.05 mM Tris-HCl, pH 7.4. The hemolysate was centrifuged (10 min, 0°C, 12,000 X g) and two-thirds of the supernatant was removed. The ghosts were resuspended and a 10 ml aliquot was incubated with 250 μl β-toxin (4.0 mg/ml, final toxin concentration 100 μg/ml) for 5 min at 0°C. The ghosts were subsequently resealed by addition of 1.5 ml of 1 M NaCl, stirring for 5 min at 0°C. The resealed cells were then stirred gently at 37°C for 1 hr and washed 4 times with 150 mM NaCl (centrifuged 10 min, 12,000 X g, 0°C). Controls were resealed in the absence of toxin.

Lysis of Intact and Resealed Cells

One ml of packed cells (either intact or resealed, treated with β-toxin or untreated controls) were suspended in 5 ml 150 mM NaCl, 5 mM $CaCl_2$ 0.05 mM Tris-HCl, pH 7.4 at 37°C while stirring. At given time intervals, 200 μl aliquots of the suspension were washed with 5 ml 150 mM NaCl, centrifuged (10 min, 12,000 X g, 0°C), and the optical density of the supernatants read at 418 nm. Further 200 μl aliquots were washed with 5 ml water and centrifuged, in order to determine 100% lysis.

Synthesis of Horseradish Peroxidase-Toxin Conjugates

The method used was essentially that of Nakane and Kawaoi (14) and Lentz et al. (15), but with three important differences: 1) Coupling of either α-bungarotoxin or β-bungarotoxin to peroxidase (1:1 molar ratio) was carried out in 50 mM potassium phosphate, pH 7.5, for 12 hr at 4°C. 2) Reduction of the intermediate Schiff's base was performed using a 10 molar excess of 0.3 M sodium cyanoborohydride (50 mM potassium phosphate pH 7.5, 4°C, 2 hr). 3) Reducing agent and protein conjugate were separated on a Sephadex G-25 column (50 mM potassium phosphate, pH 7.5, eluant) immediately after the reduction step and before application of the protein conjugate to a Sephadex G-200 column. β-Toxin conjugates were assayed for phospholipase activity as described above.

Preparation of Samples for Electron Microscopy

Cutaneous pectoris nerve-muscle preparations were dissected from small Rana pipiens, pinned down and maintained in Ringers solution (116 mM NaCl, 2 mM KCl, 2 mM $CaCl_2$, 0.5 mM NaH_2PO_4, 3 mM glucose, 5 mM HEPES, pH 7.2). After incubation with β-toxin (20 μg/ml) in the above Ringers solution for given periods of time, samples were fixed in 2% formaldehyde and 1% glutaraldehyde in a modified Ringers solution containing 30 mM HEPES buffer and 5 mM $CaCl_2$. Thin sections or freeze-fracture replicas were subsequently prepared as previously described (16). All freeze-fracture illustrations are positive images so that regions of platinum deposition appear dark while absence of platinum appears light. Prints are mounted with the source of platinum shadowing below. Horseradish peroxidase β-bungarotoxin conjugates (at concentrations of equivalent phospholipase activity to that used for β-toxin) and α-bungarotoxin conjugates were incubated with muscles in an analogous manner to that described above. Standard procedures used to localize horseradish peroxidase (17) were modified as previously described (18).

RESULTS

Purification of β-Bungarotoxin and Characterization of Phospholipase Activity on "Unnatural" Membranes

Crude venom from the krait, Bungarus multicinctus, was applied to a CM-50 Sephadex ion-exchange column and eluted with a linear ammonium acetate salt gradient (Fig. 1). Absorbances corresponding to α-bungarotoxin and β-bungarotoxin are labeled. The peak corresponding to β-toxin was subsequently purified to homogeneity on a CM-cellulose ion-exchange column. Criteria for purity include SDS-polyacrylamide gel electrophoresis, isoelectric focusing, and chromatography on phosphocellulose and Sephadex G-50 columns. Our toxin preparation has about 50% the specific activity (240 μeq fatty acid per min/mg protein in the latest preparations) of the most potent phospholipase that we have assayed (V. russellii) (12).

The phospholipase activity of β-bungarotoxin has been characterized using both soybean and saturated egg phosphatidyl choline as substrate in the presence of sodium deoxycholate as a dispersive agent (12,19). Multilamellar phospholipid liposomes, and unilamellar liposomes prepared according to Batzri and Korn (20), were equally effective physical forms of the substrates. Phospholipase activity was measured using the pH-stat technique essentially according to the procedures developed by de Haas et al. (21) and Wells (22). Under our assay conditions, the hydrolysis of phosphatidylcholine is zero order, and in the range of toxin concentrations, 0.5–20 nM, the rate of substrate hydroly-

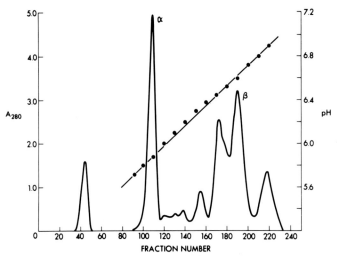

Fig. 1. CM-50 Sephadex ion exchange chromatography of Bungarus multicinctus venom. Five hundred mg of crude, lyophilized venom was dissolved in 6 ml of NH$_4$OAc buffer (0.05 M, pH 5.0) and centrifuged for 15 min (39,000 × g, 4°C). The pellet was discarded and the supernatant applied to a CM-50 Sephadex column (37 × 2 cm diam), previously equilibrated with 0.05 M NH$_4$OAc (pH 5.0). The column was eluted with 200 ml of the same buffer, and subsequently with an 800 ml linear salt gradient, 0.05 M NH$_4$OAc (pH 5.0) to 1.0 M NH$_4$OAc (pH 7.0). Five ml fractions were collected (16 ml/hr) and the absorbance of each fraction was measured at 280 nm. The fractions corresponding to β-bungarotoxin (182–197) were pooled, desalted and concentrated (Amicon UM2 membrane) and subsequently applied to a CM-cellulose ion-exchange column, whereupon 89% of the protein eluted as a single component (12). This major peak was homogeneous as evidenced by further chromatographic and electrophoretic criteria (12). All operations were carried out at 4°C.

sis is linearly related to toxin concentration (12). The phospholipase activity of β-bun-garotoxin has an ionic requirement for calcium (23), in common with phospholipases isolated from such diverse sources such as snake venom (24), mammalian pancreatic tissue or juice (25), and bee venom (26). Strontium behaves as a competitive inhibitor of calcium, whereas magnesium has no influence on the enzymatic activity in the presence of calcium (Strong and Kelly, manuscript in preparation). Using egg phosphatidylcholine specifically tritiated in the 2-acyl side chain, we have shown that β-toxin hydrolyzes only the ester linkage at the 2 position, and can therefore be characterized as a phospholipase A_2 (12,19).

Phospholipase Activity of β-Bungarotoxin on "Natural" Membranes

Although the phospholipase activity of β-toxin is measured on synthetic phospholipid membranes in the presence of the surfactant, sodium deoxycholate, the enzymatic activity is not restricted to such artificial systems. We have previously shown that β-toxin and Crotalus adamanteus phospholipase A_2 inhibit liver mitochondrial function at similar rates (19). In the experiment outlined below, we demonstrate the toxin's phospholipase activity, using erythrocyte membranes.

Van Deenen's laboratory (13,27,28) has shown that pancreatic phospholipase A_2 produces neither hemolysis nor hydrolysis of phospholipids when exposed to intact human erythrocytes. However, when this phospholipase is trapped inside resealed ghosts (in the presence of EDTA), subsequent addition of calcium (to activate the enzyme) leads to hemolysis and phospholipid hydrolysis of the resealed cell.

Figure 2 shows a time course of similar experiments using β-bungarotoxin instead of pancreatic phospholipase A_2. Erythrocytes were lysed and resealed in the presence of β-toxin and EDTA; calcium was added at zero time to activate the toxin's phospholipase activity from the inside. Intact erythrocytes were washed with EDTA, treated with β-toxin and then calcium added to the incubation medium as before. Hemolysis of resealed cells with toxin trapped inside them, proceeded linearly with time after an initial lag and was complete after 7 hr. By comparison, a control of cells resealed in the absence of toxin was only 25% lysed. Intact erythrocytes incubated with toxin showed only about 7% lysis after this time period, which is indistinguishable from a control incubation in the absence of toxin. Although the resealed ghosts are certainly more susceptible to hemolysis under these conditions than is the intact erythrocyte, the ability of the toxin, in a manner exactly analogous to pancreatic phospholipase A_2, to distinguish between the inner and outer membrane phospholipids is clearly demonstrated.

The hemolysis that we observe in our control preparation of resealed ghosts might be due to contamination by a population of ghosts that remain leaky; there is much evidence to support the notion that a ghost suspension cannot be considered homogeneous (29). Passow and collaborators have distinguished between 3 types of ghosts (30,31). Under our lysis conditions we have been optimizing for Type II ghosts, which reseal after reversal of the hemolysis procedure on the addition of alkali ions (13).

Phospholipase Activity is Responsible for Physiological Modification of Transmitter Release

Electrophysiological evidence. Before β-bungarotoxin totally blocks secretion from motor nerve terminals, it causes a small increase in the rate of spontaneous and evoked transmitter release, which we measured to be around a 5-fold increase in spontaneous miniature end plate potential (m.e.p.p.) frequency and a 10-fold increase in the

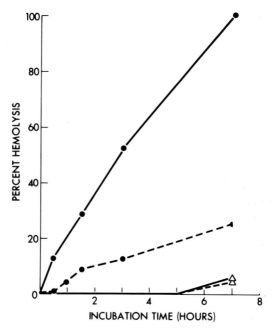

Fig. 2. The ability of β-toxin to distinguish between inner and outer membrane phospholipids. One ml of packed red blood cells in Ca^{++}-free media (intact + toxin outside ——Δ——; intact control — — —Δ— — —; resealed + toxin inside ——●——; resealed control — — —●— — —) (see the Methods section) were suspended in Ca^{++}-media (5 ml of 150 mM NaCl, 5 mM $CaCl_2$ 0.05 mM Tris-HCl pH 7.4) at 37°C at zero time. Two hundred μl aliquots of the stirred suspension were removed at given time intervals, washed with 5 ml of 150 mM NaCl at 4°C, and centrifuged for 10 min (12,000 × g, 4°C). The optical density of the supernatants was read at 418 nm. Further 200 μl aliquots were washed with 5 ml of distilled water, centrifuged, and the optical density of the supernatant read in order to determine 100% hemolysis.

quantal content of end plate potentials (e.p.p.'s) evoked in low calcium solutions (4,5,32). This transient increase in secretion did not occur in calcium-free solutions, however (9). The explanation of this could be that calcium is always necessary to trigger transmitter release and thus to reveal the toxin's effects; alternatively, the toxin might require calcium before it can act on the nerve terminal.

The following results have shown us that the latter explanation is correct. We have found that calcium, in the range of 2–10 mM, is necessary to activate the phospholipase activity of β-bungarotoxin (12,19). Other divalent cations such as magnesium and strontium cannot substitute for calcium (12). Thus we could take advantage of the fact that strontium can substitute for calcium in triggering transmitter release from motor nerve terminals (33) and design an experiment to study the effects of β-bungarotoxin in strontium-Ringers solution, in which the phospholipase activity of the toxin is blocked.

We recorded intracellularly from muscle fibers of rat phrenic nerve-diaphragm preparations and raised the extracellular potassium concentration to 15 mM in order to increase the frequency of miniature end plate potentials and so facilitate more accurate measurements. Figure 3A shows that when we added β-bungarotoxin to a normal calcium-bathed preparation, the m.e.p.p. frequency rose and subsequently slowly fell; after 2 hr the m.e.p.p. frequency was significantly below the average frequency in a control preparation analyzed simultaneously. In contrast, Fig. 3B shows that when we added

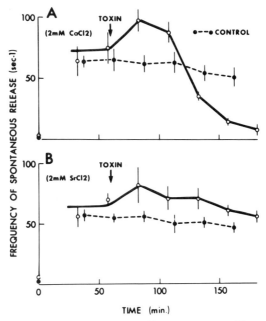

Fig. 3. Comparison of spontaneous release rates in Ca^{++} (Fig. 3A) and Sr^{++} (Fig. 3B) after treatment of a rat phrenic nerve-diaphragm preparation with β-bungarotoxin. The preparation was depolarized by K^+ to increase the m.e.p.p. frequency either in 2 mM Ca^{++} (19 mM K^+) or 2 mM Sr^{++} (15 mM K^+). Following a 15 min exposure to the toxin (20 μg/ml, application point indicated), the preparation was returned to a toxin-free solution containing the appropriate ion. Measurements of m.e.p.p. frequency of successively impaled muscle fibers were begun 30 min after transferring to depolarizing solutions and were pooled and averaged over 25 min intervals throughout the experiment (—○—○—). M.e.p.p. frequencies from control experiments (identically treated preparations except for the omission of toxin) were followed in a similar manner (– – –●– – –●– – –). Each point represents data recorded from 12–15 muscle fibers, and the bars represent the SEM.

β-bungarotoxin to a strontium-bathed preparation, m.e.p.p. frequency did not increase significantly at early times and did not decline to less than the control at long time periods. Thus in strontium, when its phospholipase activity is inhibited, β-bungarotoxin does not block secretion. Although its phospholipase activity is necessary for β-bungarotoxin's toxicity, it is not sufficient; we have previously shown that many phospholipases A_2 are not lethal when injected intraperitoneally into mice (12). Similarly, "normal" phospholipases do not modify synaptic transmission; a comparison of results from the previous experiment (Fig. 3) and from a similar experiment using purified V. russellii phospholipase A_2 is shown in Fig. 4. M.e.p.p. frequencies were compared at the end of a 2 hr exposure to either β-toxin or V. russellii enzyme. In strontium media, both phospholipases showed a m.e.p.p. frequency that was indistinguishable from a control preparation; in calcium media however, V. russellii phospholipase did not alter the m.e.p.p. frequency from the untreated control, in sharp distinction to the low levels of spontaneous transmitter release observed in the β-toxin poisoned preparation.

  Biochemical evidence. Another approach we have used to demonstrate that the phospholipase activity of β-bungarotoxin is responsible for its physiological toxicity has been to modify the toxin chemically and then determine whether it still blocks neurosecretion. In particular, we have used the specific amino acid modifying reagents

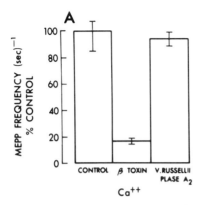
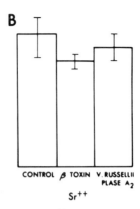

Fig. 4. Comparison of spontaneous release rates in Ca^{++} (Fig. 4A) and Sr^{++} (Fig. 4B) after treatment of a rat phrenic nerve-diaphragm preparation with either β-bungarotoxin or Vipera russellii phospholipase A_2. Firstly, the experiment in Fig. 3 was repeated using V. russellii phospholipase (20 $\mu g/ml$) instead of β-toxin. In this figure we have then compared data from the 2 experiments, viz. the m.e.p.p. frequencies 2 hr after the initial incubation with either enzyme. Each bar represents data recorded from 12–15 muscles over a 25 min period and the bars represent the SEM. M.e.p.p. frequencies in control samples after 2 hr were 50 ± 4 (2 mM Ca^{++}) and 46 ± 5 (2 mM Sr^{++}).

N-bromosuccinimide and 4-bromophenacyl bromide, which have been shown to destroy the enzymatic activity of other phospholipases A_2 (34, 35).

N-bromosuccinimide preferentially oxidizes tryptophan residues at pH 6 (36) requiring 2–4 moles of oxidizing agent per tryptophan residue. Usually, 4-bromophenacyl bromide is a nonspecific alkylating agent; however, this reagent has been shown to specifically modify histidine-53 of pancreatic phospholipase A_2 (34).

Figure 5 shows that N-bromosuccinimide, at a molar concentration 4 times that of the toxin, inhibited the phospholipase activity of β-bungarotoxin within 20 min at 37°C, while a 40-fold excess of 4-bromophenacyl bromide inhibited β-bungarotoxin more slowly. Incubating β-bungarotoxin with a 5 μl aliquot of acetone as a control did not affect its enzymatic activity. Table I shows that such chemical inhibition of β-bungarotoxin's phospholipase activity resulted in a corresponding diminution in its toxicity when injected intraperitoneally into mice. These chemical modification studies and those of others (37) provide further evidence for the idea that the phospholipase activity of β-bungarotoxin is necessary for its toxicity.

Morphological evidence. Although insufficient by itself, morphological evidence of disrupted membrane structure, hopefully specific to the nerve terminal, would provide compelling evidence for our hypothesis of enzyme-mediated neurotoxicity, when coupled with our previous biochemical and electrophysiological observations.

We have studied the effects of β-toxin on frog cutaneous pectoris neuromuscular preparations,* using both freeze-fracture replicas (Figs. 7–9) and more conventionally fixed thin sections (Figs. 10–15), in the electron microscope. In preliminary studies, we have also coupled horseradish peroxidase to both α- and β-bungarotoxins in order to examine the cellular locations of these toxins at the neuromuscular junction (Figs. 16–19).

*We have shown (Strong & Kelly, unpublished observations) that the electrophysiological responses of frog and rat neuromuscular junction preparations to the toxin are qualitatively similar. Both show a small increase in m.e.p.p. frequency prior to failure with similar time courses.

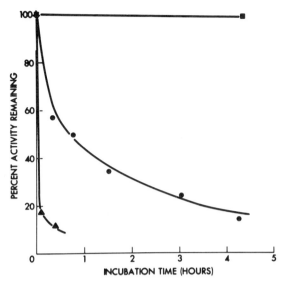

Fig. 5. Inhibition of β-bungarotoxin's phospholipase activity by chemical modification. Twenty μl of β-toxin (1.8 mg/ml) was diluted to 1 ml in buffer (100 mM NaCl, 10 mM sodium cacodylate, pH 6.0), and either 5 μl of 4-bromophenacyl bromide (14 mM in acetone, 40 molar excess, ——●——) or 5 μl of N-bromosuccinimide (1.4 mM in acetone, 4 molar excess, ——▲——) were added at zero time. Each reaction was shaken at 37°C and, at regular intervals, 20 μl aliquots were removed and assayed for phospholipase activity in the normal manner. The control (——■——) consisted of incubating the buffered toxin solution with 5 μl of acetone at 37°C. Activity of 100% represents unmodified toxin, specific activity 240 μeq/min/mg protein.

TABLE I. Toxicity and Enzymatic Activity of Chemically Modified β-Bungarotoxin

| | % Activity of unmodified toxin | |
Reagent	Phospholipase activity	Toxicity
Control	99	98
4-Bromophenacyl bromide	15	< 7
N-Bromosuccinimide	12	< 5

Chemical modification of β-bungarotoxin and determination of the phospholipase activity and toxicity of the modified derivatives was carried out as described in the Methods section and the legend to Fig. 5.

Muscles fixed a few min after the time when their twitch in response to nerve stimulation became completely blocked, contained nerve terminals with a whole range of structural changes. The more mild of these changes included an alteration in the appearance of the plasma membrane, both in thin-section and freeze-fracture views, and an alteration in the appearance of intracellular filaments. More severe changes also appeared to have occurred in some nerve terminals, which were frankly ruptured or reduced to thin skeletons of their former dimensions as a result of total dissolution of their membrane-rich secretory regions.

Figures 11–15 illustrate the range of subtle changes in nerve membranes and filaments that were the first morphological clue of nerve terminal damage by β-bungarotoxin.

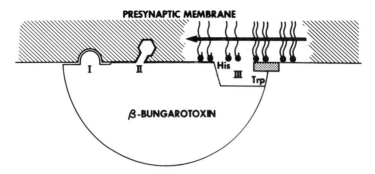

Fig. 6. A model to account for β-bungarotoxin's enzymatic action on nerve terminal membranes. Site I is a recognition site on β-toxin, specific for a receptor on presynaptic plasma membranes. Sites II and III constitute the enzymatic locus, common to β-toxin and conventional phospholipases. β-Toxin is only enzymatically active at a defined interface and this is realized in site II, a lipid-water recognition site. Site III is a catalytic site to which calcium and divalent metal ion inhibitors bind (▨); this third site possesses tryptophan and histidine residues which are essential for enzymatic activity. After β-toxin has become immobilized at the presynaptic membrane (site I), and the orientation of the toxin molecule has satisfied the lipid-water recognition site (II), the catalytic site (III) is activated by binding calcium; neighboring membrane phospholipids are hydrolyzed as they laterally diffuse across the membrane in the vicinity of site III (indicated by arrow).

The plasma membrane became progressively more electron-dense and thus apparently thicker in the thin-section image. Presumably this was because either the lipid or the protein in the membrane reacted more intensely with osmium tetroxide. Freeze-fracture (Fig. 8) of the membrane during this same time period showed many more intramembranous particles than usual. These were of the large size class which is also normally found in synaptic vesicle membranes and at the "active" secretogenous zones of the plasma membrane (Fig. 7). Possibly this increase in particles was the cause of the membrane's increased osmophilia. We do not know whether the particles are protein or lipid, or whether the particle increase was due to an addition of new particles or to the subtraction of intervening flat planar zones leading to the concentration of preexisting particles. We have some evidence that the particles are not the toxin molecules themselves, inserted in the membrane, since nerve terminals exposed to toxin for only a few min and then washed extensively still showed a progressive increase in particle concentration. This observed change was thus a consequence of toxin action.

Prolonged exposure to the toxin led to increased fragility of the presynaptic membrane as indicated by our many electron micrographs of broken membranes in thin-sections and in freeze-fractures (Figs. 8 and 9). In late stages we found complete rupture of the nerve terminal with vesicles and other membrane debris spilling out into the synaptic cleft (Fig. 9). In such freeze-fracture views, many of the membrane fragments contained no intramembranous particles at all (arrows, Fig. 9), as if they represented pure phospholipids solubilized from the presynaptic membrane by the action of the β-bungarotoxin. Often all that remained of the nerve terminal was the thin axial core of neurofilaments and microtubules (Fig. 15), surrounded by a very electron-dense membrane of extremely reduced surface area, and, again, very rich in intramembranous particles.

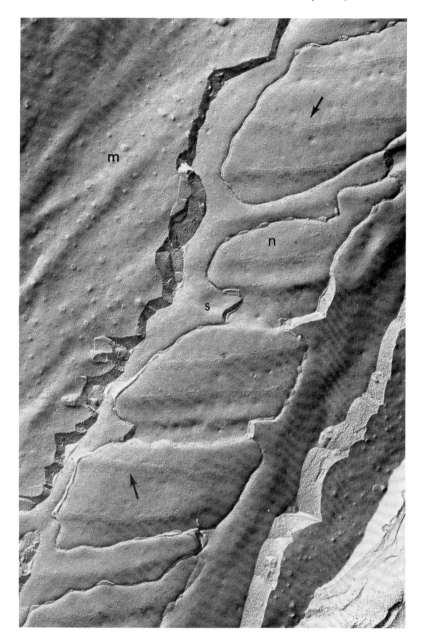

Fig. 7. Freeze-fracture of a normal motor nerve terminal (n) from an untreated frog cutaneous pectoris muscle (m). This view of the cytoplasmic leaflet of the presynaptic plasmalemma (the "A-face") reveals rows of large intramembranous particles which characterize the "active" or secreto-genous zones of this synapse (arrows) and the normal distribution of Schwann cell processes (s), which typically embrace the nerve terminal between every few active zones. Note that intramembranous particles are no more abundant in the nerve membrane, except at the active zones, than they are on the Schwann cell processes. (× 21,600.)

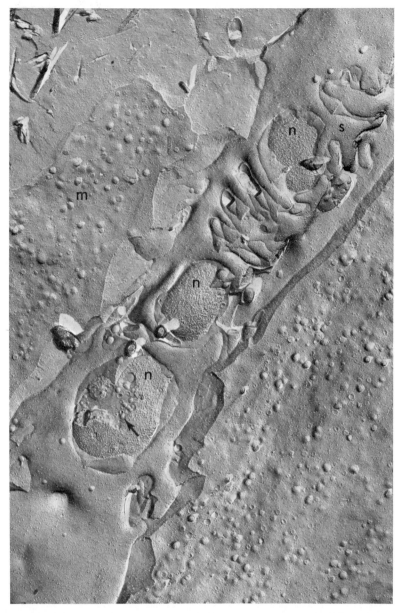

Fig. 8. Freeze-fracture of a motor nerve terminal from a muscle exposed to 20 μg/ml β-bungarotoxin for 3.5 hr, at which time its twitch became completely blocked. Schwann cell processes (s) are more abundant than usual and completely enclose the nerve in many regions, leaving only small patches of nerve membrane (n) exposed to the muscle. Since this is an "A-face" view (cf. Fig. 7), we should expect to see rows of large particles delineating active zones on the exposed patches of nerve, but no such rows are visible. Instead, large particles are scattered everywhere in the nerve membrane, in much greater abundance than normal. The nerve membrane is completely ruptured in places (arrow), exposing the underlying axoplasm with its normal complement of synaptic vesicles. (× 20,000.)

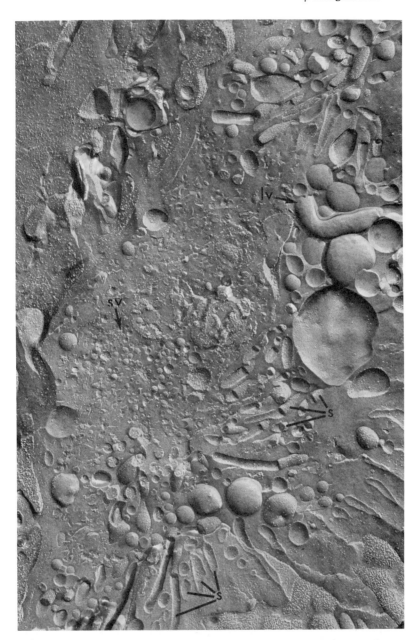

Fig. 9. Freeze-fracture of a totally disintegrated motor nerve terminal from a frog muscle exposed to 20 μg/ml β-bungarotoxin for 0.5 hr and then washed for 3 hr in normal Ringer, at which time the muscle twitch became completely blocked. There is no presynaptic membrane remaining for the fracture to travel through, and the Schwann cell processes (s) are in total disarray. The synaptic cleft is filled with diverse membranous debris, from small vesicles that have the size and particle content of normal synaptic vesicles (sv), to large vesicles which are completely devoid of intramembranous particles, and thus probably pure phospholipid (lv). (✕ 32,000.)

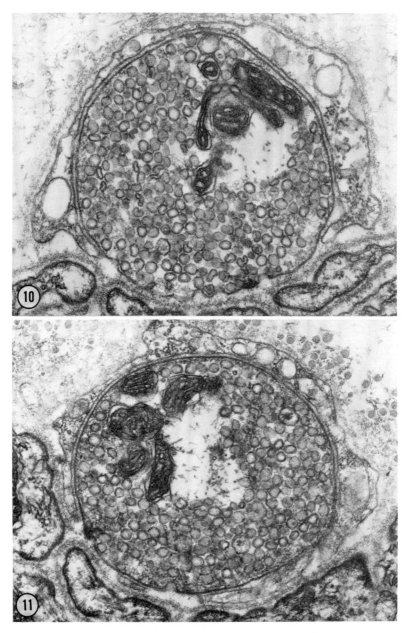

Figs. 10–15. Thin sections of cutaneous pectoris muscles exposed to 20 μg/ml β-bungarotoxin for 2 hr at 22°C (at which time their twitch was considerably weakened), and then fixed by immersion in OsO₄ in modified frog Ringer (18). All are at a magnification of × 49,600. The terminal in Fig. 10 looks essentially normal, except for some unusually-shaped synaptic vesicles and one unusually flattened mitochondrion. The terminal in Fig. 11 looks normal except that its plasma membrane is slightly more electron-dense than normal, and the delicate filamentous ectoplasm which underlies the plasma membrane looks slightly coarser and more prominent than usual. The terminal in Fig. 12 is another

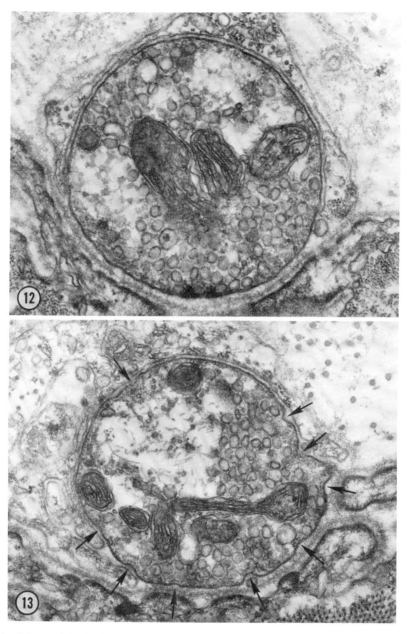

example of these subtle changes in plasma membrane and associated filaments seen with β-bungaro-toxin. Freeze-fractures of terminals at this stage show a distinct increase in concentration of intra-membranous particles of all size classes. Figure 13 is an example of terminals which display an unusual abundance of "coated pits." Such structures have previously been associated with endocytotic protein uptake and regeneration of synaptic vesicles (18). The filamentous coats underlying these plasmalemmal dimples look exactly like the coarsened filamentous ectoplasm located just inside the plasma mem-brane throughout the nerve terminals. The coarsening or increased staining of the plasma membrane

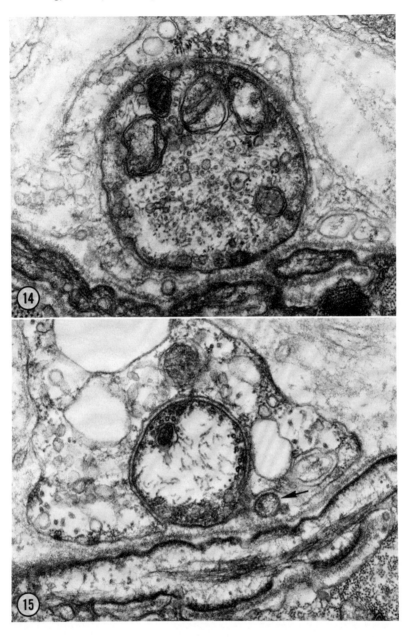

and underlying filaments has progressed even further in Fig. 14, picked randomly from another muscle of this same experiment. This nerve terminal, fixed in osmium, shows abnormally sized and shaped mitochondria which are similar to the aldehyde-fixed terminals in Figs. 17 and 19. Figure 15 shows the final stages of nerve terminals incubated with β-bungarotoxin, if the terminals do not completely disintegrate as in Fig. 9. Practically nothing is left except the terminal's axial core of neurofilaments and microtubules. These are surrounded by an unusually dense membrane which is often discontinuous or vesiculated (arrow), underlaid by a dense, flocculent precipitate of what must have been the terminal's filamentous ectoplasm. In such terminals, no vesicles or other secretory machinery remains.

The Schwann cells clearly responded to this dissolution of the nerve terminals by attempting to engulf the terminals and ingest the broken-off fragments (Fig. 8). This could have been a protective phenomenon or purely a phagocytic response to the altered nerve condition; we could not discriminate between these alternatives in the electron microscope because both happened at the same time.

We have used β-bungarotoxin labeled with horseradish peroxidase (HRP) to visualize the location of the toxin while these morphological changes were occurring. β-Bungarotoxin was conjugated to HRP by the same method used to synthesize the α-bungarotoxin-HRP conjugate which selectively stains the acetylcholine receptors of the postsynaptic membrane (Fig. 16). We found that the conjugated β-bungarotoxin bound strongly and selectively not only to the plasma membrane of the nerve terminals, but also to some of their internal membranes, including the membranes of synaptic vesicles and of mitochondria (Fig. 18). We cannot be sure whether this intracellular binding is significant physiologically or whether it is due to nonspecific fixation of conjugated toxin after rupture of the nerve terminals. However, it was clear that conjugated β-bungarotoxin was selectively accumulated by nerve terminals, either by surface adsorption or pinocytotic uptake.

We are currently attempting to determine if indeed the pinocytotic uptake mechanism is correct, by following up on the observations that β-bungarotoxin block occurs faster when the nerve is stimulated (4) and that stimulation increases the rate of pinocytosis at synapses (18).

By comparing the distribution of the intracellular binding of the HRP toxin conjugate to the distribution of free HRP which we found was sometimes trapped in nerve terminals during β-bungarotoxin action, we could see that with the supposedly specific, conjugated toxin, the density of stain was somewhat greater around mitochondria (Fig. 18 vs Fig. 19). Morphological changes in the mitochondria themselves after exposure to toxin were not very great. At first, many mitochondria were unusually condensed, even flattened (Figs. 10 and 13), which is a change we have seen before with dinitrophenol and other mitochondrial uncouplers. Later, the mitochondria were pleomorphic (Figs. 14 and 18), with some swollen, pale types and others of more normal density but still unusually rounded and swollen.

Another morphological change which accompanied those just described, was a gradual "coarsening" of the appearance of cytoplasmic filaments, both the thicker neurofilaments and the thinner microfilaments in the ectoplasm that underlies the plasma membrane and extends into the axoplasmic regions where synaptic vesicles are found (Figs. 11–15). The filaments affected included those which anchor to the plasma membrane and form "coated pits" in the process of micropinocytosis. This process must have been disturbed by toxin, since we found a distinctly abnormal abundance of coated pits in many nerve terminals (Fig. 13), prior to the grosser damage described above. We are currently investigating whether this resulted from a slowdown of endocytosis at the stage of membrane-filament interaction, or represented an actual speedup of endocytosis, in which case all stages should have been more abundant.

In conclusion, we could see in the electron microscope that β-bungarotoxin produces a progressive alteration and eventual disruption of the presynaptic plasma membrane and early signs of damage to at least one membrane function, that of endocytosis of plasma membrane. However, these morphological studies, so far, have not led to a unique explanation of why transmitter discharge is blocked by the toxin. We do not know whether the block results from the phospholipase activity directly or from the disruption of some other membrane function, such as endocytosis (18). Alternatively, it is possible that transmission failure is simply due to an abolition of the integrity of the nerve terminal membrane.

DISCUSSION

The phospholipase activity of β-toxin has properties typical of many other phospholipases A_2, with respect both to phospholipid liposomes as substrates and to natural

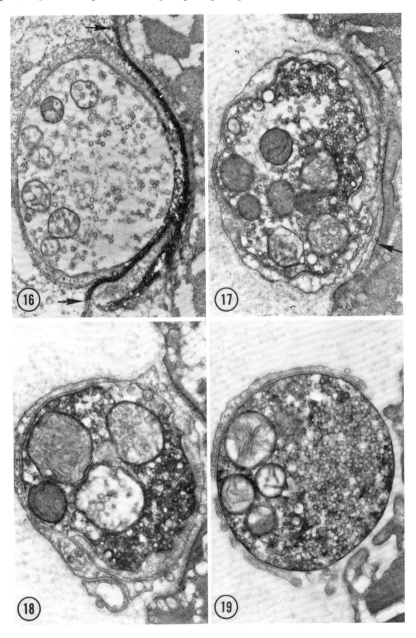

membranes. The requirements of calcium and sodium deoxycholate when pure phospho-lipid serves as a substrate are common to β-toxin and many other basic phospholipases (21,42—44). Strontium has been shown to be a competitive inhibitor of the calcium ion binding site in both pancreatic phospholipase A_2 (45) and Crotalus adamanteus phospho-lipase A_2 (46). Similarly, magnesium has been shown, from spectrophotometric evidence, not to bind to either the pancreatic or Crotalus enzyme (45,46). β-Bungarotoxin shows remarkable analogies to pancreatic phospholipase A_2 in its ability to differentiate between the inner and outer membrane phospholipids of erythrocytes (13), although the mechanism of selectivity is unknown. There is much evidence from labeling studies in favor of an asymmetric distribution of phospholipids across the erythrocyte membrane, suggesting that phosphatidylcholine and sphingomyelin are found on the outer membrane surface whereas the negatively charged lipid phosphatidylserine and phosphatidylethanolamine, reside on the inner membrane surface (47—49). However, the use of phospholipases as probes of an asymmetric phospholipid arrangement in membranes (13,27,28,50—53) has recently been questioned (54). Thus any conclusions about β-toxin's substrate specificity for anionic phospholipids from experiments with erythrocyte membranes should be treated with caution. The problem of phospholipid specificity is presently being examined in model liposome systems.

    All our present anatomical and electrophysiological knowledge regarding the effects of β-bungarotoxin on neuromuscular preparations indicate that enzymatic action is re-stricted to presynaptic nerve terminals. Even after β-bungarotoxin has blocked muscle contractions induced by nerve stimulation, muscle fibers will have normal resting poten-tials and contract vigorously upon direct electrical stimulation (5,55). Nor does the toxin affect amplitude or conduction velocities of action potentials in the rat phrenic nerve (5). Furthermore, intracellular recording from end plate regions of muscle fibers incubated with toxin demonstrate that although the frequency of m.e.p.p.'s drops to barely discernible levels, their amplitudes remain normal, indicating that the toxin has negligible postsynap-tic activity (5,9). Freeze-fracture replicas and thin-sections of muscles bathed in

---

Fig. 16. Frog neuromuscular junction treated with α-bungarotoxin-horseradish peroxidase (α-BTX-HRP) conjugate. The muscle was fixed with aldehydes and incubated with diaminobenzidine and H_2O_2 to reveal the location of α-bungarotoxin binding sites. These are seen to cover the postsynaptic membrane beneath the nerve terminal, and extend laterally as far as the arrows. There appears to have been a slight "bleeding" of the histochemical reaction product over to the adjacent nerve membrane, but there is no staining of the mitochondria or synaptic vesicles inside the nerve. (× 21,600.)

Figs. 17 and 18. Frog neuromuscular junctions treated with β-BTX-HRP conjugate and prepared for histochemistry as in Fig. 16. In contrast to the α-toxin, there is little or no staining of the postsynaptic membrane (arrows). The entire circumference of the nerve plasmalemma and its intracellular organelles is densely stained, including synaptic vesicles and especially the cytoplasmic surface of the outer mitochondrial membranes. Note that β-bungarotoxin does not appear to have actually penetrated into the mitochondria. (Fig. 17: × 24,800; Fig. 18: × 30,400.)

Fig. 19. Frog neuromuscular junction soaked in an equimolar mixture of β-bungarotoxin (20 μg/ml) and unconjugated HRP, in order to determine if the binding of HRP seen in Figs. 17 and 18 was an artifact. HRP did become trapped in this terminal during the β-bungarotoxin action, but we observed such staining only twice in 32 nerve terminals so treated. In contrast, every nerve terminal that was soaked in the β-BTX-HRP conjugate showed the staining of Figs. 17 and 18. Moreover, we had the impression, especially when the histochemical reaction was less intense than shown here, that the staining of mitochondria was more extensive and more selective with the specifically conjugated β-BTX-HRP. (× 28,800.)

β-bungarotoxin provide further morphological evidence of its selectivity. Nerve terminals shrink and become fragmented, and their mitochondria become swollen and rounded. In contrast, surrounding Schwann cell processes and postsynaptic muscle structures appear normal.

β-Bungarotoxin needs calcium, 1) to exert its phospholipase action in solution, 2) to block transmitter secretion, and 3) to disrupt the structure of motor nerve terminals in the intact tissue. Since strontium inhibits all 3 functions, we conclude that β-bungarotoxin blocks secretion by a specific enzymatic attack on the presynaptic plasma membrane.

Why the toxin should attack and enzymatically digest only membranes of motor nerve terminals remains a question. We suggest that the toxin possesses a site in addition to its enzymatic locus which permits it to recognize and selectively bind to some feature of nerve terminals.

Details of a possible model which, by analogy with the concepts of affinity chromatography (56) we have termed the affinity enzyme model, are given in Fig. 6. In addition to its nerve terminal recognition site, we propose that, like phospholipase A_2, the toxin's enzymatic locus consists of 2 spatially distinct regions; a lipid-water recognition site and a catalytic site (45). We suggest that calcium and divalent metal ion inhibitors bind to the catalytic site.

What evidence do we have for our model and what can we conclude about the nature of these 3 sites from presently held information? Chemical modification studies indicate that β-toxin has catalytically important residues common to both Crotalus and pancreatic phospholipases A_2. Modification of the toxin with N-bromosuccinimide rapidly destroys enzymatic activity in an analogous fashion to inactivation of the Crotalus enzyme. N-bromosuccinimide preferentially oxidizes tryptophan residues, and indeed Wells (35) has shown that 2 such residues in Crotalus phospholipase A_2 are destroyed by this reagent. Modification of the toxin with 4-bromophenacyl bromide again leads to elimination of enzymatic activity, but at a much slower rate. We believe that the modified amino acid is probably a histidine residue; although 4-bromophenacyl bromide is usually a nonspecific alkylating agent, this reagent has been shown to selectively modify histidine residues of both pancreatic phospholipase A_2 (34) and another presynaptic neurotoxin with phospholipase activity, notexin (57,58). In both cases, modification results in a loss of enzymatic activity. Because of the increasing evidence for amino acid sequence homologies between pancreatic and snake venom phospholipases with presynaptic neurotoxins (58), we suggest that both tryptophan and histidine residues are located near the catalytic site of β-bungarotoxin.

The postulation of a lipid-water recognition site, an intrinsic part of the enzymatic locus but spatially distinct from the catalytic site, is derived from models formulated to explain the mechanism of pancreatic phospholipase A_2 (45). It is necessary to postulate these 2 additional membrane binding regions (common to other phospholipases) on β-bungarotoxin, distinct from the specific presynaptic receptor locus, to account for the conventional phospholipase activity of β-toxin which is observed with liver mitochondria (19) and red blood cells. The enzymatic requirement for deoxycholate in model phospholipid liposome systems suggests that, as with the pancreatic enzyme, β-toxin requires a defined interface (lipid-water recognition site) and that this requirement must be satisfied before the catalytic site can be activated.

Evidence for a nerve terminal recognition site is derived from studies with radioactively labeled toxin (41). ^{125}I-labeled β-bungarotoxin binds specifically and with high affinity to a limited number of receptor sites on synaptosomal membranes (13 pmole/mg protein, K_d = 2 nM) (41). Since neither calcium nor strontium affect β-toxin binding, the receptor locus may be distinct from the catalytic (metal binding) site (41). As yet we have not been able to demonstrate specific binding of labeled β-bungarotoxin to neuro-muscular junctions, and it is possible that the binding described above is not physiologi-cally significant. It is also possible that the postulated recognition site does not exist; an alternative we have not eliminated is that an unusual phospholipid or an arrangement of phospholipids is concentrated in nerve terminals and is an especially good substrate for the toxin's phospholipase activity.

Even if selective recognition and binding of the toxin occurs, the optimal interaction of toxin and membrane at the interfacial recognition site could be critically dependent on the physical state of the phospholipids within the membrane. There is some evidence that saturated phosphatidylcholines dispersed as liposomes can only be hydrolyzed near the transition temperature of the lipid (59). It has been shown that irregularities in the packing of lipid molecules at this temperature (where gel and liquid crystalline phases coexist) would favor insertion of enzymes into the interface at the border of the frozen lipid domains (60–62). More recently Van Deenen's group have shown that pancreatic phos-pholipase A_2 hydrolyzes unsaturated phosphatidylcholines at temperatures above, as well as at, their lipid transition temperature (61). This gives rise to the idea that phospholipase A_2 preferentially hydrolyzes those lipids that are in the most fluid environment, although greatest enhancement of enzymatic activity still occurs when the lipid system is in a phase transition equilibrium. Several laboratories (63–65) have shown that synaptic plasma membranes contain an unusually large proportion of phosphatidylserine and phosphati-dylethanolamine possessing very long chain fatty acids with a high degree of unsaturation (e.g., 22:6 fatty acid). These longer chain fatty acids are not prominent in phospholipids from either liver cell plasma membranes (66) or from erythrocytes (67). The resultant in-creased regions of fluid pools within synaptic plasma membranes, as compared with membranes from other cell types, could well contribute to β-bungarotoxin's selectivity for nerve terminals. Alternatively, the nature of the polar head group may be important in regulating membrane fluidity (68).

Finally, we would like to consider possible explanations of the electrophysiological results (4,5,9,32) in terms of the toxin's phospholipase activity. The reaction products of phospholipase A_2 hydrolysis of phospholipids are fatty acids and lysophospholipids; fatty acids have been shown to stimulate the fusion rate of synthetic liposomes (69), and Lucy and his coworkers have provided evidence for the increased probability of cell fusion in the presence of lysophospholipids (70). Elevation of levels of fatty acid and lysophospho-lipid in the presynaptic plasma membrane as a result of phospholipase activity might well increase the probability of synaptic vesicles fusing with this membrane, leading to an increase in transmitter release. This provides a plausible explanation for β-bungarotoxin's initial stimulation of spontaneous, evoked and delayed release (9). We cannot, however, rule out the possibility of more indirect mechanisms, such as some modification of calcium metabolism (6,26,71). Intraterminal mitochondria have been proposed as the primary locus of β-bungarotoxin (71), but the morphological data presented here shed no light on this alternative hypothesis. To explain the eventual failure of transmission in the presence of the toxin, we like to think that as a result of phospholipase activity, the nerve terminal membrane finally disintegrates. At present, however, we cannot determine whether the toxin blocks synaptic transmission before or after lysis of the terminal membrane.

We have demonstrated that it is possible for a toxin that binds to a membrane re-ceptor with high affinity to possess a potent enzymatic activity that is involved in its physiological function. Although toxins have been conventionally regarded as interacting passively with their target receptors, we wonder whether our observations might be part of a more generalized phenomenon and that other protein molecules that bind to membrane sites with high affinity might also have enzymatic activity. Preliminary evidence indicating that other presynaptic neurotoxins might possess phospholipase activity (3), and the established ADP-ribosylating properties of diphtheria toxin (72–74), provide support for our speculations.

ACKNOWLEDGMENTS

We thank Louise Evans and Ignacio Caceres for their excellent technical assistance, Dr. J. Goerke for making available facilities in his laboratory to assay phospholipase activities, and Dr. S. G. Oberg for some of the electrophysiological experiments in Sr^{++} solutions. This work was supported by National Institutes of Health grant NS-09878-2 (RBK) and a grant to JEH from the Muscular Dystrophy Associations of America; PNS is a fellow of the Muscular Dystrophy Association of America.

REFERENCES

1. Habermann, E. and Heller, I., Naun-Schmiedeberg's Arch Pharmakol. 287:97 (1975)
2. Frontali, N., Ceccarelli, B., Gorio, A., Mauro, A., Siekevitz, P., Tzeng, M.-C., and Hurlbut, W. P., J. Cell Biol. 68:462 (1976).
3. Eaker, D., Halpert, J., Fohlman, J. and Karlsson, E., in "Animal, Plant and Microbial Toxins" vol. 2. A. Ohsaka (Ed.). New York: Plenum Press, pp. 27–45 (1976).
4. Chang, C. C., Chen, T. F., and Lee, C. Y., J. Pharmacol. Exp. Ther. 184:339 (1973).
5. Kelly, R. B., and Brown, F. R. III, J. Neurobiol. 5:135 (1974).
6. Wernicke, J. F., Oberjat, T., and Howard, B. D., J. Neurochem. 22:781 (1974).
7. Lau, Y. H., Chiu, T. H., Caswell, A. H., and Potter, L. T., Biochem. Biophys. Res. Commun. 61:460 (1974).
8. Sen, I., and Cooper, J. R., Biochem. Pharmacol. 24:2107 (1975).
9. Oberg, S. G., and Kelly, R. B., J. Neurobiol. 7:129 (1976).
10. Selinger, Z., Sharoni, Y., and Schramm, M., in "The Cytopharmacology of Secretion." B. Ceccarelli, F. Clementi, and J. Meldolesi, (Eds.). New York: Raven Press, p. 23.
11. Rahamimoff, R., Erulkar, S. D., Alnaes, E., Meiri, H., Rotshenker, S., and Rahamimoff, H., Cold Spring Harbor Symp. Quant. Biol. 40:107 (1975).
12. Strong, P. N., Goerke, J., Oberg, S. G., and Kelly, R. B., Proc. Nat. Acad. Sci. USA 73:178 (1976).
13. Zwaal, R. F. A., Roelofsen, B., Comfurius, P., and Van Deenen, L. L. M., Biochim. Biophys. Acta 406:83 (1975).
14. Nakane, P. K., and Kawaoi, A., J. Histochem. Cytochem. 22:1084 (1974).
15. Lentz, T. L., Rosenthal, J., and Mazurkiewicz, J. E., Neuroscience Abst. 1:627 (1975).
16. Heuser, J. E., Reese, T. S., and Landis, D. M. D., J. Neurocytol. 3:109 (1974).
17. Graham, R. C., and Karnovsky, M. J., J. Histochem. Cytochem. 14:291 (1966).
18. Heuser, J. E., and Reese, T. S., J. Cell Biol. 57:315 (1973).
19. Kelly, R. B., Oberg, S. G., Strong, P. N., and Wagner, G. M., Cold Spring Harbor Symp. Quant. Biol. 40:117 (1975).
20. Batzri, S., and Korn, E. D., Biochim. Biophys. Acta 298:1015 (1973).
21. De Haas, G. H., Postema, N. M., Nieuwenhuizen, W., and Van Deenen, L. L. M., Biochim. Biophys. Acta 159:103 (1968).
22. Wells, M. A., Biochemistry 11:1030 (1972).
23. Wernicke, J. F., Vanker, A. D., and Howard, B. D., J. Neurochem. 25:483 (1975).
24. Habermann, E., Biochem. Z. 328:474 (1957).
25. Figarella, C., Clemente, F., and Guy, O., Biochim. Biophys. Acta 227:213 (1971).
26. Shipolini, R. A., Callewaert, G. L., Cottrell, R. C., Doonan, S., Vernon, C. A., and Banks, B. E. C., Eur. J. Biochem. 20:459 (1971).

27. Roelofsen, B., Zwaal, R. F. A., Woodward, C. B., and Van Deenen, L. L. M., Biochim. Biophys. Acta 241:925 (1971).
28. Zwaal, R. F. A., Roelofsen, B., and Colley, C. M., Biochim. Biophys. Acta 300:159 (1973).
29. Hoffman, J. F., J. Gen. Physiol. 42:9 (1958); 45:837 (1962).
30. Bodemann, H., and Passow, H., J. Memb. Biol. 8:1 (1972).
31. Schwoch, G., and Passow, H., Mol. Cell. Biochem. 2:197 (1973).
32. Alderdice, M. T., and Volle, R. L., Neuroscience Abst. 1:622 (1975).
33. Dodge, F. A., Jr., Miledi, R., and Rahamimoff, R., J. Physiol. 200:267 (1969).
34. Volwerk, J. J., Pieterson, W. A., and De Haas, G. H., Biochemistry 13:1446 (1974).
35. Wells, M. A., Biochemistry 12:1086 (1973).
36. Spande, T. F., and Witkop, B., Methods Enzymol. 11:498 (1967).
37. Truog, R., and Howard, B. D., Fed. Proc. 35:1356 (1976).
38. Tsai, M.-C., Ph.D. Thesis, National Taiwan University, Taipei, Taiwan (1975).
39. Clark, A. W., Hurlbut, W. P., and Mauro, A., J. Cell Biol. 52:1 (1972).
40. Okamoto, M., Longenecker, H. E., Jr., Riker, W. F., Jr., and Songs, S. K., Science 172:733 (1971).
41. Oberg, S. G., and Kelly, R. B., Biochim. Biophys. Acta 433:662 (1976).
42. Goerke, J., De Gier, J., and Bonsen, P. P. M., Biochim. Biophys. Acta 248:245 (1971).
43. Magee, W. L., Gallai-Hatchard, J., Sanders, H., and Thompson, R. H. S., Biochem. J. 83:17 (1962).
44. Van Deenen, L. L. M., De Haas, G. H., and Heemskerk, C. H. Th., Biochim. Biophys. Acta 67:295 (1963).
45. Pieterson, W. A., Volwerk, J. J., and De Haas, G. H., Biochemistry 13:1439 (1974).
46. Wells, M. A., Biochemistry 12:1080 (1973).
47. Bretscher, M. S., Science 181:622 (1973).
48. Bordesky, S. E., and Marinetti, G. V., Biochem. Biophys. Res. Commun. 50:1027 (1973).
49. Whiteley, N. M., and Berg, H. C., J. Mol. Biol. 87:541 (1974).
50. Colley, C. M., Zwaal, R. F. A., Roelofsen, B., and Van Deenen, L. L. M., Biochim. Biophys. Acta 307:74 (1973).
51. Verkleij, A. J., Zwaal, R. F. A., Roelofsen, B., Comfurius, P., Kastelijn, D. and Van Deenen, L. L. M., Biochim. Biophys. Acta 323:178 (1973).
52. Gul, S. and Smith, A. D., Biochim. Biophys. Acta 367:271 (1974).
53. Kahlenberg, A., Walker, C., and Rohrlick, R., Can. J. Biochem. 52:803 (1974).
54. Martin, J. K., Luthra, M. G., Wells, M. A., Watts, R. P., and Hanahan, D. J., Biochemistry 14:5400 (1975).
55. Chang, C. C., and Lee, C. Y., Arch. Int. Pharmacodyn. 144:241 (1963).
56. Cuatrecasas, P., and Anfinsen, C. B., Ann. Rev. Biochem. 40:259 (1971).
57. Halpert, J., and Eaker, D., J. Biol. Chem. 250:6990 (1975).
58. Halpert, J., Eaker, D., and Karlsson, E., FEBS Letts. 61:1 (1976).
59. Op den Kamp, J. A. F., De Gier, J., and Van Deenen, L. L. M., Biochim. Biophys. Acta 345:253 (1974).
60. Phillips, M. C., and Chapman, D., Biochim. Biophys. Acta, 163:301 (1968).
61. Op den Kamp, J. A. F., Kauerz, M. Th., and Van Deenen, L. L. M., Biochim. Biophys. Acta 406:169 (1975).
62. Linden, C. D., Wright, K. L., McConnell, H. M., and Fox, C. F., Proc. Nat. Acad. Sci. USA 70:2271 (1973).
63. Cotman, C., Blank, M. L., Moehl, A., and Synder, F., Biochemistry 8:4606 (1969).
64. Breckenridge, W. C., Gombos, G., and Morgan, I. G., Biochim. Biophys. Acta 266:695 (1972).
65. Kishimoto, Y., Agranoff, B. W., Radin, N. S., and Burton, R. M., J. Neurochem. 16:397 (1969).
66. Pfleger, R. C., Anderson, N. G. and Snyder, F., Biochemistry 7:2826 (1968).
67. Ways, P., and Hanahan, D. J., J. Lipid. Res. 5:318 (1964).
68. Demel, R. A., Geurts Van Kessel, W. S. M., Zwaal, R. F. A., Roelofsen, B., and Van Deenen, L. L. M., Biochim. Biophys. Acta 406:97 (1975).
69. Kantor, H. L., and Prestegard, J. H., Biochemistry 14:1790 (1975).
70. Poole, A. R., Howell, J. I., and Lucy, J. A., Nature 227:810 (1970).
71. Wagner, G. M., Mart, P. E., and Kelly, R. B., Biochem. Biophys. Res. Commun. 58:475 (1974).
72. Honjo, T., Nishizuka, Y., Kato, I., and Hayaishi, O., J. Biol. Chem. 246:4251 (1971).
73. Collier, R. J., and Kandel, J., J. Biol. Chem. 246:1496 (1971).
74. Gill, D. M., and Dinius, L. L., J. Biol. Chem. 246:1485 (1971).

Factors Influencing Monolayer Cell Culture Morphology and Survival of Cerebellar Granule Cells From Wild-Type and Mutant Mice

Anne Messer

Department of Neuroscience, Children's Hospital Medical Center, and Department of Neuropathology, Harvard Medical School, Boston, Massachusetts 02115

A distinction must be made between genetic factors intrinsic and extrinsic to a specific degenerating cell type if neurological mutants that show such effects are to be used to assess cause-and-effect correlations of neural development. When the growth of granule cells from cerebella of staggerer mutant mice is investigated in monolayer cell cultures using modified Hams F12 medium plus fetal calf serum, cells from the mutant are found to clump less and survive longer than their wild-type counterparts. Thus, the degeneration of granule cells observed in these mutants in vivo cannot be a function of irreversibly programmed cell death before postnatal day 7, the age at which cells are dissociated. The possibility that the increased survival is simply a function of initial cell-cell interactions is examined by comparing normal cells grown on glass, plastic, or polylysine-coated glass to each other, and then comparing the behavior of staggerer vs control cells under the same conditions. Although the polylysine coating both reduces the amount of initial clumping and increases the survival of normal cells, it does not completely eliminate the difference between mutant and control. Mutant and control cultures exhibit the same behavior only when culture conditions are changed to include supplementation with horse serum instead of fetal calf serum in addition to the substrate coating.

Key words: tissue culture, cerebellar mutants, cerebellar granule cells

INTRODUCTION

A distinction must be made between genetic factors intrinsic and extrinsic to a specific degenerating cell type if neurological mutants that show such effects are to be used to assess cause-and-effect correlations of neural development. This is a particularly perplexing question in the case of neurological mutant staggerer (sg/sg). It was initially described as a cerebellar granule cell degeneration mutant (1), but several reports subsequently established that the Purkinje cells are definitely abnormal by a variety of criteria (2–5), giving rise to a theory that a normal population of granule cells may be degenerating after failing to make proper postsynaptic contacts. However, Yoon (6) had found a reduced rate of granule cell proliferation and premature migration from the external granule layer; and, more recently (7) he has observed that in sg/sg—reeler double mutants, the Purkinje cells are identical to those in sg/sg Purkinje cells, while the external granule layer is completely destroyed. He therefore proposes that the mutation may have an early direct effect on granule cells, even though their actual degeneration later may be due to the Purkinje abnormality.

We have shown (8) that sg/sg cerebellar granule cells will survive in a monolayer culture in vitro, and that such cells can be distinguished from wild-type cells by both a decrease in the intracellular adhesion (i.e., clumping) shortly after plating and by an increased capacity to survive in culture. The sg/sg cultures grow optimally (judged by the complexity of the process outgrowth and the number of cells surviving with intact morphology for at least 3 weeks) in about 80% of the preparations, while wild-type do so in only 30% (9). Optimal preparations of both types are very similar. These results rule out hypotheses of mutant gene action that require that the granule cells be irreversibly committed to cell death prior to 7 days postnatally (the time of dissociation). However, since the decrease in initial clumping could itself lead to the increase in survival, these results do not distinguish between a change in the granule cells themselves (either intrinsic, or extrinsic due to some early interaction with another cell type) and a change in some other cell type that, in turn, changes the behavior of the entire mixed cerebellar cell culture system (e.g., glial cells upon which granule cells can be seen growing).

This work examines the effect of substratum and serum on initial clumping and subsequent survival of cells. Yavin and Yavin (10) have shown that embryonic rat cerebral cells will spread out evenly on a substratum coated with polylysine; a similar effect is seen here with mouse cerebellar cells. However, while extreme initial clumping is not compatible with eventual survival in this system, simply spreading the cells out is not sufficient to eliminate the differences seen with the mutant cells. A change in serum is required as well.

MATERIALS AND METHODS

Techniques of dissociation (1% trypsin, 0.1% deoxyribonuclease), plating (1.5×10^6 cells/35 mm dish) (media modified Hams F12), and serum (fetal calf and horse) are the same as in Messer (9). Polylysine (p-Lys) coating is a combination of the methods of Yavin and Yavin (10) and Letourneau (11) with the actual concentration used determined empirically. Sigma poly-L-lysine (type 1-B P-1886) is dissolved at 2 mg/100 ml in double-distilled water and filtered to sterilize. Three 15mm glass coverslips in a 35 mm dish are incubated overnight with 1.5 ml p-Lys solution, then detoxified over the course of a week by washing and incubating with calcium-magnesium-free Tyrodes — 3 changes the first day, one each the next 2 days, and every 3 days subsequently.

Observations of dishes for evaluation of growth and survival are made on living cultures using an inverted phase microscope. At least 10 fields are viewed. If gross differences are apparent among these fields, cultures are recorded as "patchy." Qualitative evaluation of intact appearance of cells, plus number, length, and complexity of processes, is designated by "poor" through "excellent" (the latter representing fields similar to Fig. 3) and further described if necessary. (Age is considered in evaluating process outgrowth in cultures less than 7 days in vitro.)

Mutant sg/sg mice are obtained by crossing C57B1 sg++/+dse, originally from the Jackson Laboratory and maintained here for about 8 generations. Controls are heterozygous littermates, sg++/+dse (designated +/sg here).

RESULTS

Previous work has shown (8) that the majority of the neuronal cells from sg/sg cerebella that survive when plated in modified F12 plus fetal calf serum are granule cells. There are differences between mutants and control cells, however, both in the survival times and in the morphologies of cell interactions in cultures as a whole. The former is shown in Table I, which charts the time course for 7 experiments comparing sg/sg with +/sg cell in vitro. Although the variability discussed previously (9) is obvious, the mutant cultures are notably hardier than their controls. The clumping phenomenon is difficult to prove in just a few pictures, since individual fields on the same dishes are not identical, but there is relatively less clumping in sg/sg than +/sg cultures. Figure 1 shows 2 pairs of fields from cultures at 1 and 2 days in vitro, demonstrating this point.

Under the same culture conditions (modified F12 plus fetal calf serum), differences in the degree of clumping initially observed varies consistently with substrate for wild-type cells. Figure 2 shows sister cultures 3 days in vitro (3 DIV) plated on glass and on plastic. The enormous clumps in the culture plated on plastic are seen in about 50% of preparations, and are incompatible with survival beyond a week. In most remaining cases, there will be larger clumps on plastic than on glass, although neither the morphological difference nor the survival difference is as large. If the glass is coated with p-Lys, an even better spreading of cells is obtained, along with some increase in survival. Figure 3 shows cells 3 DIV on p-Lys, with a characteristic, even distribution of cells. Table II compares the effects of glass vs p-Lys-coated glass on survival. The amount of clumping varies from preparation to preparation, but within this variation there is less clumping on p-Lys than plain glass. Polyornithine was also tested, with comparable results.

TABLE I. Comparison of Staggerer and Control Cultures on Glass

Preparation	Genotype	Appearance at 3 DIV	Survival (DIV)*
197	sg/sg	Excellent network of cells and processes	35†
	+/+	Very poor, mostly debris	3
208	sg/sg	Excellent cells	23
	+/sg	Patchy, fairly good clumps ± outgrowth	13
218	sg/sg	Patchy, some good areas	6
	+/sg	Poor, very clumped	6
227	sg/sg	Very good, small clumps with outgrowth	37
	+/sg	Patchy, good areas with some clumps	21
232	sg/sg	Very patchy, fair	10
	+/sg	Patchy, fair, some outgrowth from clumps	10
255	sg/sg	Patchy, some excellent areas	17+ (used for experiment)
	+/sg	Very poor, few neurons	3
259	sg/sg	Patchy, some good areas	13+ (used for experiment)
	+/sg	Very poor, mostly debris	3

*Remaining neurons, if any, very sparse.

†This survival is particularly notable, since all other cell cultures in this 10-day period failed to survive at all.

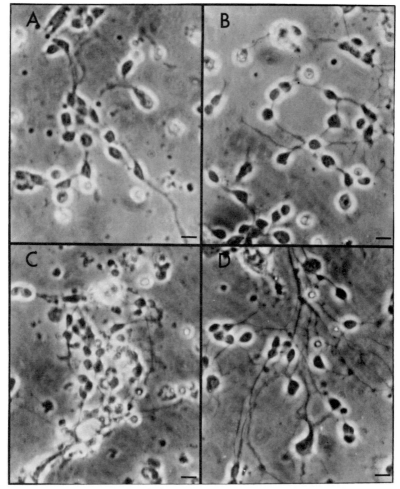

Fig. 1. Phase contrast morphology of living cells grown from sg/sg and +/sg cerebella, showing differences in the degree of initial clumping of cells. (A) +/sg and (B) sg/sg, sister cultures, 1 DIV; (C) sg/sg and (D) +/sg, sister cultures, 2 DIV. Bar = 10 μ.

Staggerer and control cells were grown on plastic and p-Lys-coated glass to examine the effects of substratum on the differences that had been observed with uncoated glass. On plastic, sg/sg cells were much more spread out and survived much longer than controls on plastic, particularly since the latter often clumped excessively. In 2 experiments where sg/sg and +/sg cells were simultaneously compared on both glass and plastic, survival and clumping were inversely related, sg/sg on plastic showing the least clumping, followed by sg/sg on glass, +/sg on glass, and +/sg on plastic. Thus the plastic substratum tends to maximize the difference between cell types. On the other hand, p-Lys reduces the difference somewhat. Table III shows fewer dramatic differences between sg/sg and +/sg preparations than Table I, mostly due to an improvement in the survival of controls. However, the 2 can still be distinguished in many cases, suggesting that substratum alone cannot change the behavior of the normal cells enough to eliminate the differences.

Horse serum was found superior to fetal calf serum as a supplement in this system after one feeding (based on optima as described above), but it could not be used at the

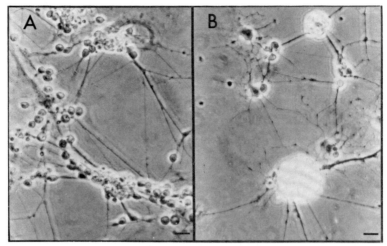

Fig. 2. Phase contrast microscopy of wild-type cells, 3 DIV, showing differences in amount of cell clumping with different substrata. (A) Glass surface and (B) plastic surface, sister cultures, 3 DIV. The large phase-bright areas in (B) represent large clumps of cells that cannot be focused in a single plane. Bar = 10 μ.

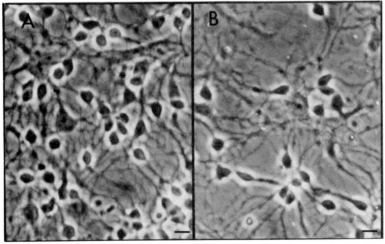

Fig. 3. Phase contrast microscopy of wild-type cells grown on p-Lys substrata, 3 DIV. Bar = 10 μ.

time of plating on glass or plastic because it caused the cells to clump very greatly (9). However, the p-Lys coating allowed an even spreading of cells even in the presence of horse serum, giving results similar to Fig. 3 at 3 DIV. Wild-type cells grown on horse serum from the time of plating are far more consistent in their growth and survival characteristics than cells started on fetal calf serum (even with the same bottle of lot-tested fetal calf serum). Table IV shows a comparison of sg/sg and +/sg cells grown on p-Lys using modified F12 medium plus horse serum from the time of plating. This combination of surface coating and horse serum allows mutant and control cells to survive equally well.

TABLE II. Growth of Wild-type Cells on Plain Glass vs Polylysine-Coated (p-Lys) Glass

Preparation No.	Surface	Appearance at 3 DIV	Survival time (DIV)*
234	glass	Patchy, debris, clumping	8 a
	p-Lys	Very good, some debris	15 b
235	glass	Somewhat clumped	10 a
	p-Lys	A bit clumped, mostly spread out	13 b
236	glass	Patchy, mostly debris	3 b
	p-Lys	Better, many good cells	19 a
237	glass	Patchy, some good areas	15 b
	p-Lys	Sparse, spread out	15 b
251	glass	Clumps and many single cells	19 a
	p-Lys	Very uniform	29 b
260	glass	Mostly debris	3 a
	p-Lys	Mostly debris	3 a
265	glass	Clumps, some outgrowth	14 a
	p-Lys	Good – spread out	14 b
274	glass	Debris and moderate clumps	16 b
	p-Lys	Excellent, some debris	23 a

*Note: a) mostly debris; b) sparse neurons.

TABLE III. sg/sg vs Control on Polylysine-Coated Glass

Preparation	Genotype	Appearance at 3 DIV	Survival time (DIV)*
266	sg/sg	Very good	16 b
	+/sg	Some clumping, but overall good	16 a
261	sg/sg	Good, but some debris	9+
	+/sg	Only a few neurons	6a
268	sg/sg	Excellent cells, but some debris	10 b
	+/sg	Patchy, fewer cells than above	10 b
275	sg/sg	Very good	19 b
	+/sg	Occasional neurons	6 b
277	sg/sg	Excellent	47 b
	+/sg	Good, slightly lower density	47 a
278	sg/sg	Excellent	39 c
	+/sg	Good, somewhat more death	14 b
280	sg/sg	Fairly good, some debris	25 b
	+/sg	Very poor, mostly debris	3 a
281	sg/sg	Fair, cells sparse	10 b
	+/sg	Fair, a bit worse than above	10 a

*Note: +) used for exp.; a) mostly debris; b) sparse neurons; c) not recorded.

DISCUSSION

These studies show that a reduction in excessive clumping is necessary, but not sufficient, to ensure optimal growth of mouse cerebellar cells in this system of monolayer culture. In order to attain the quality of cultures seen using cells from the staggerer mutant, it is necessary to change both the cell substratum and the serum used to supple-

TABLE IV. sg/sg vs +/sg Grown on Polylysine-Coated Glass Using Horse Serum

Preparation	Genotype	Appearance at 3 DIV	Survival time (DIV)*
326	sg/sg	Good, moderate density, moderate debris	10
	+/sg	Good, a bit denser than above, debris again	10
327	sg/sg	Very good	23
	+/sg	Good, a bit less dense in patches	23
334	sg/sg	Very good, some debris	27
	+/sg	Very good, some debris	27

*Remaining neurons very sparse.

ment the medium for wild-type. Therefore, the difference seen between mutant and control cannot be explained by postulating that the increase in cell survival is simply a function of altered cell interaction.

These results support theories of action of the mutant gene in which the granule cells at postnatal day 7 differ from their wild-type counterparts, whether because of intrinsic differences or prior interactions with another altered cell type. However, it is not possible to entirely rule out the hypothesis that a change in the glial cells changes the environment in a manner equivalent to changing both the substratum and the serum for the normal cells. Additional data (not shown here) indicate that the factor excreted by the rat glial tumor line C_6, which causes neuroblastoma cells to elaborate processes (12), somewhat reduces the clumping and greatly enhances the survival of otherwise poor or mediocre preparations of mouse cerebellar cells, while having no effect on optimal preparations. Further experiments to examine the effect of this factor on sg/sg and +/sg granule cells directly will be necessary to solve this problem.

ACKNOWLEDGMENTS

I thank Mr. David M. Smith for expert technical assistance, and Dr. Frank Solomon for his generous gift of C_6 factor. This work was supported by USPHS Research grant No. NS 11237 and fellowships from the Helen Hay Whitney Foundation and the Medical Foundation of Boston.

REFERENCES

1. Sidman, R. L., Lane, P. W., and Dickie, M. M., Science 137:610 (1962).
2. Sidman, R. L., In "Physiological and Biochemical Correlates of Nervous Integration" (F. D. Carlson, ed.) Englewood Cliffs, N. J.: Prentice-Hall, 1968.
3. Sotello, C., and Changeaux, J-P., Brain Res. 67:519 (1974).
4. Mallet, J., Huchet, M., Pougeois, R., and Changeaux, J-P., Brain Res. 103:291 (1976).
5. Herrup, K., and Mullen, R. J., Abstr. Soc. for Neuroscience Ann. Meeting, Vol. 2 #141 (1976).
6. Yoon, Chai H., Neurology 22:743 (1972).
7. Yoon, Chai H., Brain Res. 109:206 (1976).
8. Messer, A., and Smith, D. M., Brain Res., in press.
9. Messer, A., Brain Res., in press.
10. Yavin, E., and Yavin, F., J. Cell. Biol. 62:540 (1974).
11. Letourneau, P. C., Develop. Biol. 44:77 (1975).
12. Monard, D., Solomon, R., Rentsch, M., and Gysin, R., Proc. Nat. Acad. Sci. USA 70:1895 (1973).

Regulation of Release From Isolated Adrenergic Secretory Vesicles by ATP-Mediated Changes in Transmembrane Potential and Anion Permeability

Harvey B. Pollard*, Christopher J. Pazoles*, Philip G. Hoffman §, Oren Zinder‡, and Olga Nikodijevik**

*Reproduction Research Branch, National Institute of Child Health and Human Development, National Institutes of Health, Bethesda, Maryland 20014; §Department of Obstetrics and Gynecology, University of California, School of Medicine, San Francisco, California 94122; ‡Department of Clinical Biochemistry, Rambam Hospital, Haifa, Israel; and **Department of Physiology, University of Skopje, Skopje, Yugoslavia

Isolated chromaffin granules release their contents when exposed to calcium, magnesium, ATP, and high levels of chloride ions. The mechanism of release is not well-understood, but changes in anion permeability may be involved. We found that another anion, thiocyanate (SCN^-), also activated release in a fashion similar to chloride, while isethionate ($HO\text{-}CH_2\text{-}CH_2SO_3{}^-$) an impermeant anion, was inactive. Mg^{++}-ATP was found to activate the uptake of ^{36}Cl and $^{14}C\text{-}SCN$, leading us to conclude that activation of anion uptake might be involved in the release process. The ^{36}Cl and the $^{14}C\text{-}SCN$ compartments were then compared by studying displacement of the trace anions by excess cold mass. Chloride and SCN displaced large amounts of both ^{36}Cl and $^{14}C\text{-}SCN$, while isethionate displaced little of either tracer anion. We suggest, on the basis of these data, that ATP-mediated anion uptake may be the basis for the release mechanism. Release may occur as a consequence of anion and subsequent water uptake into granules, resulting in osmotic imbalance and osmotic shock. This may also be of physiologic importance, and we propose a cellular model for secretion based on the biochemical properties of the isolated chromaffin granule.

Key words: secretion, anions, membrane potential, chromaffin granules, secretory vesicles, epinephrine

INTRODUCTION

Isolated adrenergic secretory vesicles (chromaffin granules) from the adrenal medulla are able to release their contents in an all or none fashion when exposed to Mg^{++}-ATP and chloride ions (1–6). Small amounts of calcium are also required (7). This reaction, found in many types of secretory vesicles, has attracted the attention of ourselves (5, 6, 8) and others (1–4, 9–13) as a possible model for chemical events associated with the process of secretion from cells by exocytosis.

It has been assumed, either implicitly or explicitly, that release is mediated by an ATPase on the granule membrane (3, 12, 13). However, we have recently shown that ATP analogs that were not substrates for myosin-like ATPase [e.g., AppNHp, (14)] would also support release from chromaffin granules (5, 6). As an alternative, we considered that both ATP and AppNHp could function as substrates for adenylate cyclase. We found that releasing granules synthesized cAMP (5), with an enzyme intrinsic to the granule membrane (15, 16). However, GTP could also support release, and we concluded that cyclase activity was not essential for the release event. Thus, the mechanism of how ATP promoted release from veiscles remained a significant unsolved problem.

More recently it has been shown that ATP can regulate the transmembrane potential of chromaffin granules (8, 17), and we have suggested that this process might be related to ATP-evoked release (8). In our own studies, the pH gradient was monitored by ^{14}C-methylamine distribution, while the electrical component of the potential was monitored by ^{35}S-SCN. Upon the addition of ATP the granule took up ^{35}S-SCN and the granule interior became markedly alkaline (8). Several important parallels between ATP-evoked release and changes in potential were noted. For example, the pH optimum for both events was approximately 6.2 (6, 8). In addition, GTP was nearly as active as ATP, while AppNHp was also active (8).

However, in spite of these parallels, it was still not apparent mechanistically how ATP-evoked changes in membrane potential could be coupled to ATP-evoked release. An important point not previously emphasized here is that chloride (or some other permeant anion, such as thiocyanate) is absolutely required for ATP-evoked release (1–7). The concentration of chloride required is greater than 20 mM, and is optimal at chloride concentrations approaching that of the extracellular space. We have already shown that ATP could regulate the entry of tracer levels of thiocyanate (8), and it was thus possible that ATP could also regulate the entry of chloride in a similar fashion. A plausible consequence of anion entry would be concommittant influx of water leading to osmotic imbalance and shock.

In this communication, we have tested the hypothesis that ATP regulates release by affecting anion permeability. The ATP-dependence of release has been compared with both chloride and SCN, and we have inquired whether both ^{14}C-SCN and ^{36}Cl enter the same compartment within the granule when exposed to ATP.

MATERIALS AND METHODS

Preparation of Granules

Chromaffin granules were prepared by a modification of the differential centrifugation method of Taugner (18), as described by Hoffman et al. (6) and Pollard et al. (8).

Measurement of Labeled Anion Distribution

Anion distribution was measured in an incubation mixture containing granules (0.2–0.5 mg protein), variable amounts of KCl, KCN or K-isethionate, 50 mM HEPES-NaOH buffer, pH 6.2, ^{14}C K-SCN (4 μM) or ^{36}Cl (2 mM), ^{3}H-Dextran to mark the extragranular water, and variable amounts of sucrose to make a final volume of 1 ml containing 335 mOsm. The granules were added to the incubation mixture at 4°C and allowed to equilibrate for 15 min. The granules were then centrifuged at 20,000 × g × 30 min and the pellets were assayed for bound radioactivity (8).

Release of Epinephrine

Granules in 0.5 ml isotonic sucrose (4°C) were added to 3.5 ml prewarmed medium (37°C) and incubated for 10 min. Release medium consisted of 50 mM HEPES-NaOH buffer, pH 6.0, 1 mM $MgSO_4$, variable amounts of KSCN, KCl, and ATP and enough sucrose to adjust the solution to 335 mOsm. The reaction was terminated by the addition of 2 ml of ice cold 0.335 M sucrose, and tubes were centrifuged at 20,000 rpm × 30 min at 4°C to sediment the granules. Released epinephrine in the supernatant was assayed by the method of Anton and Sayers (19). The protein was determined by the Lowry method (20). The release rates were linear over a 20 min incubation, as long as 10% of the epinephrine remained within the granules at the end of the time period.

RESULTS

Activation of Release by Chloride and Thiocyanate

Chloride and thiocyanate were compared with regard to their ability to promote release as a function of magnesium-ATP concentration. As shown in Fig. 1, the rate of release was a saturable function of the ATP concentration in the presence of either 60 mM chloride or 60 mM thiocyanate. Lineweaver-Burke plots of the data were linear, and revealed similar $K_{1/2}$ values for ATP with both anions (data not shown). Figure 1 also shows that release was completely dependent upon the presence of the anion.

Isethionate ($HO-C_2H_4-SO_3^-$), an impermeant anion (21), did not support release (6). As shown in Fig. 1, 30 mM isethionate actually reduced baseline release levels below the zero ATP level, even when tested at higher ATP concentrations. We concluded that SCN and chloride were able to support Mg^{++}-ATP-dependent release in a similar fashion in the presence of ATP.

Activation of Anion Uptake by ATP

We have previously shown that ATP enhanced [35]SCN uptake by granules at pH 7.2 (8). As shown in Table I, Mg^{++}-ATP also activated ^{14}C-SCN uptake by over 3-fold at pH 6.2. The actual amount of the thiocyanate taken up was rather small since only tracer amounts of thiocyanate were included. It thus became important to know if ATP could also regulate the uptake of chloride.

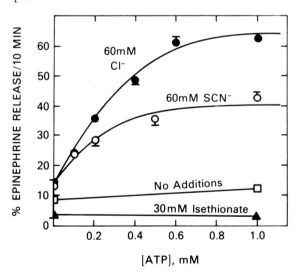

Fig. 1. Activation of release by ATP and permeant anions. The release reaction was carried out as described in the Materials and Methods section.

TABLE I. Activation of Anion Uptake by Mg^{2+}-ATP

Anion	1 mM Mg^{++}-ATP	cpm/mg protein	pmoles/mg protein	Fold activation after ATP
^{14}C-SCN[a]	—	24,651 ± 50	65.7	—
(4 μM)	+	76,322 ± 200	200.8	3.04
^{36}Cl[b]	—	993 ± 200	110 × 10^3	—
(2 mM)	+	1,626 ± 150	180 × 10^3	1.63

[a]S.A. =   375 cpm/pmole
[b]S.A. = 9,000 cpm/μmole

Chloride uptake by granules was in fact also increased by exposure to Mg^{++}-ATP (Table I). However, the results were not nearly as dramatic as those for thiocyanate since the specific activity of the chloride was quite low, and activation was only about 1.5-fold. Nonetheless, as indicated in Table I, the actual amounts of chloride taken up were quite high. We concluded that both chloride and thiocyanate ions could be taken up into granules in an ATP-dependent fashion.

Displacement of Labeled SCN by Unlabeled Anions

In many cases radioactive ligands can be displaced from specific compartments by adding excess unlabeled ligand to the system. The relative ability of ligand analogs to displace the labeled ligand can provide information about the size and location of the specific compartment. We have used this approach to analyze the distribution of labeled anions in chromaffin granules.

As shown in Table II, the relative ability of unlabeled anions (90 mM; 27.5 × 10^3-fold greater mass) to displace bound ^{14}C-SCN was SCN > Cl ≫ ISETH. Isethionate (90 mM) was extremely poor at displacing the trace anion, implying that isethionate had poor affinity for the permeant anion compartment. This seemed consistent with the observation that isethionate could not support release and was, in general, an impermeant anion.

An important observation was that while granule-associated counts were reduced in the presence of greater unlabeled mass, the increment from added ATP was still generally observed. This suggested that the ^{14}C-SCN did not enter a new compartment when ATP was added. Rather, the preexisting compartment was probably expanded.

Displacement of ^{36}Cl by Unlabeled Anions

As shown in Table III, both SCN and Cl (90 mM; 45-fold greater mass) were also able to displace ^{36}Cl from granules. The relative ability of the anions to displace ^{36}Cl from granules followed the pattern, Cl > SCN ≫ ISETH. As in the case of ^{14}C-SCN, the impermeant anion isethionate proved to be quite poor at displacing ^{36}Cl. In addition, the percent displacement was independent of the presence or absence of ATP, when compared to the relevant control incubation. In the chloride experiments, there appeared to be a relatively larger amount of nonspecifically associated ^{36}Cl as compared to the experiments with ^{14}C-SCN. However, this could probably be traced to the smaller amount of mass used to displace ^{36}Cl. We interpret these results to suggest that SCN and Cl, but not isethionate, go into analogous compartments within the granule.

TABLE II. Displacement of ^{14}C-SCN by Other Anions

^{14}C-SCN, 4μM + additions	1 mM Mg^{2+}-ATP	cpm/mg protein	% Displaced counts relative to presence or absence of Mg^{2+}-ATP
None	−	24,650 ± 50	−
	+	78,300 ± 200	−
SCN$^−$, 90 mM	−	1,400 ± 50	94.4
	+	820 ± 200	98.9
Cl$^−$, 90 mM	−	6,310 ± 1,000	74.4
	+	16,720 ± 780	77.8
Isethionate, 90 mM	−	21,130 ± 400	14.2
	+	87,530 ± 170	0

TABLE III. Displacement of ^{36}Cl by Other Anions

^{36}Cl, 2 mM + additions	1mM Mg^{2+}-ATP	cpm/mg protein	% Displaced counts relative to presence or absence of ATP
None	−	990 ± 200	−
	+	1,625 ± 150	−
Cl$^−$, 90 mM	−	140 ± 100	86%
	+	565 ± 120	65%
SCN$^−$, 90 mM	−	300 ± 70	70%
	+	520 ± 70	68%
Isethionate, 90 mM	−	1,580 ± 90	0
	+	2,440 ± 140	0

DISCUSSION

These results show that ATP stimulates epinephrine release from secretory granules in the presence of permeant anions such as chloride and thiocyanate. Concomitantly, ATP also supports the uptake of ^{36}Cl and ^{14}C-SCN into granules. It is thus likely that these 2 processes are closely linked. Further evidence for a connection between release and anion uptake is that isethionate did not support release, and was unable to displace ^{36}Cl or ^{14}C-SCN from granules. The latter result probably reflects the impermeant character of isethionate. As indicated earlier, a reasonable consequence of anion influx would be an accompanying water influx. This would lead to osmotic imbalance and subsequent lysis. This concept is consistent with earlier reports that hypertonic sucrose or salt solutions were able to suppress ATP-stimulated release (6). These suggestions are summarized in Fig. 2.

It is important to note that the uptake of ^{36}Cl and ^{14}C-SCN was studied at 4°C, as in previous studies, in order to minimize release. The Arrhenious plot for ATP-mediated release was linear between 41°C and 4°C (6). This led us to conclude that events studied at 4°C gave valid information on events occurring at 37°C.

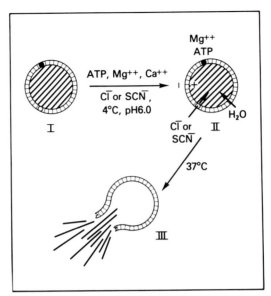

Fig. 2. Role of ATP and permeant anions in the regulation of internal osmotic pressure and subsequent release of granule contents. (I) represents the intact, stable granule. The solid circle represents the ATP binding site, while the open circle represents an anion permeation site. (II) represents the granule in the process of ATP binding, and anion and water uptake. The generation of a membrane potential positive on the inside by the addition of magnesium ATP is indicated on the ± signs on opposite sides of the membrane. (III) represents the releasing granule. Release only occurs if the temperature is raised to 37°C. The empty granule then reseals to form an osmotically intact ghost (8).

The studies with displacement of ^{14}C-SCN and ^{36}Cl by excess mass supported the concept that thiocyanate and chloride occupied analogous compartments within the granule. Both thiocyanate and chloride displaced large amounts of labeled SCN and Cl, respectively (94% and 86% for each homologous pair). Yet, both SCN and Cl displaced significant amounts of ^{36}Cl and ^{14}C-SCN, respectively (75% and 70% for each heterologous pair). The ability of large amounts of unlabeled mass to displace labeled anions suggests that the capacity of the anion compartment is limited. The specificity of these compartments for anions that support release is emphasized by the observation that isethionate, which does not support release, displaced only negligible amounts of either ^{36}Cl or ^{14}C-SCN.

An important question is how this anion-dependent osmotic mechanism might relate to exocytosis from cells. We have suggested a plausible hypothesis to account for release by exocytosis in terms of the biochemistry of release from isolated secretory vesicles (Fig. 3). A fundamental assumption in pursuing this analysis is that the chemistry of the "fusion" complex of secretory vesicle and plasma membrane is defined in part by the chemistry of the secretory vesicle. This may be why a release mechanism can be demonstrated with isolated secretory vesicles but without added plasma membranes. Evidence for formation of such a "fusion" complex in other cells prior to the actual loss of locale granule and cell membrane integrity in the "fission" step is discussed by Palade et al. (22).

It is likely that the sensitive ATP, Cl-mechanism underlying vesicle release may also be intimately involved in the actual physiological events of secretion. One approach to

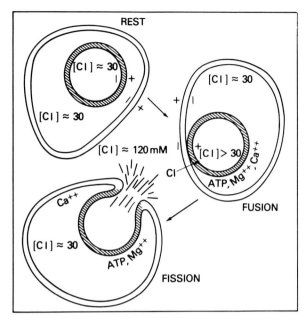

Fig. 3. Model for exocytosis based on regulation of anion permeability of granules by ATP. The granule membrane is represented by the cross-hatched profile, while the chromaffin cell plasma membrane is blank. In the resting chromaffin cell (REST) the chloride concentration within and outside the granule is similar (approximately 30 mM). By contrast, the extracellular chloride concentration is approximately 120 mM. The chromaffin cell has a resting potential of −35 mV while the granule at pH 7 also has a negative potential for ^{35}S-SCN (8). FUSION represents a state in which the granule and plasma membranes become closely juxtaposed. This concept serves to indicate that an interaction between membranes must occur before the release event occurs, and is further elaborated in an accompanying paper by Heuser (22). Upon the introduction of ATP into the system, the granule membrane potential becomes relatively positive inside, and chloride can move down the local gradient: FISSION represents formation of an exocytotic complex, possibly through local osmotic rupture of the granule membrane.

analyzing the relationship of vesicle chemistry to secretion is to consider the relative concentration of chloride in different chromaffin cell compartments. As summarized in Fig. 3, the concentration of chloride is approximately 120 mM in extracellular fluid. By contrast, it is only 30 mM both within the cell (6) and within the granule (6). However, when a "fusion" complex is established, a new chloride gradient is also established across the "fusion" site between the extracellular fluid and the granule interior. The role of ATP in this model would be to activate anion uptake and to allow chloride to move down the concentration gradient.

The most important part of this model is the molecular insight regarding conversion of the "fusion" state to the "fission" state. We have presented evidence here for an osmotic imbalance hypothesis in which ATP, divalent cations, and permeant anions play a major role in this conversion. The major assumption in this analysis is that the mechanism of ATP-mediated release from vesicles is the same as that for the cellular process of secretion. However, the strength of our hypothesis is that it only invokes components and conditions found in the in vivo secretory system. It is worthwhile noting that high speed cinematographic observations of releasing mast cells show the histamine granules rapidly "swelling" evidently just prior to their release by exocytosis (23). This result is seemingly consistent with the osmotic imbalance mechanism presented here.

REFERENCES

1. Oka, M., Ohuchi, T., Yoshida, H., and Imaizumi, R.: Biochim. Biophys. Acta 97:170–171 (1965).
2. Oka, M., Ohichi, T., Yoshida, H., and Imaizumi, R.: J. Pharmacol. 17:199 (1967).
3. Poisner, A. M., and Trifaro, J. M.: Molec. Pharm. 3:561–571 (1967).
4. Lishajko, F.: Acta Physiol. Scand. 75:255–266 (1969).
5. Hoffman, P. G., Zinder, O., Nikodijevik, O., and Pollard, H. B., J. Supramol. Struct. 4:181–184 (1976).
6. Hoffman, P. G., Zinder, O., Bonner, W. M., and Pollard, H. B.: Arch. Biochem. Biophys., 176:375–388 (1976).
7. Oka, M., Ohuchi, T., Yoshida, H., Imaizumi, R.: Japan J. Pharm. 15:348–365 (1965).
8. Pollard, H. B., Zinder, O., Hoffman, P. G., and Nikodijevik, O.: J. Biol. Chem. 251:4544–4550 (1976).
9. Poisner, A. M., and Douglas, W. W.: Molec. Pharm. 4:531–540 (1968).
10. Matsuda, T., Hata, F., and Yoshida, H.: Biochim. Biophys. Acta 150:739–741 (1968).
11. Yoshida, H., Ishida, H., Miki, N., and Yamamoto, I.: Biochim. Biophys. Acta 158:489–490 (1968).
12. Berl, S., Puszkin, S., and Nicklas, W. J.: Science 179:441–444 (1973).
13. Putzkin, S., and Kochwa, S.: J. Biol. Chem. 249:7711–7714 (1974).
14. Yount, R. G., Ojala, D., and Babcock, D.: Biochemistry 10:2490–2496 (1971).
15. Zinder, O., Nikodijevik, O., Hoffman, P. G., and Pollard, H. B.: J. Biol. Chem. 251:2179–2181 (1976).
16. Nikodijevik, O., Nikodijevik, B., Zinder, O., Wu, M-Y. W., Guroff, G., and Pollard, H. B.: Proc. Natl. Acad. Sci. USA 73:771–774 (1976).
17. Bashford, C. L., Radda, G. K., and Richie, G. A.: FEBS Letters 50:21–24 (1975).
18. Taugner, G.: Biochem. J. 130:969–973 (1972).
19. Anton, A. H., and Sayer, D. F.: J. Pharm. Exptl. Therap. 138:360–375 (1962).
20. Lowry, O. H., Rosebrough, N. J., Farr, A. L., and Randall, R. J.: J. Biol. Chem. 193:265–275 (1951).
21. Deffner, R. J.: Biochim. Biophys. Acta 47:378–388 (1961).
22. Palade, G.: Science 189:347–358 (1976).
23. Douglas, W. W.: Personal communication (1976).

Analysis of Spastic: A Neurological Mutant of the Mexican Axolotl

C. F. Ide and N. Miszkowski

Biology Department, Princeton University, Princeton, New Jersey 08540

C.B. Kimmel and E. Schabtach

Biology Department, University of Oregon, Eugene, Oregon 97403

R. Tompkins

Biology Department, Tulane University, New Orleans, Louisiana 70118

O. Elbert and M. Duda

Jenkins Biophysical Laboratories, The Johns Hopkins University, Baltimore, Maryland 21218

The spastic mutation induces swimming coordination and equilibrium deficiencies in the Mexican axolotl, Ambystoma Mexicanum. Behavioral ontogeny studies determined that spastics fail to develop behavior trains of sinusoidal flexures necessary to mediate escape swimming at the time of onset of cerebellar function. Behavior analysis, after lesioning different cranial nerve roots and CNS areas in wild-type animals, confirmed the "behavioral focus" of the mutation to lie in the auricle or vestibulocerebellum. Unit recordings determined that the mutant auricle and adjacent area acousticolateralis (AAL) maintain a full complement of functional vestibular unit types found in wild-type. However, the topographical distribution of vestibular units in these areas changed under the influence of the spastic gene. Seventy percent of all mutant vestibular units were encountered in a small zone defined by the ventral auricle and adjacent tissue connecting auricle and AAL; only 41% appeared in this zone in wild-type, a statistically significant difference (P < .001). Correlated with this translocation of spastic vestibular units, mutant Purkinje cells and allied afferent and efferent fiber tracts are also translocated into the ventral auricle. Moreover, boundaries between cerebellar granule cell and Purkinje cell zones are less precise in mutants. At the time of onset of spasticity (feeding stage larvae), the mutant cerebellum and adjacent midbrain are reduced dorsally and laterally; mutant cells appear disoriented and are clustered about the cerebellar ependymal zone. These and other findings indicate that faulty morphogenetic movements and/or altered cell-cell recognition may underlie spastic behavioral and neurological deficiencies.

Key words: behavior, phenocopy, vestibular function, cerebellum, Purkinje cell

With pleasure we dedicate this paper to Dr. R. R. Humphrey, who discovered the spastic mutant and many other mutants of the Mexican axolotl.

Address all correspondence to C. F. Ide, Jenkins Department of Biophysics, The Johns Hopkins University, Baltimore, MD 21218.

INTRODUCTION

The analysis of behavior mutants provides unique opportunities for combining techniques of behavior, anatomy, physiology, and embryology into understanding how a single gene can influence basic morphogenetic processes during neurogenesis (1). Cerebellar mutants found in the mouse have been instructive in categorizing developmental abnormalities in CNS morphology which accrue from single genetic changes. Most of these mutants show degeneration of particular cerebellar cell types: granule cells degenerate in both the staggerer (2, 3, 4) and the weaver (5, 6) mutants; Purkinje cells in both the Nervous (7, 8) and Pcd (9) mutants. Unlike these mutants, all cerebellar cell types are present in the Reeler mutant; however, the cerebellum, cerebral isocortex, and hippocampus are severely malformed due to the inability of migrating cells to attain their proper positions during development (10, 11, 12).

Mutant analysis has also added new dimensions to neuroethology by providing a tool for categorizing how genetic contributions shape functional circuitry underlying behavior. For example, in the hyperkinetic[1P] mutant in Drosophila, abnormal leg shaking during anesthetization correlates with abnormal burst activity in thoracic motoneurons (13). Another Drosophila mutant, stripe, cannot fly due to abnormal motor output bursts (14). In the filiform mutant found in the cricket, changes in form and function of identifiable interneurons result from the absence of sensory hairs (15). Among vertebrate mutants, the visual system of the Siamese cat shows anomalous rewiring (16, 17, 18). In the staggerer mouse, cerebellar Purkinje cells exhibit changes in antidromic activation as well as the absence of spontaneous climbing fiber responses (19).

A behavior mutant of the amphibia has recently become available which, like the mutants described above, lends itself to studies of both neurogenesis and neuroethology. The spastic gene found in the Mexican axolotl shows mendelian recessive inheritance (20, 21, 22, 23). The phenotype includes bizarre coiling and thrashing locomotor patterns, and failure to maintain equilibrium. The following report traces the focus of spastic gene expression through: 1) behavioral ontogeny where locomotor and equilibrium deficiencies occur at a discrete stage of development; 2) alterations in the regional distribution of vestibular units in the cerebellum and other areas; 3) alterations in the anatomical organization of cerebellum and midbrain; and, finally, to 4) the possibility that faulty morphogenetic movements occur during neurogenesis.

MATERIALS AND METHODS

Behavior

Procedures used to quantitatively describe the locomotor ontogeny of wild-type and spastic axolotls have been detailed elsewhere (23). These techniques were modified for analysis of spastic behavior phenocopies created by surgically lesioning different CNS areas of known vestibular projection in wild-type animals. Both before and after lesioning, animals were placed in a 30 cm diameter bowl containing Steinberg's saline; 2 Ag/AgCl wires connected to a Grass S-44 stimulator (with isolation unit) were placed each on 1 side of the bowl; the bowl remained permanently positioned beneath a Bolex 16 mm movie camera. After triggering the camera (32 frames/sec), a series of 10 msec shocks (3 pps) were delivered to the bath until the animal showed the first sign of movement. A shock voltage sufficient to induce the axolotl to swim, but not intense enough to directly induce muscle contraction, was determined phenomonologically on the 1st day of the study and utilized in all studies thereafter. Each bout of locomotor activity was analyzed in its entirety. Of 45 bouts filmed after cerebellar lesioning, 41 were composed of 90 frames or more; all 45 bouts filmed before lesioning contained 90 frames or more. The behavioral criteria employed for analysis of locomotor responses were essentially those of Coghill (24). Coghill described an early response in embryos capable of reacting to external stimuli as a thrashing or "coiling" response which, later in development, gradually gives rise to true swimming or the "sinusoid" response. Still, larvae and even adult wild-type axolotls show low levels of coiling during vigorous swimming, and, as shown below, spastic and spastic phenocopies coil repeatedly during strong locomotor bouts. Thus, the "coil," the "sinusoid," and the "straight" positions were chosen as locomotor elements used for analysis.

Each locomotor bout was scored by recording the locomotor element the animal showed for each frame in a particular bout; either "coil" (Fig. 1b), "sinusoid" (Fig. 1c), or "straightout." The mean "coil/frame" and the mean "sinusoid/frame" were then computed for each bout: these 2 variables were then averaged on the one hand, for un-lesioned animals, and on the other, for lesioned animals; means for lesioned and un-lesioned were subjected to statistical analysis employing a modified t-test which does not assume the population variances for both lesioned and unlesioned to be equal, but esti-mates each separately (25). Most animals contributed 4 pre- and 4 postlesion bouts.

Behavior Phenocopies

The study encompassed behavioral analysis of more than 30 wild-type axolotls (5–10 cm in length). After behavioral testing (above) each axolotl was anesthetized in 1:1,000 Finquel (MS-222) for 5–10 min. A craniotomy was then performed which exposed the brain from the level of the optic tectum to the spino-bulbar junction. A choroid plexus covering the hindbrain was carefully removed to allow visualization of the cerebellar auricle, the V, VII, and VIIIth cranial roots, and the posterior medulla. Cerebellar auricle, cranial root, midbrain, and medullar lesions were accomplished by cutting through these structures with microscissors and then completely separating the cut pieces with a tungsten probe. For cerebellar lesions, similar results were obtained by using the end of a sharp syringe needle as a microknife. Several sham operated animals served as additional controls.

The animal was allowed to recover for 12 hr in Steinberg's saline and then tested behaviorally (above). The axolotl was then re-anesthetized and fixed in Bouin's fluid for 4–7 days. The heads were paraffin embedded, sectioned at 10 μm in the horizontal plane, and stained with hematoxylin-metanil yellow-alcian blue according to Humason (26). All lesions were confirmed histologically.

Electrophysiology

Data are presented for 11 wild-type and 5 spastic animals, although more than 30 animals were examined, including the pilot study. Adult axolotls ranging in length from 20–30 cm were anesthetized by immersion in either a 4% urethan solution or a 1:500 (w/w) Tricaine (MS-222) solution for 30–50 min. The anesthetized animal was then placed in a small plexiglass bath. The animal was held in place by adjustable brass rods (covered with plastic) which were form-fitted to the curvature of the axolotl's neck. The rods were applied on both sides of the animal directly behind the gills to clamp the mid-line axis of the body in line with the longitudinal center line of the bath. A small Teflon clip was applied to the upper jaw on one side of the animal. Moist cotton was then tightly packed around the trunk of the animal to facilitate integumental respiration, and to steady the axolotl during rotation. The bath was then filled with cold Steinberg's saline containing 0.5% Dextrose, to a level just covering the axolotl. The bath temperature was maintained at $12°C$, during surgery by a cooling plate fixed beneath the bath.

A craniotomy was performed exposing the brain from the level of the diencephalon to the level of the first spinal segment. Since a choroid plexus, covering the hindbrain from the posterior cerebellum to the calamus scriptorius, obscured both the area acousticolateralis and the cerebellar auricle, portions of it were removed or pushed to the side to expose these areas. The pial membrane was opened above the optic tectum to allow placement of the electrodes in the cerebellum. The axolotl was then immobilized with a 1 ml injection of d-tubocuraine (5mg/ml), and kept in the cooled bath for 3–6 hr before recording was initiated. The bath was transferred to a table designed to rotate from $0°$ to a maximum of $20°$ to either side about the longitudinal axis. Up to 4 micromanipulators were clamped onto bars mounted on the rotating table to serve as electrode carriers. A Trent-Wells hydraulic microdrive was utilized for stereotaxic recording. Extracellular single and multiunit recordings were accomplished with either 4M NaCl or tungsten microelectrodes. The tip of the NaCl electrode was carefully broken off under a compound microscope to lower the tip resistance to 2–5 megaohms. The electrode tip was dipped in India ink to aid visualization of the tip near the brain surface.

A coordinate system composed of grids was superimposed on the cerebellum and adjacent area acousticolateralis. The brain areas where sufficient responses were found for analysis in both wild-type and spastic are pictured in Figs. 3 and 4. Extracellular potential changes were recorded with a WPI AC coupled DAM-5 preamplifier (gain = 100) and displayed on a model 5103 Tektronix oscilloscope at 2 different sweep speeds.

To mark the table position at any given instant, a 1 kHz sine wave was applied through a variable potentiometer mounted on the center rod of the turntable such that the amplitude of the wave changed with the degree of rotation. In several experiments a DC current was applied through the potentiometer such that the vertical deflection of an extra oscilloscope trace marked the degree of rotation.

To avoid inaccuracies of depth measurement due to surface dimpling, the initial penetration for each transect was carried out via the coarse drive on the electrode carrier. Once the electrode penetrated the surface tissue, it was carefully returned to the surface (a 10–20 μm excursion), and then lowered with the fine microdrive. Most unit types encountered during electrode descent were reencountered at the same position on electrode ascent. To be considered a valid transect, the "zero" or surface position after ascent had to match the "zero" position before descent. The response criteria employed for categorization of unit types were determined phenomenologically in pilot studies.

Neuroanatomy: Adult Brains

Adult brains were removed from 5 mutant and 10 wild-type animals studied in electrophysiology experiments described above. Two mutant and 5 wild-type brains were fixed in 10% formalin for 1 week and then transferred to a 1:1 formol-saline:gum arabic solution for 3 days. They were then incubated in 5% gelatin ($52°C$) for 8 hr followed by 10% gelatin and soaked in 1:1 formol-saline:gum arabic solution for 3 days. The blocks were mounted on a freezing microtome with sliding knife and sectioned in the sagittal plane at 35 μm; sections were floated onto albumenized slides, stained for 8 hr in 0.1% Luxol fast blue (1.0 gram): 95% Ethanol solution (1 liter): 10% acetic acid (5.0 ml) followed by differentiation in lithium carbonate (0.5 g/liter). Sections were then stained in 0.5% cresyl violet solution (1 molar acetic acid, 34%; 1 molar sodium acetate, 6%) for 4 min. Slides were mounted with permount.

An additional 3 mutant and 5 wild-type brains were fixed in Bouin's solution for 1 day, washed 4 times in 70% alcohol, dehydrated in an alcohol series, cleared for 12 hr in methyl salicylate, and embedded in paraplast. Of these, 2 mutant and 4 wild-type brains were cut at 15 μm in the sagittal plane; 1 mutant wild-type pair was sectioned in the transverse plane. Alternate sections from each brain were divided into 2 sets; 1 set was silver stained either by the Guillery method (27) or by a modification of the Rowell method (28).

Two mutant brains and 2 wild-type brains were photographed serially at 30 μm; negatives were printed on 4 × 5 film sheets. These "transparencies" were superimposed upon one another at 60 μm intervals to allow reconstruction of tracts and nuclei for each hemicerebellum. The remaining 3 mutant cerebella, together with the 3 matched wild-type cerebella, were reconstructed from tracings via a Leitz drawing tube.

Neuroanatomy: Light and Electron Microscopy of Early Larvae

Spastic and sibling wild-type larvae were obtained from 3 different matings of adult axolotls known to carry the spastic gene heterozygously. At the early feeding stage (Harrison stage 46, 13—18 mm length), the time of onset of spasticity, larvae were anesthetized in 1:1,000 MS-222, and the heads were removed with a single transverse slice just caudal to the otic capsules; the heads were than placed in 1% OsO_4 buffered with 0.16 M sodium phosphate, pH 7.2 and containing 0.005% $CaCl_2$ and 0.54% glucose. After fixation for 1 hr the specimens were thoroughly washed in buffer, dehydrated through alcohols and propylene oxide, and embedded in epon-araldite.

The hindbrain and midbrain was sectioned in the transverse plane at 5 μm, using glass knives with the Reichert OMU-2 ultramicrotome. The sections were saved in serial order, each being laid on a small drop of water and dried at 45°C on slides previously treated with Dupont "slip-spray." Sections were stained for 5 min with 1% paraphenylene diamine in 70% methanol, covered with a drop of resin and a coverslip, and either examined immediately or stored at 0°C.

Representative 5 μm sections through cerebellar areas were photographed using phase optics, and the photographs were subsequently used to identify areas studied with the electron microscope. These sections were then re-embedded after removal of the coverslip, by inverting a resin-filled capsule over each individual section.

After polymerization the block was snapped away from the slide; it contained the 5 μm slice of the cerebellum near its surface in proper orientation for thin sectioning. These were cut and groups of sections were saved on serially numbered grids. This re-embedding technique has been described in detail elsewhere (29). The sections were subsequently stained with uranyl acetate (30) and lead citrate (31) and examined with a Philips 300 electron microscope.

RESULTS

The data to be presented here represent a panoramic overview of the principal findings from 5 very different studies concerned with how the spastic gene affects neurogenesis. Since full documentation of data from each of these studies in one paper is unfeasible, the salient features of each are presented here; each study will be described in detail elsewhere.

Behavior Ontogeny

A quantitative study of the development of locomotor behavior patterns in mutants and sibling controls discerned the first functional expression of the spastic gene (23).

Approximately 6,000 movie frames were scored for, among other variables, the incidence of 2 elements of swimming behavior: embryonic coiling (Fig. 1b), and sinusoid (Fig. 1c) or true swimming. Homozygous mutants show bizarre patterns of behavior, as may be seen in the cinematographic records of larval escape responses in Fig. 1a. Wild-type larvae swim in a straight line and remain dorsal-side up (D). The spastic mutant exhibits circular coiling, and frequently turns ventral-side up (V) (Fig. 1a). Figures 1b and 1c show the ontogeny of behavioral deficiencies; early embryos of either genotype exhibit coil (Fig. 1b) responses, and later begin to show sinusoidal (Fig. 1c) movements which are the precursors of patterned swimming. In these graphs the ordinate on the left measures the percent occurrence of either coil or sinusoidal responses: the responses of mutant and wild-type are shown as overlapped bars with the bar shaded when wild-type values exceed mutant values; asterisks and the right-hand ordinate plot the t-test probability that normal and mutant means differ by chance (values between 0.05 and 0.0 are statistically significant).

A major difference is first observed at day 18 in development, which corresponds to the early larval feeding stage. At this time, and at later times, the wild-type is seen to exhibit many more sinusoid responses than the mutant. Prior to day 18, through Harrison's swimming stages (H38–44), both mutants and controls respond to strong tactile or electrical stimulation by interspersing coils and sinusoids. At the early feeding stage (H46), wild-type animals abruptly decrease coiling behavior and begin coupling sinusoid elements into strong "escape swimming" patterns; mutants fail to generate such "escape" patterns; solitary sinusoid elements persist, interspersed with coil elements, into adult life (Fig. 1). Previous studies by Coghill (32, 33) ascribed such changes in wild-type behavior seen at the early feeding stage (e.g., strong swimming, orientation) to the onset of function in midbrain and cerebellum.

Behavior Phenocopies

To test the hypothesis that cerebellar deficiencies can account for altered locomotor and equilibratory patterns such as those seen in mutants, "spastic phenocopies" were created by surgically ablating different brain areas in wild-type larvae (Elbert et al., in preparation). Previously, phenocopies were made by bilaterally sectioning the ascending projection of the VIII (vestibular) cranial nerve (34, 35). These fibers are the main afferent projection to the cerebellum in early larval stages. Sectioning the descending vestibular projection or the V, VII, or X cranial nerves failed to create phenocopies. In recent studies, lesioning the cerebellar auricle (vestibulocerebellum) created phenocopies; removing the entire brain anterior to the level of the cerebellum failed to make phenocopies. Moreover, this ablation failed to disrupt phenocopy behavior of previously cerebellectomized or VIII-sectioned animals. Thus, the "phenocopy circuit" involves the VIII projection to the cerebellum, the cerebellum, and possibly the motor tegmentum ventral to the cerebellum.

Quantitative behavioral measurements for the 3 most instructive lesions appear in Fig. 2. Where unlesioned animals perform sinusoidal movements 68.9% of the time during

Fig. 1. Behavioral ontogeny of wild-type and spastic mutant axolotls. 1a. In cinematographic records of larval escape responses, a wild-type animal swims in a straight line and remains dorsal-side up (d); a spastic animal exhibits circular coiling, and frequently turns ventral-side up (v). Figs. 1b and 1c show the ontogeny of behavioral deficiencies; coil (1b) and sinusoid (1c) frequencies are plotted as a function of days of development; responses of mutant and wild-type appear as overlapped bars with the bar shaded when wild-type values exceed mutant values; asterisks and the right-hand ordinate plot the t-test probability that normal and mutant means differ by chance (values between 0.05 and 0.0 are statistically significant).

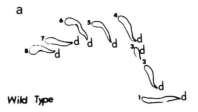

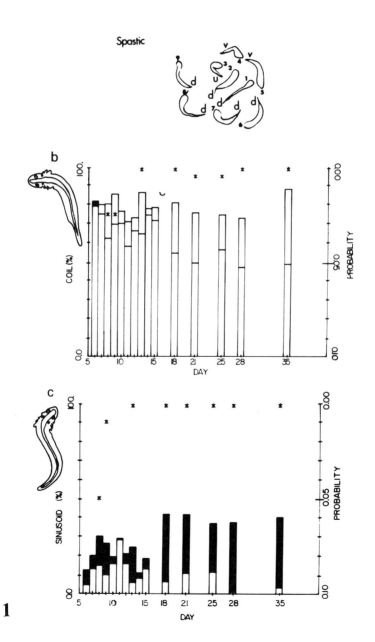

1

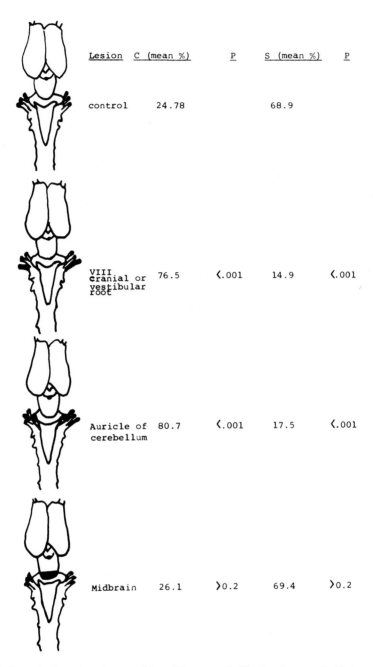

Lesion	C (mean %)	P	S (mean %)	P
control	24.78		68.9	
VIII cranial or vestibular root	76.5	<.001	14.9	<.001
Auricle of cerebellum	80.7	<.001	17.5	<.001
Midbrain	26.1	>0.2	69.4	>0.2

Fig. 2. This figure depicts selected areas of the wild-type axolotl brain where surgical lesions did or did not produce spastic behavioral phenocopies. Frequencies of occurrence of coil and sinusoid responses during locomotor bouts appear with their respective lesion sites. "P" represents the t-test probability that the responses for lesioned animals differ by chance from unlesioned animals.

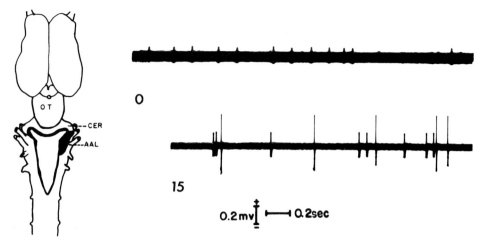

Fig. 3. Small "level" units found in the wild-type AAL discharge when the table is held at 0° ("0"). Two ipsilateral tonic units ("+ tonic") become active after the table is tilted about the longitudinal axis to a sustained tilt of 15° ("15").
Abbreviations: AAL = area acousticolateralis; CER = cerebellum, OT = optic tectum.

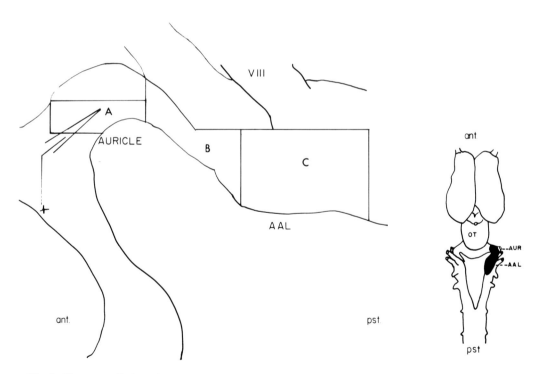

Fig. 4. Mutant vestibular units show a statistically significant topographical "translocation" into the zone defined, rostrally, by the ventral (below 300 μm) auricle (A) and, caudally, by tissue (B) joining auricle and AAL (C). Two by two contingency analysis comparing the number of units in this zone (deep A and B) vs the remaining analysis area (shallow A and C) reveals a difference between spastic and wild-type significant at the 0.001 level. Sampling was accomplished by dividing the length of the AAL plus the auricle into 7 contiguous zones, each of which was characterized by sampling an equal number of times. Abbreviations: AUR = auricle; AAL and OT as in Fig. 3; ANT = anterior; PST = posterior.

locomotion, both vestibular nerve-sectioned and cerebellar-lesioned animals perform sinusoidal movements only 14.9% and 17.5% of the time, respectively. Both values are significantly different from the value for unlesioned animals at the 0.001 level. These differences occur concommitant with increases in coiling behavior. Unlesioned animals coil 24.7% of the time; vestibular nerve-sectioned animals coil 76.5% of the time; cerebellar auricle-lesioned animals 80.7% of the time. Older spastic larvae show coil frequencies of 89% and sinusoid frequencies of 4% (Fig. 1b, c; day 35). Thus, both lesions create quantitative phenocopies with respect to spastic locomotor behavior. Interestingly, the coil and sinusoid behavior of animals with complete isolation of the entire brain anterior to the level of the cerebellum is equivalent to that of unlesioned animals (Fig. 2). Although these axolotls lack spontaneity and vigor during locomotor bouts, their swimming pattern (many sinusoid elements, few coils) remains unchanged. It appears, then, that the "behavioral focus" of the mutation may be an exclusive property of hindbrain structures.

Focus of Functional Lesions in Vestibular Circuitry: Electrophysiology

Physiological studies were undertaken to further localize the focus of functional lesions in the cerebellum and other vestibular areas in the mutant. Initial experiments determined that a full complement of vestibular unit types found in the wild-type also appears in the spastic.

The data presented below were gathered with the primary goal of comparing vestibular function in the spastic and wild-type axolotl. Because the normal axolotl had not been studied, it was first necessary to obtain some baseline data before the effects of the spastic gene on vestibular physiology could be assessed. This goal necessarily restricted the scope of the wild-type analysis to a broad classification to which the mutant could be conveniently compared.

Microelectrode recordings were taken from the area acousticolateralis (AAL, primitive vestibular nucleus) and the cerebellar auricle (vestibulocerebellum) (36) while the preparation was tilted to either side of the longitudinal body axis. A variety of vestibular unit types previously described for other vertebrate groups were encountered in both animal types. Units responding to the level position (tonically = "level units," phasically = "0° burst units"), phasic units responding during ipsilateral ("+ phasic") or contralateral ("− phasic") tilting, and tonic units responding to ipsilateral ("+ tonic") or contralateral ("− tonic") tilts were mapped in areas known from anatomy to contain vestibular projections.

Individual units were tested by a series of rotations (0° to ipsilateral, ipsilateral back through 0° to contralateral, contralateral back to 0°) performed in sequence. This sequence was repeated as many as 5 times during isolation and tuning of individual units. All units were tested at least twice, e.g., a + tonic unit showing tonic activity at ipsilateral tilt had to cease firing after rotation to contralateral tilt and retain its former tonic activity after rerotation through 0° to ipsilateral tilt. All units which could not be repeatedly tested were discarded.

Thus, units were selected with considerable care with regard to vestibular response criteria. Application of these rigorous response criteria made it impossible to also obtain information concerning average amplitudes, firing rates, and other discharge parameters of the 5 unit types, and such information awaits further analysis.

A further constraint was imposed by the survival to adulthood of only 5 of 300 spastic embryos embracing several spawnings by adults heterozygous for the spastic gene. In addition to the problem of limited experimental material, it must be recognized that the 5 survivors may represent a minority in which the spastic gene shows incomplete penetrance. Thus, these adult mutants used in physiology studies may represent the "most anatomically and physiologically organized" spastics.

Table I depicts the frequency of occurrence of the different unit types as a percentage of total units encountered for the AAL and cerebellar auricle. Unfortunately, sample sizes are too small to permit statistical comparisons between wild-type and mutant for different individual unit types. However, individual distributions do form several interesting patterns which, although tentative, are worth pointing out. First, when compared to wild-type, mutants showed 15% more units spontaneously active in the level position in the AAL, and again, 15% more in the auricle ("level" plus "$0°$ burst" units). In the same light, units recorded in the trochlear (IV) motor nerve of the mutant showed more spontaneous activity in the level position; in addition, where wild-type trochlear units cease firing on contralateral rotation, mutant trochlear units remain active at contralateral tilt (37). Increases in spontaneous discharge in AAL, auricle, and trochlear nucleus suggest the absence of an inhibitory influence in the mutant, possibly due to a reduced Purkinje cell efferent projection.

Second, concommitant with increases in spontaneous activity, the data suggest that mutants show a reduction in relative numbers of predominant unit types found in both AAL and cerebellum of wild-type animals. The unit type most frequently encountered in the wild-type AAL discharges continuously at sustained ipsilateral tilt ("+ tonic" units, Fig. 3); these units remain silent during tilting to either side, at sustained contralateral tilt, or in the level position. In the wild-type AAL, 52% of all units encountered were "+ tonic" units, compared to 33% in mutants, a difference of 19%.

Curiously, a similar pattern emerges in the cerebellar auricle. Here the most frequently encountered unit type increases its discharge rate during tilting to ipsilateral ("+ phasic" units). Forty-five percent of wild-type cerebellar units are of this type, compared to 32% for spastics, a difference of 13%. In both cerebellum and AAL, the remaining 3 unit types responding during tilting or at sustained tilt occur in similar numbers in both mutant and wild-type. Thus, in both AAL and cerebellar auricle, mutants show apparent decreases in frequency of occurrence of the predominant unit type, apparent increases in occurrence of spontaneously active units, and roughly equivalent percentages of remaining unit types. These findings, although provocative, must be repeated and extended by statistical testing, when and if more adult mutants become available.

TABLE I. Distribution of Unit Types Found in AAL and Auricle

	Unit type	"+ tonic"	"+ phasic"	"− tonic"	"− phasic"	"level"	"0° burst"
AAL	Wild-type (% total units) (n = 87)	52.	26.	3.	6.	13.	
	Spastic (% total units) (n = 33)	33.	18.	9.	12.	28.	
	Δ%	+ 19.	+8.	− 6.	− 6.	− 15.	
Auricle	Wild-type (% total units) (n = 44)	21.	45.	5.	11.	7.	11.
	Spastic (% total units) (n = 40)	20.	32.	5.	10.	13.	20.
	Δ%	+1.	+ 13.	0	+ 1.	− 6.	− 9.

Perhaps the most compelling evidence pointing to differences in neurophysiology between mutant and wild-type lies in the topographical distribution of vestibular units in AAL and cerebellum. Anatomical studies described below point out obvious changes in mutants in the gross morphology of auricle and of adjacent tissue separating auricle from anterior AAL (Figs. 5a, b). In addition to these macroscopic changes in structure, a population of Purkinje cells and allied afferent and efferent tracts are "translocated" ventrally in the mutant auricle. Comparison of the distribution of vestibular units between mutant and normal in this anatomically distinct zone (ventral auricle plus adjacent caudal tissue, Fig. 4) vs the rest of the AAL and auricle is instructive; mutant vestibular units show a ventral and caudal "translocation" similar to cell and fiber translocations. Where 70% (N = 73) of all units encountered in the mutant AAL and auricle appeared in this ventro-caudal auricular area, only 41% were encountered here in the wild-type (N = 131). Statistical analysis showed this difference to be significant at the 0.001 level [2 × 2 contingency test (25), x^2 = 14.3].

Thus, electrophysiology studies revealed:1) that mutants maintain a full complement of vestibular unit types found in wild-type AAL and auricle; 2) that the incidence of occurrence of different unit types may be influenced by the spastic gene; and 3) that a significant difference between wild-type and spastic in the topographical distribution of vestibular units in AAL and auricle correlates with observed anatomical differences.

Neuroanatomy: Adult Cerebellum

Anatomically, the urodele cerebellum consists of 3 major parts: 1) the median body, or corpora, activated from the spinal cord, trigeminal nerve (Vth cranial root), and the tectum; 2) the lateral auricles, which are enlargements of the anterior area acoustico-lateralis (AAL); and 3) ventrally of the median body, a nucleus cerebelli (38). Vestibular (VIIIth) and lateral-line (VIIth, Xth cranial roots) fibers terminate in the auricle; the spino-cerebellar tract and Vth sensory root terminate in the median body (38).

Examination of brains previously characterized electrophysiologically revealed dramatic changes in both gross and fine anatomy of the mutant cerebellum (39). Obvious differences between spastic and wild-type in the gross anatomy of the cerebellum appear in Figs. 5a and b. Viewed from the side, the wild-type shows an acute flexure at the junction between the area acousticolateralis (AAL) and the cerebellum. The same area in the mutant gently rises from the AAL to the midbrain, inferior colliculus, at an obtuse angle (Fig. 5a). When viewed from the dorsal aspect, the cerebellar auricle (vestibulo-cerebellum) flares anterodorsally in the wild-type; the same area in the mutant is thickened ventrolaterally and fails to flare anterodorsally (Fig. 5B). Moreover, an area of the median body, the corpora, of the mutant cerebellum bulges medially where the equivalent area in the normal cerebellum forms a smooth ridge (Fig. 5b). In addition, the cerebellum of the spastic, when viewed from both aspects, appears to lack structural support. The cerebellum is limited in its dorsal extent and fails to show distinct boundaries between cerebellum and AAL. The midbrain bordering the cerebellum is also limited in its dorsoventral extent. Detailed changes in midbrain structure will be presented at another time.

Figures 5c and d are reconstructions of wild-type and spastic hemicerebella which plot the lateromedial position of Purkinje cells encountered every 60 μm. Although Purkinje cells are present in the mutant, their physical location is changed under the influence of the spastic gene. Auricular Purkinje cells are "crowded" ventrally in the cerebellar auricle, and caudally in the median body (Fig. 5c). These "crowded"

Purkinje cells occur in the auricular area which , when viewed from the gross aspect (Fig. 5b), fails to flare anterodorsally in the mutant; in like manner, median body Purkinje cells are "translocated" caudally toward the AAL. It is important to note that the external morphology of the reconstructed cerebella seen in Figs. 5c and d matches the gross morphology of the cerebella photographed directly in Figs. 5a and b.

By matching the cerebellar commissures and most dorsal points of the respective median bodies of spastic and wild-type reconstructions, superimposition of the 2 cerebella was effected (Fig. 5d). Differences in Purkinje cell distribution (ventrolateral and caudal translocations of Purkinje cells) are even more obvious after this superimposition. Purkinje cells fail to appear in the superficial auricle (above 200 μm), but do appear in a tight group below 200 μm.

The changes observed in Purkinje cell location are mirrored in changes in the distribution of other cell types and fiber tracts. Cerebellar granule cells are present in the mutant internal to the Purkinje cell zone and molecular layer (Fig. 6); however, more mutant granule cells appear to encroach further and in greater numbers into the Purkinje cell zone.

Moreover, all spastic preparations show radical changes in orientation and distribution of fibers and fascicles appearing in the molecular layer and cerebellar white matter. The wild-type molecular layer contains fibers oriented in the dorsoventral plane, many emanating from the Purkinje cell zone. Afferent tracts form recognizable fascicles in the white matter. The mutant molecular layer contains few fibers oriented dorsoventrally. White matter afferent tracts, such as VIII (vestibular) root fibers show varying degrees of disorientation (Fig. 6). Thus, the distribution and orientation of Purkinje cells, granule cells, and allied fiber tracts and fascicles are radically altered by the action of the spastic gene.

Neuroanatomy: Light and Electron Microscopy of Early Larvae

The onset of spastic behavioral deficiencies occurs very early, in terms of cerebellar development namely, in young feeding larvae (Fig. 1). Deficiencies in cerebellar morphology are also present at this stage (Ide et al., in preparation). Figure 7 compares cross-sections of the cerebellum of the wild-type (left) and mutant (right) at 3 levels — from the most rostral (Fig. 7a) to the most caudal (Fig. 7c). Gross defects in the form of the brain are encountered at each of these levels. Rostrally (Fig. 7a), the midbrain (M) is much smaller in the mutant, and the auricle (A) is less extended laterally. The same is observed at the intermediate level (Fig. 7b) and, in addition, the usually prominent isthmic sulcus (S) is nearly absent in the spastic. In the wild-type, ependymal cells are highly oriented with respect to this sulcus, while, in the mutant, the corresponding cells are arranged in disorganized clusters. At the caudalmost level of the cerebellum (Fig. 7c), the median body (B) is seen to be very reduced in size in the mutant; and, as shown above, the ventricular sculpturing is less pronounced (S), and ependymal cells are disoriented.

Electron microscopic examination of the cerebellum and midbrain of young feeding larvae also showed the gross defects described in Fig. 7. However, preliminary examination of the cerebellar neuropil has so far revealed no major defects in the mutant. In both the wild-type (Fig. 8a) and spastic (Fig. 8b), numerous presynaptic (axons) and postsynaptic profiles are present; chemical synapses (arrows) are numerous.

In like manner preliminary montage maps (constructed from electron micrographs of small areas of auricular neuropil) from matched spastic-wild-type pairs show no clear differences in the distribution of chemical synapses (Figs. 9a and b). However, extending

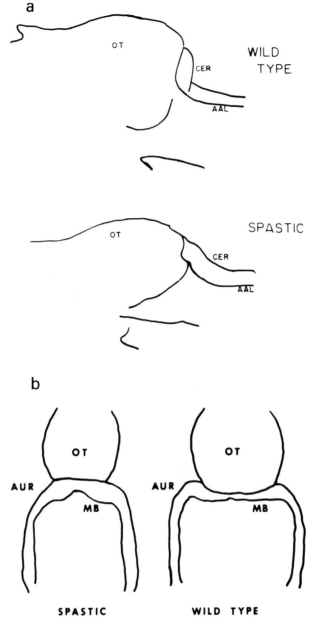

Fig. 5. In the mutant cerebellum, neuroanatomical differences correlate with physiological differences. 5a. Sagittal view of wild-type and spastic midbrain and cerebellum (tracings from stereophotomicrographs). Note the acute flexure between cerebellum (CER) and area acousticolateralis (AAL) in wild-type (upper) compared to the obtuse flexure between the 2 areas in the spastic (lower); OT = optic tectum. 5b. Dorsal view of whole brains described in Fig. 1 — where the wild-type cerebellar auricle flares rostrally (AUR), that of the mutant slopes caudally. Note the thickened cerebellar median body (MB) near the midline in the spastic. 5c. Reconstructions of wild-type and spastic hemicerebella from

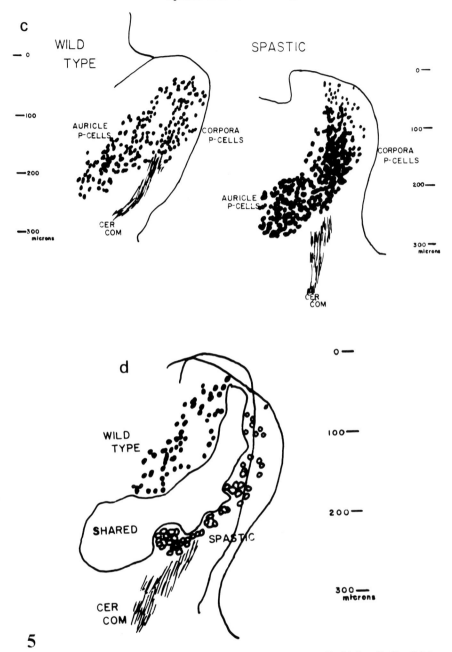

5 sagittal sections sampled every 60 μm. Note the "crowding" of auricular Purkinje cells (P-cells) between 200 and 300 μm in the spastic; CORPORA = median body; CER COM = cerebellar commissure. 5d. Spastic and wild-type hemicerebella are superimposed by rotating the spastic hemicerebellum 30°. Superficial Purkinje cells found exclusively in wild-type are shaded; Purkinje cells occurring caudoventrally exclusively in the spastic appear as open circles, and the area where Purkinje cells occur in both is outlined (shared).

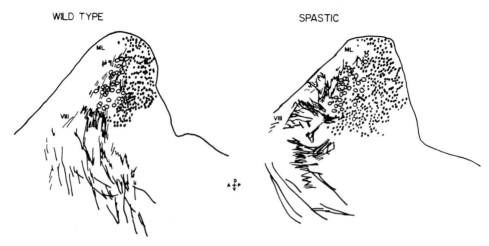

Fig. 6. Purkinje cells (open circles), granule cells (shaded), and molecular layer (ML) of mutant and wild-type cerebellar auricles – tracings from representative sections. In the spastic, granule cells encroach into the Purkinje cell zone, the molecular layer is smaller, and vestibular fibers (VIII) are disoriented with respect to the Purkinje cell zone (silver stained preparations; sagittal sections).

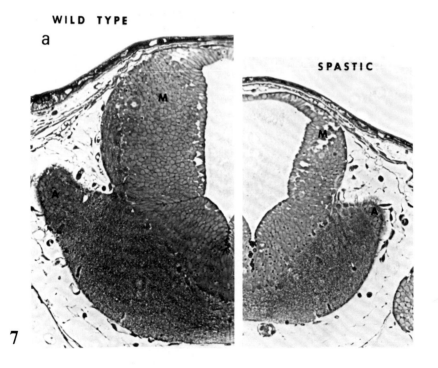

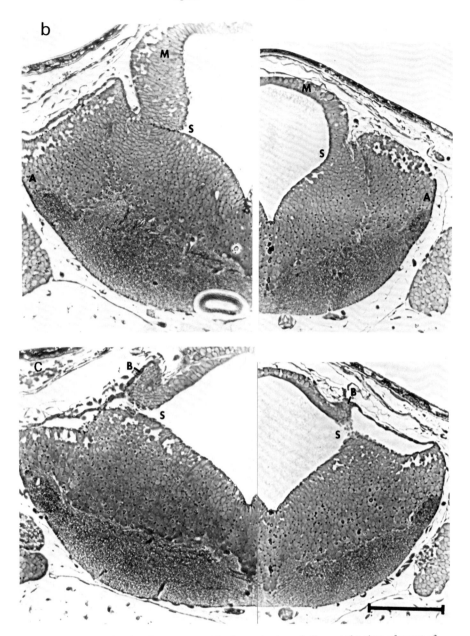

Fig. 7. Morphological deficiencies are present in the mutant cerebellum at the time of onset of spasticity. This figure compares cross-sections of the cerebellum of the wild-type (left) and the mutant (right) at 3 levels; from the most rostral (Fig. 7a) to the most caudal (Fig. 7c). Gross defects in the form of the brain are encountered at each of these levels. Rostrally (Fig. 7a), the midbrain (M) is much smaller in the mutant, and the auricle (A) is less extended laterally. The same is observed at the intermediate level (Fig. 7b), and, in addition, the usually prominent isthmic sulcus (S) is nearly absent in the spastic. In the wild-type, ependymal cells are highly oriented with respect to this sulcus, while, in the mutant, the corresponding cells are arranged in disorganized clusters. At the caudalmost level of the cerebellum (Fig. 7c), the median body (B) is seen to be very reduced in size, in the mutant; and, as shown above, the ventricular sculpturing is less pronounced (S) and ependymal cells are disoriented. The dimension marker indicates 200 μm.

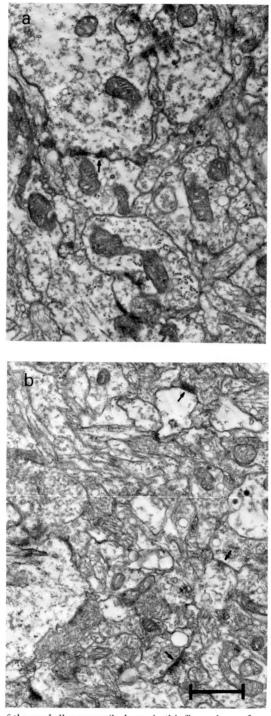

Fig. 8. Examination of the cerebellar neuropil, shown in this figure, has so far revealed no major defects in fine structure in the mutant. In both the wild-type (Fig. 8a) and spastic (Fig. 8b), numerous presynaptic (axons) and postsynaptic profiles are present; chemical synapses (arrows) are numerous. The dimension marker indicates 1 μm.

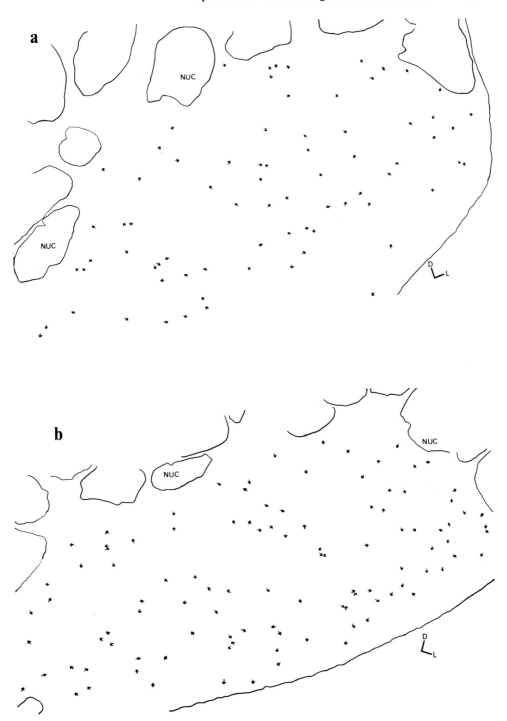

Fig. 9. Montage maps of 1 level of auricular neuropil made from electron micrographs indicate no obvious differences in the distribution of "synaptic" profiles (arrows) between normal and mutant. Arrows point in the direction of transmission. Fig. 9 a = wild-type; Fig. 9b = mutant; NUC = cell nucleus; D = dorsal; L = lateral.

these studies to include other areas of auricular neuropil, other planes of section, and material from adult animals may reveal ultrastructural correlates to the obvious cerebellar disorganization defined by light microscopy.

DISCUSSION

Many details of spastic neurogenesis remain to be elucidated before the story is complete at even the cellular level. For the present, however, it is clear that, during behavioral ontogeny, the spastic fails to develop behavior trains of sinusoidal flexures necessary to mediate escape swimming. These deficiencies appear at the time the cerebellum wires into the neuroaxis. Behavior analysis after lesions suggested that the "phenocopy circuit" for spastic behavior involves the vestibulocerebellar pathway and the cerebellar auricle. Thus, sectioning the VIIIth (vestibular) root or lesioning the cerebellar auricle produced genetic wild-type animals with spastic behavior. Remarkably, sectioning the other major sensory projections to the cerebellum (V, VII 1.1, X 1.1. cranial roots, spinocerebellar tract, tectocerebellar tract) had little effect on the coil vs sinusoid composition of locomotor behavior. Preliminary data even suggest that section of the cerebellar median body fails to create spastic phenocopies. The behavioral focus of the mutation apparently lies in the connectivity between the sensory vestibular projection and the vestibulo-cerebellum.

Electrophysiologic studies of the vestibular projection to the interneurons of the sensory medulla (AAL) and the cerebellar auricle revealed a full complement of vestibular unit types in the mutant. Notwithstanding the limited characterization of the units, and the possibility that the study focused on the least drastic of spastic phenotypes, both wild-type and spastic AAL and auricles contain burst units, units responding to the level position, and units responding during and after ipsilateral tilt, as well as during and after contralateral tilt. Interestingly, mutants show more spontaneously active units in AAL, cerebellar auricle, and trochlear nerves. Such activity increases can be explained by a testable model attributing them as due to a diminished Purkinje cell efferent projection; Purkinje cells fail to inhibit target neurons; these neurons are permanently "disinhibited," leading to feedback facilitation of primary sensory neurons, AAL interneurons, and cerebellar neurons. The lack of Purkinje cell inhibition on motoneurons leads to abnormal behavior output, perhaps mirrored in activity changes observed in spastic trochlear moto-nerves (36, 37, 39).

Mutants also showed a significant "crowding" of vestibular units reaching from ventral auricle into adjacent tissue connecting auricle and anterior AAL. Concomitant with this redistribution of functional vestibular units, this area contains both "translocated" cerebellar cells and afferent and efferent fiber tracts. Thus, the "translocated" vestibular units may represent responses of malpositioned cerebellar cells or, perhaps, the activity of vestibular afferents arborizing in the area of the "translocated" cells.

Neuroanatomically, the spastic gene is compatible both with differentiation of cerebellar cell types and with morphogenesis of the basic cerebellar pattern. However, the gene appears to influence either interactions between cells, or between cells and the external milieu such that all cell types fail to attain their proper positions. Auricular Purkinje cells are "crowded" ventrally, median body Purkinje cells caudally. Mutant granule cells and Purkinje cells overlap each other. Thus, the condition of the cerebellum of the adult spastic axolotl resembles that of another neurological mutant, the reeler mouse (10, 11, 12). Although all cell types are present in the reeler cerebellum, they fail to organize into precise neuronal networks due to faulty morphogenetic movements during neurogenesis.

Similarly, the cerebellum of the spastic axolotl contains a disorganized complement of all cerebellar cell types, and may also reflect aberrations in specific processes of cerebellar development.

The character of the mutant cerebellum at the time of onset of spasticity provides insight into the nature of these morphogenetic aberrations. At the early feeding stage, the time when spastic larvae can be clearly distinguished from wild-type siblings, the mutant cerebellum and caudal midbrain show gross defects. The auricles fail to extend laterally, and the median body is reduced dorsally. Preliminary autoradiographic studies indicate that, in wild-type embryos, the ependymal zone bordering the IV ventricle at the level of the cerebellum gives rise to cells which enter the cerebellum medially. Older cells appear to be pushed anterolaterally and dorsally by these new medial cells. The failure of the mutant cerebellum to grow laterally and dorsally may be linked to clustering of mutant cells about this ependymal germinal zone. Where medial wild-type cells appear to be oriented in rows which extend from this medial zone into the cerebellum, mutant cells appear to be clustered in this area (Fig. 7b). Cell-cell recognition may be involved. In wild-type, a prominent isthmic sulcus borders the germinal zone and medial cerebellum; ependymal cells are highly oriented with respect to this sulcus. In mutants, the isthmic sulcus is often absent; cells which are clearly ependymal cells are clustered about one another in the general area of missing sulcus. These cells never align, as if they fail to recognize one another via altered cell surface, or, possibly, simply lack extracellular cement.

Data from electron-microscopic studies are consistent with the idea that the mutant lacks no particular cerebellar element, but, rather, suffers from disorganization of existing elements. Examination of the cerebellar neuropil of wild-type and mutant larvae described above revealed the presence of pre- and postsynaptic elements. These findings corroborate physiological data (above), and point to deficiencies in gross rather than fine structure as primarily responsible for spastic syndrome.

In an attempt to further localize the focus of the mutation, anatomical, physiological, and cell-movement analyses performed on mutants are now being applied to chimeric animals containing both wild-type and mutant tissues. Such animals are created by grafting small areas of presumptive brain tissue, cerebellum, AAL, trochlear nucleus area, etc., from normal donors into mutant hosts on 1 side of the body axis only. Grafts are labelled with 3H-thymidine or the albino gene. In initial experiments, presumptive tissue containing wild-type cerebellum and AAL grafted into mutant hosts "rescues" the behavior of the mutant on the grafted side. Chimera analysis represents a truly powerful technique similar to that used to map the histotypic focus of mutations in the fruit fly (40).

In summary, all roads of investigation into the neurogenic abnormalities subserving the abnormal behavior of spastic lead to the cerebellum, and provide insights into interrelated processes of neurogenesis and also into the neural control of locomotion and balance in the axolotl. Yet the function of the wild-type gene product may be much more fundamental, and the consequences of its absence much more widespread. The malpositioned cerebellar cells and misaligned tegmental cells arise from nearby loci in the neural plate; behaviorally inconsequential cells, which are also abnormal in spastic (e.g., cartilage flexures of eye sockets and face), arise from adjacent neural crest and mesoderm. This suggests that a basic defect may exist in positional information or local inductions. Still, data from the different experimental approaches outlined above have defined the pathology of spastic syndrome at many levels. These studies in conjunction with chimeric studies should add to our understanding of how single genes control the orderly progression of morphogenetic events which give rise to the fantastic complexity of the vertebrate brain.

ACKNOWLEDGMENTS

We thank Dr. Masakazu Konishi for advice, Dorothy Goldman, Reida Kimmel, and Leslie Gardiner for technical assistance, Dr. R. K. Hunt for advice and materials, and for reviewing the manuscript, and Ms. Patricia Burck for preparing the manuscript. We are indebted to Dr. A. Janice Brothers and the Zoology Department of the University of Indiana for providing many of the axolotls used in these studies. This work was supported by NSF Grant GB30599, NIH Grant NS-12606, NSF Grant 75-05473, the Spencer Foundation, the Eugene Higgins Trust Fund, and NIMH Postdoctoral Fellowship MH05286.

REFERENCES

1. Benzer, S., Sci. American 229:24 (1973).
2. Sidman, R. L., in "Cell Interactions." L. G. Silvestri (Ed.). North Holland, Amsterdam, p. 1 (1972).
3. Sotelo, C., and Changeux, J. P., Brain Res. 67:519 (1974).
4. Hirano, A., and Dembitzer, H. M., J. Neuropath. Exp. Neurol. 34:1 (1975).
5. Rakic, P., and Sidman, B. I., J. Comp. Neurol. 152:133 (1973).
6. Sotelo, C., and Changeux, J. P., Brain Res. 77:484 (1974).
7. Sidman, R. L., and Green, M. C., in "Les Mutants Pathologiques chez l'Animal, Leur Interet dans la Recherche Biomedicale." M. Sabourdy (Ed.). CNRS, Paris, p. 69 (1970).
8. Landis, S., J. Cell Biol. 57:782 (1973).
9. Mullen, R. J., Eicher, E. M., and Sidman, R. L., Proc. Nat. Acad. Sci., U.S.A. 73:208 (1976).
10. Sidman, R. L., in "Physiological and Biochemical Aspects of Nervous Integration." F. D. Carlson (Ed.). Prentice-Hall, Englewood Cliffs, New Jersey, p. 163 (1968).
11. Hamburgh, M., Develop. Biol. 8:165 (1963).
12. Meier, H., and Hoag, W. G., J. Neuropath. Exp. Neurol. 21:649 (1962).
13. Ikeda, K., and Kaplan, W. D., Proc. Nat. Acad. Sci., U.S.A. 66:765 (1970).
14. Levine, J. D., and Wymann, B. J., Proc. Nat. Acad. Sci., U.S.A. 70:1050 (1973).
15. Bentley, D., Science 187:760 (1975).
16. Berman, N., and Cynader, M., J. Physiol. 224:363 (1972).
17. Guillery, R. W., Casagrande, V. A., and Oberdorfer, M. D., Nature 252:195 (1974).
18. Hubel, D. H., and Wiesel, T. N., J. Physiol. 218:33 (1971).
19. Crepel, F., and Mariani, J., Brain Res. 98:135 (1975).
20. Humphrey, R. R., in "Handbook of Genetics," Vol. IV. R. C. King (Ed.). Plenum Press, New York (1975).
21. Briggs, R., in "Genetic Mechanisms of Development," 31st Symp. Soc. Develop. Biol. F. Ruddle (Ed.). p. 169. Academic Press, New York (1973).
22. Malacinski, G. M., and Brothers, A. J., Science 184:1142 (1974).
23. Ide, C. F., and Tompkins, R., J. Exp. Zool. 194:467 (1975).
24. Coghill, G. E., "Anatomy and the Problem of Behavior," Cambridge University Press, Cambridge (1929).
25. Blalock, H. M., "Social Statistics." McGraw-Hill Book Co., New York (1960).
26. Humason, G. I., "Animal Tissue Techniques." W. H. Freeman and Co., San Francisco (1967).

27. Guillery, R. W., Shira, B., and Webster, K. E., Stain Technology 36:9 (1961).
28. Rowell, C. H. F., Quart. J. Micr. Sci. 104:81 (1963).
29. Schabtach, E., and Parkening, T., J. Cell Biol. 61:261 (1974).
30. Watson, M. L., J. Biophys. Biochem. Cytol. 4:475 (1958).
31. Reynolds, E. S., J. Cell. Biol. 17:208 (1963).
32. Coghill, G. E., J. Comp. Neurol. 37:71 (1924).
33. Coghill, G. E., J. Comp. Neurol. 40:47 (1926).
34. Prewitt, V., Unpublished Senior Thesis, Princeton University (1971).
35. Ide, C. F., Unpublished Ph.D. Dissertation, Princeton University (1975).
36. Ide, C. F., (Submitted for review) (1976).
37. Ide, C. F., Biophys. Journal 16:215a (1976).
38. Herrick, C. J. "The Brain of the Tiger Salamander." University of Chicago Press, Chicago (1948).
39. Ide. C. F., (Submitted for review) (1976).
40. Hotta, Y., and Benzer, S., Nature 240:527 (1972).

Permeability and Phase-Boundary Potentials Determined From Conductance in a Transmitter-Activated Potassium Channel in Aplysia Californica in the Absence of a Constant Field

Tobias L. Schwartz

Biological Sciences Group, The University of Connecticut, Storrs, Connecticut 06268

Raymond T. Kado

Laboratoire de Neurobiologie Cellulaire, C.N.R.S., 91190 Gif sur Yvette, France

A potassium-selective, chemically excitable channel, whose characteristics cannot be accurately described by "constant field" theory, is studied using a new approach based on diffusion theory but having no need for the classical assumptions of constant field, homogeneous membrane, and equal phase-boundary potentials at both interfaces. Permeability is defined, free of these constraints, and the Goldman coefficient is demonstrated to be a special case useful only when the constraints apply. Permeability can be evaluated directly from chord conductance, and it is found not to be a parameter in this channel, but rather a function of both the voltage and the concentration of the permeant ion. However, it becomes concentration-independent when the membrane voltage is equal to the sum of the phase-boundary potentials. That sum can therefore be determined from these data, and it is -65 mV in this channel. The permeability at that potential is a channel parameter, and equal to $8.77 (10)^{-6}$ cm/sec for this channel. A constant field is shown not to exist in this channel, and the Goldman coefficient not to be a parameter but a function of potential and concentration. Although errors introduced into this coefficient by nonconstant field and unequal surface potentials partially cancel each other, the coefficient is nevertheless not a correct measure of permeability.

Key words: aplysia, boundary potential, channel conductance, channel permeability, cholinergic channel, constant-field, Goldman coefficient, intrachannel concentration effects, partition coefficient, potassium channel

INTRODUCTION

Investigations of ionic permeability in biological membranes generally start from the premises provided by the Goldman-Hodgkin-Katz theory (Goldman, 1943; Hodgkin and Katz, 1949). Ginsborg and Kado (1975), however, have reported discrepancies between rectification in a potassium-selective channel as predicted by this theory and as actually observed. The channel is cholinergic and occurs in the somatic membrane of the medial cells of Aplysia californica (Kehoe, 1972a, b). The reversal potential for potassium is sufficiently negative (-70 to -80 mV) in these cells to allow the membrane to be clamped to a wide range of potentials without initiating an action potential, and the channel is selectively activated under certain conditions of agonist application (Ascher and Kehoe, 1975; Ginsborg and Kado, 1975). These features, coupled with its single-ion selectivity, make this channel most convenient for investigating problems relating to ionic permeability.

The passive flow of ions through a biological membrane is usually described as diffusion through a regime in contact with aqueous media at both of its faces. This approach yields descriptive differential equations which, to be useful, must be integrated across the thickness of the membrane. But the integrands generally contain unknown functions of potential or concentration. Integration is therefore impossible without several somewhat arbitrary assumptions as to the nature of these functions. The most widely used of these assumptions are that the electrical field in the membrane is constant, that the membrane regions through which diffusion occurs are macroscopically homogeneous so that mobilities may be taken to be constant in space,* and that the phase-boundary potentials at the two membrane-solution interfaces are equal (Goldman, 1943; Hodgkin and Katz, 1949).

The expressions derived in this way have proven extremely useful. But contradictions between experiment and theory have also been noted in several permeability systems other than the one we have studied (Jaffe, 1974; Hille, 1975). The problem is thus more general than this specific channel. Its source may lie either in the simplifying assumptions indicated above or, more basically, in the diffusion approach itself. The question thus merits investigation.

Its resolution requires an approach that is still based on diffusion, but avoids the suppositions necessary to the Goldman-Hodgkin-Katz theory. One of us had previously developed such an approach (Schwartz, 1971a, b), and we have extended it for the purposes of this paper. An integral expression for the permeability had been obtained. We demonstrate that this integral can, for a single-ion channel, be evaluated directly from experimentally determined conductances without the assumption of either a constant field or a homogeneous membrane, and neither the phase-boundary potentials nor the partition of ions need be taken to be identical at the two membrane-solution interfaces. The analysis then yields three channel properties: 1) its permeability as a function of membrane potential, 2) the sum of the two phase-boundary potentials, and 3) a permeability factor that is a constant, characteristic of the channel. The values of both the phase-boundary potentials and the permeability factor are consistent with estimates obtained by other methods. The Goldman coefficient is, by contrast, shown not to describe the permeability of this channel. These findings seem to confirm the continued applicability of diffusion theory as well as the usefulness of this new, more physically exact solution of this problem.

This preliminary report was presented to the ICN–UCLA 1976 Winter Conference on Neurobiology, and at the meetings of the Biophysical Society (Schwartz and Kado, 1976), and a full report has been published elsewhere (Schwartz and Kado, 1977).

METHODS

Either the right or left pleural ganglion of Aplysia californica (obtained from Pacific Biomarine Laboratories, Inc., P.O. Box 536, Venice, Ca.) was isolated, connective tissue

---

*These two constraints have been shown to be more stringent than required as concerns the expression for the zero-current potential, but they are still necessary for the flux equations (see, for instance, Schwartz, 1971a, b).

was dissected away so that the cell bodies were entirely exposed, and the ganglion was firmly pinned to the transparent 'Sylgard' bottom of a chamber by utilizing connective tissue remaining on the nerves. The ganglion was positioned so that single cells in the medial group (Kehoe, 1972b) could be impaled with two electrodes, one to measure voltage and the other to pass current.

Carbamylcholine was applied to the somatic membrane of the impaled cell by iontophoresis from a point sufficiently distant that only the potassium-selective response was observed (Ascher and Kehoe, 1975), and located in a region of rapid solution flow so that the drug could be quickly washed away. The iontophoresing electrode system was composed of one double-barreled electrode, both of whose barrels were filled with 0.1 M carbamylcholine and then electrically connected in parallel, and a second pipette with a larger tip to provide a return electrical path. The paralleled, double-barreled electrode was found to minimize tip blockage and variations in drug application during the long iontophoresing times used in this study. Drug was generally applied until the membrane's response began to decrease. The iontophoresing current was held constant by either a large series resistance, or an active constant-current source. It was necessary to very carefully isolate this current source with regard to both resistance and capacitance in order to avoid artifactual transients in the voltage-clamp current measuring circuit.

A fast voltage-clamp composed of operational amplifers and having a high-voltage output stage (Kado, 1971) was used. The bath was grounded through an agar-seawater salt bridge connected to a current-to-voltage converter. Total resistance to ground was 800 ohms, sufficiently low that at the currents encountered (up to 100 nA) the error in voltage measurement was negligible. Ginsborg and Kado (1975) have demonstrated that this method of voltage-clamping holds the entire region of the cell membrane that is reached by the carbachol at the clamping potential.

All electrodes were pulled with a DeFonbrune microforge so as to yield resistances between 5 and 20 megohms, depending on their purpose. Finer-tipped electrodes were used for measuring voltage, and were filled with 3 M KCl. Coarser-tipped electrodes were used to pass current, and were filled with 0.6 M $K_2 SO_4$. The iontophoresing electrodes have already been described.

Artificial seawater, formulated as follows, was used as the standard bathing medium: NaCl, 480 mM; KCl, 10 mM; $CaCl_2$, 10 mM; $MgCl_2$, 50 mM; and pH was held at 7.7 at $25°C$ by adding Tris-Cl, 10 mM. Alterations of potassium concentration always involved an equimolar exchange for sodium. Bath temperature was held between 12 and $18°C$ by a Peltier cell under the chamber. A constant flow, gravity-feed system changed the chamber contents approximately once per minute.

RESULTS

1. Current-Voltage Characteristics

The steady-state currents required to hold the membrane at a series of voltages were determined, first in the absence and then in the presence of the drug (Ginsborg and Kado, 1975). Steady-state was generally reached within 1 sec at a given voltage. Each cell was exposed to at least two concentrations of external potassium.

The I–V characteristic of the drug-activated channel was then obtained by plotting the change in the clamping current produced by the drug, against the membrane potential. I–V plots for three concentrations of external potassium, and typical of this channel, are shown in Fig. 1.

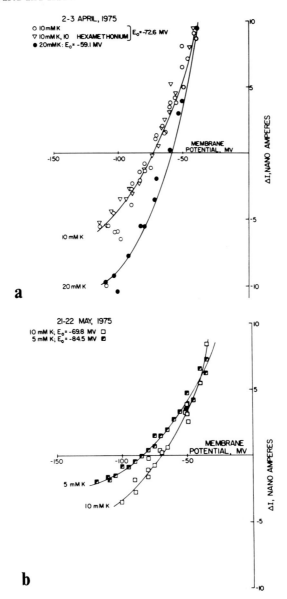

Fig. 1. Current-voltage relationships for the carbachol-activated K channel. ΔI is the change in current under voltage-clamp following drug application. Outward currents are taken as positive, and potential is referenced to the bath. Lines were drawn by eye. a) 5 and 10 mM external potassium. b) 10 and 20 mM external potassium. Some 10 mM points were obtained in the presence of 10^{-4} M hexamethonium, an agent known to block the excitatory response in these neurons, but which has no effect on the inhibitory response of this channel (Kehoe, 1972b).

These current-voltage characteristics are nonlinear and, as was pointed out by Ginsborg and Kado (1975), have a curvature opposite to that in the neuromuscular junction for iontophoretically applied carbamylcholine or acetylcholine (Magleby and Stevens,

1972; Dionne and Stevens, 1974). In the neuromuscular junction the nonlinear I–V plots have been attributed to voltage-dependent parameters in the receptor-agonist channel-gating mechanisms. We shall demonstrate that the conductance characteristics of this Aplysia channel may, by contrast, be entirely due to shifting intrachannel concentration profiles.

2. Channel Selectivity

Channel reversal potential (E_0) was determined after prolonged exposure to various external potassium concentrations. The pooled results of all experiments followed the Nernst equation (Fig. 2). In a few individual experiments the change of potential with concentration was less than that predicted by theory (Fig. 2). This was probably caused by potassium leakage into the cell when external K was higher than that in seawater, and out of the cell when it was lower (Ginsborg and Kado, 1975; Ascher, Kunze, and Neild, 1976; Ascher, personal communication). Our results are thus in agreement with Kehoe's: This channel is highly selective for potassium.

Calculating from E_0 with an assumed intracellular activity coefficient of 0.68 (Baker, Hodgkin, and Shaw, 1962), we obtain an average K activity of 126.8 mM inside the cell. Kehoe (1972a) calculated 167.3 mM for these cells; and Russell and Brown (1972) have reported 165.3 mM in the related giant cell of the abdominal ganglion.

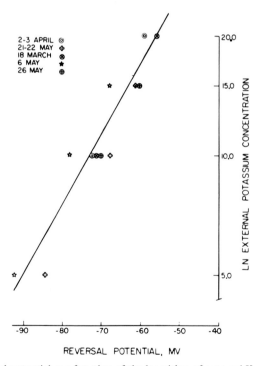

Fig. 2. Channel reversal potential as a function of the logarithm of external K concentration. The line was drawn at the slope of F/RT, with T = 15°C – an approximate average temperature for these experiments.

ANALYSIS AND DISCUSSION

1. Channel Conductance

Channel chord conductance can easily be calculated from the I–V characteristics as $I/(E - E_0)$. Analysis requires the comparison of conductances calculated for different cells. This, however, is impossible without normalization because one cannot determine how many channels or, stated otherwise, how much membrane area has been activated by the applied drug. For a constant iontophoretic current, this area will vary with iontophoresing-electrode tip characteristics, distance from the cell of the drug injection point, ganglion geometry, and the rate and pattern of flow of the perfusion solution. With great care these parameters can be maintained constant within a single experiment; but generally not between separate experiments with different cells. We have normalized all conductances for any one cell with a single normalization factor: the chord conductance of that cell at its reversal potential in seawater. All experiments were thus placed on an equal footing, and their results could be combined.

Normalized conductances (conductance always means chord conductance in this paper) obtained at 5, 10, and 20 mM external K were plotted as functions of membrane potential (Fig. 3a). Two features stand out. First, conductance is a strong function of external K concentration, increasing with rising concentration. Second, at all concentrations the conductance increases nonlinearly, and with no evidence of saturation, as the membrane is depolarized.

The conductance of an ensemble of channels of this sort would be expected, on theoretical grounds, to depend on intrachannel concentration (Finkelstein and Mauro, 1963). However, other factors may also be involved. For instance, the voltage dependence of the conductance may be attributed to either of two mechanisms: intrachannel concentration shifts sensitive to the driving force, $E - E_0$, and hence to changes in either E or E_0; or "gating" processes sensitive to E – which reflects the electrical field in the channel – but not to E_0. Their different properties with regard to E_0 may be used to decide which of these mechanisms is actually operative.

Reversal potentials differed somewhat from cell to cell in our experiments even when at the same external potassium concentration. In the case of intrachannel concentration shifts, the normalized conductances measured with different cells should consequently correlate better with each other when viewed as functions of $E - E_0$ than as functions of E. In the case of gating, this change of independent variable is not expected to matter.

In actuality, this correlation is considerably better with $E - E_0$ than with E (Figs. 3a and 3b). This suggests that diffusion controlled intrachannel concentration shifts, and not gating, produce the voltage dependence of this conductance. Its strong dependence on external K concentration is also consistent with this sort of mechanism.

We have probed this question in still another, though less direct manner. The relationship between conductance and external concentration is linear when the membrane is held at E_0 (Fig. 4). Furthermore, this relationship displays qualitative symmetry about the E_0 line for any other pair of voltages $E_0 + V$ and $E_0 - V$. Some simple connection between conductance, external potassium concentration, and the net diffusive driving force, $E - E_0$, must therefore exist, and a strong role for diffusion in the control of this conductance is once again implied.

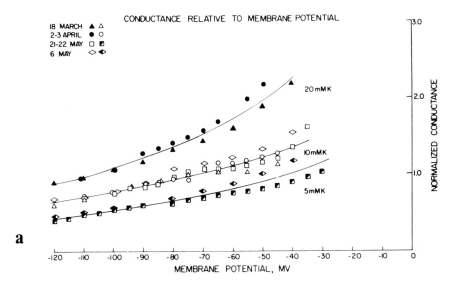

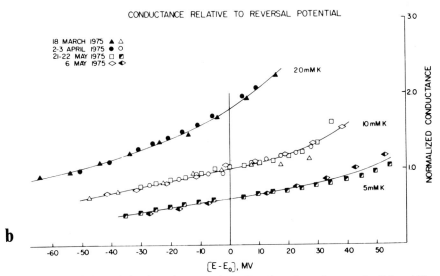

Fig. 3. Normalized channel chord conductance a) as a function of membrane potential, and b) as a function of the departure of the membrane potential from the reversal potential. Data have been pooled from several experiments, and lines drawn by eye.

2. Channel Permeability

The two forces that produce simple ionic diffusion — an electrical gradient and an activity gradient — give rise to two ways of defining "permeability." The definition will differ depending upon which force is chosen as reference (Appendix A). Terminology is such that only when the activity gradient is chosen does one speak of permeability; when

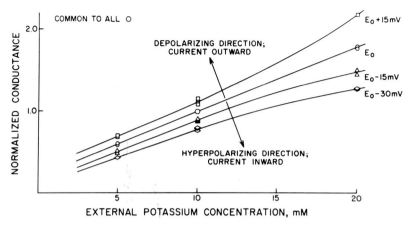

Fig. 4. Normalized conductances at several fixed values of E − E$_0$, as functions of external potassium concentration. This figure contains the pooled data of all experiments.

the electrical gradient is chosen one speaks instead of conductance. But, terminology notwithstanding, they both remain "permeabilities" and therefore bear a relationship to each other. Just as conductance can be evaluated from electrical measurements even though the mathematical integration involved in its definition (Eq. 3A) cannot in general be performed, so also can the permeability be evaluated. In this section we utilize the relationship between conductance and permeability to deduce the latter from the former, as a function of membrane potential.

A general expression relating the steady-state current due to a univalent cation to the driving force has been derived for the case in which the concentration gradient is reference, thereby defining a generalized permeability (Schwartz, 1971a, b). When that expression is modified to deal with measureable quantities in the solutions instead of unmeasurable ones interior to the membrane (Appendix B), and with activities instead of with concentrations, we obtain

$$I = \frac{ARTF}{Q'}\left[a(s2)\exp\left(\frac{F}{RT}E\right) - a(s1)\right]$$

where

$$Q' = \frac{1}{\beta}\int_0^\delta \frac{\gamma}{\omega}\exp\left\{\frac{F}{RT}\ [\varphi - \varphi(m1)]\right\}dx, \qquad (1)$$

and

$$E \equiv \varphi(s2) - \varphi(s1).$$

Integration is across the membrane, whose thickness is δ. The extracellular and intracellular compartments are denoted, respectively, by the numbers 1 and 2. The letter m indicates a point just inside the membrane bordering on the appropriate compartment, while the letter s similarly indicates points in the bulk external solutions. The activity coefficient γ, as well as the mobility ω, may be functions of x, a is activity, φ is electrical potential, A is activated area, and

$$\beta \equiv \frac{a(m1)}{a(s1)} \tag{2}$$

is the equivalent of a partition coefficient. R, T, and F have their usual meanings.

The quantity, ART/Q' is the permeability*. As we indicated earlier, the integration necessary to determine Q' from first principles cannot be performed because the integrand is unknown. If, in order to solve this problem, constant field, equal phase-boundary potentials, and a homogeneous membrane are assumed, Eq. 1 yields a Goldman flux equation, and the permeability is given by a Goldman coefficient (Appendix C). The Goldman-Hodgkin-Katz equations are therefore a special case of Eq. 1, and the Goldman coefficient is a special case of the more general permeability, ART/Q'.

ART/Q' can, however, be determined without an integration and, hence, without assuming the nature of the integrand. If I is eliminated between Eq. 1 and

$$I = G (E - E_0) \tag{3}$$

and $a(s2)$ is taken into account with the help of Eq. 6D, we obtain

$$\frac{A}{Q'} = \frac{G}{F^2\,a(s1)} \left[\frac{\frac{F}{RT}(E - E_0)}{\exp\left\{\frac{F}{RT}(E - E_0)\right\} - 1} \right], \tag{4}$$

a relationship between A/Q' and the chord conductance G in which all other parameters are known.

We have calculated A/Q' according to Eq. 4, and have plotted the normalized results as a function of membrane potential (Fig. 5). A/Q' is, as expected (Eq. 1), voltage-dependent. It increases with hyperpolarization in an S-shaped manner, and approaches zero for large depolarizations (Eq. 4). Its voltage dependence, however, is itself a function of external potassium concentration, being steeper for lower concentrations. Permeability is thus not a channel parameter but, rather, a complex function of both potential and concentration and dependent on conditions inside the channel. Indeed, even in the case of constant G, permeability cannot be constant.

3. Phase-Boundary Potentials

    a. **Determining the potentials.** There are, however, two channel parameters that can be determined from the permeability by a somewhat different approach to the diffusion equation. We describe the first in this section, and the second in Section 4.

    An alternate expression for A/Q' is (Appendix D)

$$\frac{A}{Q'} = A \left(\frac{\overline{\omega}}{\gamma}\right)\left(\frac{\beta}{\delta}\right) [1 - f] ,$$

where

$$f = \frac{\exp\left[\frac{F}{RT}(E - E_0)\right] - \exp\left[\frac{F}{RT}(\eta - E_0)\right] - \frac{\overline{a(m)}}{a(m1)}\frac{F}{RT}(E - \eta)}{\exp\left[\frac{F}{RT}(E - E_0)\right] - 1} , \tag{5}$$

*Kimizuka and Koketsu (1964) have defined a related permeability.

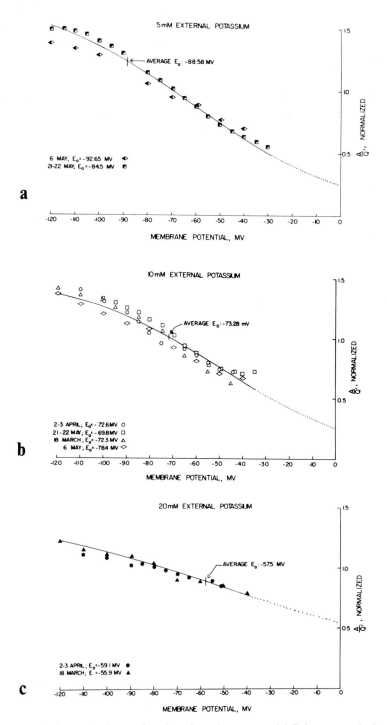

Fig. 5. Normalized permeability as a function of membrane potential. Points were calculated from conductance data as described in the text. Lines were calculated as described in Appendix E. The normalization factor for each cell was A/Q' at reversal in seawater. a) 5 mM external potassium, b) 10 mM external potassium, and c) 20 mM external potassium.

$\overline{\omega/\gamma}$ and $\overline{a(m)}$ are averages inside the membrane, and η is the sum of the two phase-boundary potentials so that

$$\eta = E - \Delta\varphi, \tag{6}$$

where $\Delta\varphi$ is the potential difference across the membrane interior (Eq. 2C).

The function, f, has the important property that it is zero when $E = \eta$. Consequently, when the membrane potential is equal to the sum of the phase-boundary potentials,

$$\left[\frac{A}{Q'}\right]_{\eta} = A_{\eta} \overline{\left(\frac{\omega}{\gamma}\right)} \left(\frac{\beta}{\delta}\right). \tag{7}$$

It is reasonable to suppose $\overline{(\omega/\gamma)} \, (\beta/\delta)$ to be a parameter characteristic of the channel and independent of concentration and voltage. A is a function of applied drug, and there is no reason to believe it to be dependent on potassium concentration. Therefore A/Q' at $E = \eta$ should be concentration-independent (Eq. 7), and graphs of A/Q' at different potassium concentrations should all intersect at that voltage.

An overlay of Figs. 5a, 5b, and 5c shows such an intersection to occur between -60 and -70 mV. To smooth the data and simplify further calculation, a function of the form suggested by Eq. 5 was fitted to the data at all three concentrations (Appendix E), yielding the solid lines in Figs. 5a, b, and c. A single graph of these fitted curves shows a common point of intersection at -65.4 mV (Fig. 6a).

We have eliminated the possibility that this is an artifact of the normalization by examining nonnormalized results for three cells, each of which was exposed to two concentrations of external potassium (Fig. 6b). The two resulting curves for each cell again intersect, and all three intersections lie between -67.6 and -70.0 mV.

This common permeability point can, furthermore, be tested in still another manner, and that directly from the I–V plots and without calculating A/Q'. Using Eq. 6D, Eq. 1 may be rewritten for $E = \eta$, and normalized by I_{η} in seawater. If the subscript SW denotes seawater, and c denotes concentration, we then have

$$\left[\frac{I_{\eta}}{I_{\eta,\text{SW}}}\right] \frac{\left[\exp\left\{\frac{F}{RT}(\eta - E_0)\right\} - 1\right]_{\text{SW}}}{\left[\exp\left\{\frac{F}{RT}(\eta - E_0)\right\} - 1\right]} = \frac{c(\text{sl})}{c(\text{sl})_{\text{SW}}} \tag{8}$$

provided $(A/Q')_{\eta}$ is not a function of concentration. If the intersection has been properly identified, a graph of the left side of this equation against concentration must yield a straight line with a slope of 0.10, passing through the origin. Excepting a negligible difference in the slope, it does (Fig. 7).

Thus, the sum of the phase-boundary potentials can be directly determined for such a single ion channel from the common intersection of graphs of A/Q' for different external concentrations of the permeant ion. In this particular channel the phase-boundary potential sum is approximately -65 mV. It should be noted that this method of determining these potentials is a direct consequence of diffusion theory, and does not require additional modeling of events at the membrane-solution interfaces.

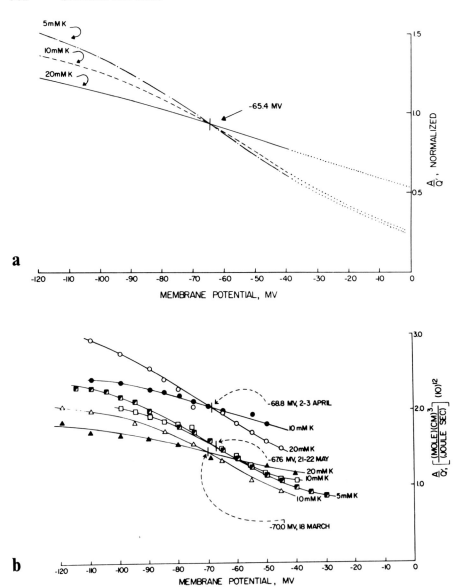

Fig. 6. Permeability as a function of membrane potential. a) An overlay of the curves in Fig. 5. b) 3 different experiments, data not normalized. Lines drawn by eye.

b. Asymmetric conditions in the channel. The fact that η is not zero has the consequence that conditions at the inner and outer boundaries of the channel must be asymmetric. This can be more clearly seen if we define, for the membrane boundary facing the inside of the cell,

$$\beta' = \frac{a(m2)}{a(s2)} \tag{9}$$

analogous to β at the membrane boundary facing the extracellular medium. It follows from Eqs. 2, 2A, 6D, and Appendix B, that

$$\frac{\beta}{\beta'} = \exp\left(-\frac{F}{RT}\eta\right) \tag{10}$$

Calculating for the average temperature of 15°C maintained during these experiments, and for a value of η of -65.4 mV, β/β' is 13.9. Thus, for a given potassium activity in the extra or intracellular solutions, a much higher activity would result in the region inside the channel but close to the outside of the cell than in a comparable region close to the inside of the cell. Barring large activity coefficient differences, the implication is that of a much higher concentration of fixed anionic charges at the outer than at the inner channel surface.

We can, by our method, determine only the sum of the two phase-boundary potentials. The separate potentials remain unknown. Individual surface potentials and their related surface charges have, however, been estimated for various excitable cells by a quite different method. The voltage dependence of the parameters of membrane excitation can be shifted by altering the ionic composition of the extra or intracellular solutions. Through models, these shifts can be related to the phase-boundary potential at the appropriate membrane surface (see, for instance, Chandler, Hodgkin, and Meves, 1965; Gilbert and Ehrenstein, 1969; Mozhayeva and Naumov, 1970; Brismar, 1973; Drouin and Neumcke, 1974; Hille, Woodhull, and Shapiro, 1975). Although this method yields information about the individual phase-boundary potentials, it suffers from a lack of uniqueness with regard to the calculated results due to a surfeit of parameters (Hille, Woodhull, and Shapiro, 1975). Nevertheless, estimates of 8.3 (10)^{13} (Gilbert and Ehrenstein, 1969), and 1.4 (10)^{13} electronic charges/cm^2 (Chandler, Hodgkin, and Meves, 1965) have been obtained for the external and internal surfaces of the squid axon, respectively. Thus, in agreement with our conclusion, this very different approach also suggests that a higher charge density exists at the outer than the inner surface.

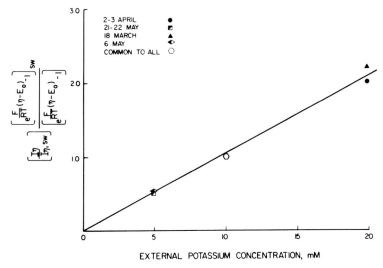

Fig. 7. Left-hand side of Eq. 8 as a function of external K concentration. Slope is 0.105 L/mM. I_η was read directly from the I–V plots; E_0 was taken as the value found in the corresponding experiment, and η was assumed to be -65.4 mV.

As a result of the asymmetry of the channel, boundary potentials and activities are quite different from what one would otherwise have assumed (Fig. 8). It is particularly striking that between 10 and 20 mM K, the transchannel interior activity difference reverses; that is, it becomes higher at the outer than at the inner edge. This occurs in spite of the fact that the exterior transmembrane activity difference maintains its orientation: inside higher than outside. The potential relationships (Fig. 8a) of course also reflect the internal shift in direction. It follows that making the external solution equimolar in K with the internal will not generate symmetrical boundary conditions across the membrane's interior. Actually $\Delta\varphi_0$ will then be 65.4 mV, precisely because E_0 is zero. Symmetrical internal conditions will, in fact, occur at reversal at an external K concentration between 10 and 20 mM, when $E_0 = \eta$.

The boundary potentials at 10 mM external potassium calculated by our method are remarkably similar to those calculated by Hille, Woodhull, and Shapiro (1975) for their model I using the method of shifting excitability parameters described above. Two points must be noted to make this comparison easier. Firstly, Hille, Woodhull, and Shapiro have depicted the electrical double layer as external to the membrane, while we have shown it as just inside the membrane; the two pictures are, of course, equivalent. Secondly, β, regarding which a degree of arbitrariness exists (see legend for Fig. 8), is here rechosen for purposes of comparison to yield a potential of −91 mV just inside the membrane's outer surface instead of the −114.3 mV used in Fig. 8a. The remaining potentials are then calculated from the data to yield 0, −91, −99, and −73.3 mV reading in the direction outside to inside. Hille, Woodhull, and Shapiro obtained, by comparison, 0, −91, −100, and −75 mV. It is possible that this agreement consititutes an independent confirmation of the parameters assumed in their model I as opposed to model II, despite the fact that different cell types as well as channels have been examined in the two investigations. Indeed, even though they have different physical bases, our method and the method of shifting excitability parameters seem to yield encouragingly similar picitures of membrane surface phenomena.

4. Permeability at the Potential η

When the membrane potential is held at η, the steady-state channel permeability is equal to $A_\eta RT\overline{(\omega/\gamma)}(\beta/\delta)$ (Eq. 7). This quantity is the product of the activated area A, and precisely the permeability factor that has generally been estimated by calculating Goldman coefficients. That factor should therefore now be available without the necessity of making the usual Goldman-Hodgkin-Katz assumptions.

TABLE I. Channel Permeability Factor

Experiment	Normalizing factor [(mole cm^3)/(joule sec)] $(10)^{12}$	$A_\eta RT \overline{(\omega/\gamma)} (\beta/\delta)$ (cm^3/sec) $(10)^9$
18 March	2.21	4.97
2–3 April	3.16	7.12
6 May	2.11	4.75
21–22 May	2.31	5.21
Average	— —	5.51

The normalized value of $A_\eta\overline{(\omega/\gamma)}(\beta/\delta)$ was read from Fig. 6a as 0.94. Column 3 was calculated as the product of 0.94, RT, and the individual normalizing factors, at 15°C. Variations between experiments probably mainly reflect variations in activated area.

The average value of $A_\eta RT \, (\omega/\gamma) \, (\beta/\delta)$ for this channel is $5.51 (10)^{-9}$ cm^3/sec (Table I). In the absence of voltage-sensitive gating, A may be presumed constant with membrane potential. Even so, in a preparation of this sort A is not known; but it may be estimated and the permeability factor may then be deduced.

A typical medial cell has an approximate diameter of 200 μm. We have applied the agonist to a spherical cell body in a manner such that only approximately half of the somatic membrane can be readily reached by the drug. An average A can therefore be estimated as $6.28 (10)^{-4}$ cm^2, and $RT(\overline{\omega/\gamma}) \, (\beta/\delta)$ is $8.77 (10)^{-6}$ cm/sec. In comparison,

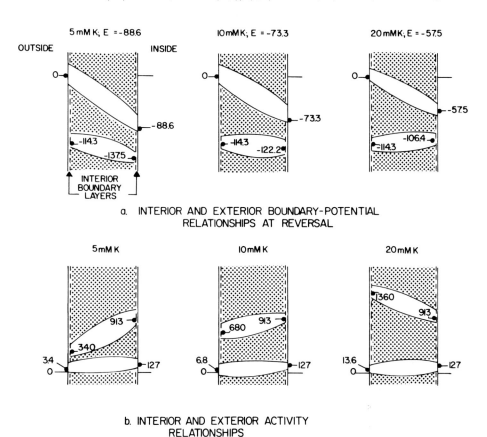

a. INTERIOR AND EXTERIOR BOUNDARY-POTENTIAL RELATIONSHIPS AT REVERSAL

b. INTERIOR AND EXTERIOR ACTIVITY RELATIONSHIPS

Fig. 8. The effect of channel asymmetry on potentials and concentrations at the boundaries. Only the ratio β/β' can be determined in these experiments; the individual coefficients remain unknown. β must therefore be fixed at a physiologically reasonable value for purposes of illustration; it was chosen as 100 to construct this figure. The effect of a possible difference between the standard chemical potentials in the bulk external solution and the channel interior has been ignored. Other choices regarding either β or the standard chemical potential simply cause linear shifts of all potentials relative to the external reference potential, and proportional changes in both interior activities. Neither of these effects are relevant to the point at hand. Drawings are approximately to scale. a) Boundary potentials at reversal. Numbers are in mV. Temperature: 15°C. Passage of current will leave the exterior-interior relationship at each boundary unchanged, but will shift the potentials at one boundary relative to those at the other. b) Boundary activities. Numbers are in mM. The intracellular activity is 127 mM, as determined from reversal potentials in these experiments. The activity coefficient in the extracellular medium was taken as 0.68. These relationships will be undisturbed by current; current can affect only the interior concentrations away from the boundaries.

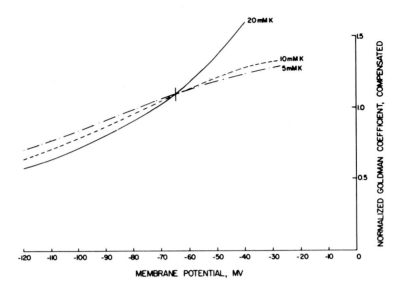

Fig. 9. Normalized Goldman coefficients as a function of membrane potential for 5, 10, and 20 mM external potassium. These coefficients have been compensated to take into account that $\eta = -65.4$ mV. Calculation was made from the smoothed curves fitted to the normalized plots of A/Q' (Figs. 5 and 6). The normalization factor for each cell was PA at reversal in seawater. The vertical bar indicates the voltage η.

Hodgkin and Katz (1949) obtained a Goldman coefficient of $1.8 \, (10)^{-6}$ cm/sec for the resting potassium system in squid axon.

5. Goldman Coefficients

We have shown how channel permeability can be determined from the ordinary data of electrophysiology without resort to certain assumptions regarding the membrane's interior. It remains possible, however, that the classical Goldman-Hodgkin-Katz approach also "works" for this channel. In that case a Goldman coefficient would also yield the correct value of the permeability factor. Since we now know the Hodgkin-Katz assumption of a zero sum of phase-boundary potentials to be incorrect, it would then have to follow that the effect of this nonzero sum would have to be exactly counterbalanced by a non-constant electrical field. Ginsborg and Kado's observation (1975) that the Goldman-Hodgkin-Katz theory predicts a rectification smaller than that actually observed in this channel makes this sort of phenomenon doubtful, but the question should be explored.

To this end, we have first examined the possibility that the electrical field may actually be constant. Assuming constant field and membrane homogeneity to exist in the channel, and allowing η to assume its true value, it follows from Eq. 6C, 3, and 6D that

$$PA = \frac{G}{Fa(s1)} \left[\frac{E - E_0}{\exp\left\{ \frac{F}{RT}(E - E_0) \right\} - 1} \right] \left[\frac{\exp\left\{ \frac{F}{RT}(E - \eta) \right\} - 1}{\frac{F}{RT}(E - \eta)} \right], \qquad (11)$$

where P is the Goldman coefficient under these circumstances (Eq. 7C). In the absence of voltage-sensitive gating this coefficient shouldn't vary with voltage, nor, in any case,

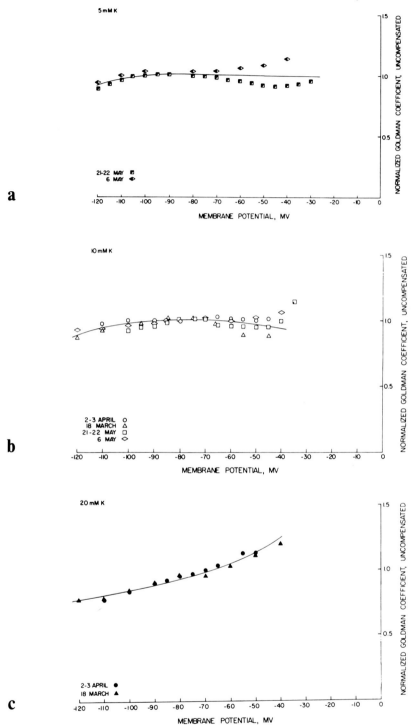

Fig. 10. Normalized Goldman coefficients as functions of membrane potential, uncompensated in that the phase boundary potentials are assumed equal and opposite, so that their sum is zero. a) 5 mM external potassium. b) 10 mM external potassium, and c) 20 mM external potassium. Normalization was as for Fig. 9.

should it vary with concentration if the above description of the channel is correct.

We have calculated PA according to Eq. 11, and plotted the normalized results as a function of membrane potential (Fig. 9). The coefficient is a function of both membrane potential and external K concentration, although its concentration dependence becomes less severe for voltages more hyperpolarized than η. At $E = \eta$, $(PA)_\eta$ is concentration-independent, and it can be shown to equal $(ART/Q')_\eta$. This is a consequence of the existence of a constant field at that potential (Appendix D). However, a constant field appears not to exist at any other membrane potential.

We therefore returned to the possibility that the effects of the nonconstant field and of the nonzero boundary potential sum cancel each other. That possibility may be examined by taking η to be zero in Eq. 11, yielding

$$PA = \frac{G}{Fa(s1)} \left[\frac{E - E_0}{\exp\left\{\frac{F}{RT}(E - E_0)\right\} - 1} \right] \left[\frac{\exp\left(\frac{F}{RT} E\right) - 1}{\frac{F}{RT} E} \right]. \tag{12}$$

This expression is analogous to the one used by Dodge and Frankenhaeuser (1959) to calculate sodium permeability coefficients. If the effects do indeed cancel, the coefficient should, once again, not vary with either membrane potential or external K concentration.

We calculated PA according to Eq. 12 and plotted the normalized results (Fig. 10). At 5 mM K the coefficient is constant except for a dip at potentials more hyperpolarized than -90 mV. At 10 mM K it is somewhat more voltage-dependent than at 5 mM K; but comparing these two sets of coefficients shows the effect of the concentration change to be small and within the scatter of the data. At 20 mM K, however, both the voltage and concentration dependencies are pronounced.

It appears, then, that the effects of non-constant field and nonzero boundary potential sum do partially cancel each other, and that in the range 5–20 mM K the degree of cancellation decreases as external potassium concentration increases. If the observed rectification is compared with that predicted by the Goldman-Hodgkin-Katz theory, one finds, in agreement with this observation, that the discrepancy between them increases with increasing external K (Table II). In agreement with Ginsborg and Kado (1975), we find the observed rectification to be greater than that predicted by the theory (Table II). Ginsborg and Kado noted, also, that at 50 mM external K this disparity

TABLE II. Comparison of Observed Rectification With That Predicted by the Goldman-Hodgkin-Katz Theory

Concentration mM K	Normalized G -40 mV	Normalized G -100 mV	$\frac{G_{-100}}{G_{-40}}$ Observed	$\frac{G_{-100}}{G_{-40}}$ Calculated
5	1.02	0.54	0.529	0.529
10	1.42	0.79	0.556	0.594
20	2.31	1.09	0.472	0.673

Rectification is measured as the ratio of the chord conductance at -100 mV to that at -40 mV. The closer the ratio is to unity, the less the rectification. Normalized conductances were read from Fig. 3b. The calculated ratios are from Eq. 12, with PA assumed constant.

appeared to decrease. Our data do not extend to that concentration. In general, permeability cannot be calculated for this channel by determining Goldman coefficients.

ACKNOWLEDGMENTS

This work was supported by grants to T. L. Schwartz from NIH (NS08444), the European Molecular Biology Organization, the University of Connecticut Research Foundation, and to both authors from the DGRST in France.

APPENDIX A: "PERMEABILITY" DEPENDS ON THE CHOICE OF A REFERENCE FORCE

1. Electrical Force is Reference

The reference force is stated as a simple gradient. Hence, when the Nernst-Planck equation for the flux density due to a single univalent cation is written as

$$j = -\frac{\omega}{\gamma}\, aF\left[\frac{RT}{F}\,\frac{d}{dx}\,\ln a + \frac{d\varphi}{dx}\right], \tag{1A}$$

the reference force is electrical, and the driving force due to the activity appears as an additive term. Symbols are as defined for Eq. 1 in the main text. Integration, in the steady-state, then yields a total driving force of $\Delta\varphi - \Delta\varphi_0$, where

$$\Delta\varphi_0 = \frac{RT}{F}\,\ln\frac{a(m1)}{a(m2)}, \tag{2A}$$

and a force-flux proportionality factor, or "permeability," of

$$\frac{G}{F} = \frac{A}{\int_0^\delta (1/F\omega c)dx}, \tag{3A}$$

where G is the chord conductance (Finkelstein and Mauro, 1963). Since the phase-boundary potentials are taken to be invariant with current (Appendix B),

$$\Delta\varphi - \Delta\varphi_0 = E - E_0 \tag{4A}$$

where E includes the phase-boundary potentials (Eq. 1).

2. Activity Gradient is Reference

When the Nernst-Planck equation is written as

$$j = -RT\left(\frac{\omega}{\gamma}\right)\left[\frac{da}{dx} + \frac{F}{RT}\,a\,\frac{d\varphi}{dx}\right] \tag{5A}$$

the activity term appears as a simple gradient with the electrical term more complex, and additive. However, the expression is not useful in this form because the electrical term cannot be integrated to yield a force dependent only on boundary conditions. This difficulty can be circumvented, since

$$\frac{da}{dx} + \frac{F}{RT} \, a \, \frac{d\varphi}{dx} = \exp\left(-\frac{F}{RT}\varphi\right)\frac{d}{dx}\left[a \, \exp\left(\frac{F}{RT}\varphi\right)\right] \tag{6A}$$

so that

$$j = -RT\left(\frac{\omega}{\gamma}\right)\exp\left(-\frac{F}{RT}\varphi\right)\frac{d}{dx}\left[a \, \exp\left(\frac{F}{RT}\varphi\right)\right] \tag{7A}$$

In this form the driving force $\dfrac{d}{dx}\left[a \, \exp\left(\dfrac{F}{RT}\varphi\right)\right]$ is the gradient of an electrically modified activity. It returns to its unmodified, Fickian, form when either the diffusing species uncharged or φ is constant in x. The same modified activity occurs in the derivations by Ussing (1949) and Teorell (1949) of the unidirectional flux ratio. Integration of Eq. 7A and correction for phase-boundary effects yields a permeability of ART/Q' (Eq. 1 and Schwartz, 1971a, b). In the case of uncharged species this coefficient is analogous to AD, where D is Fick's diffusion coefficient.

APPENDIX B

Assuming local equilibria at the membrane-solution interfaces (Kirkwood, 1954),

$$\beta \, \frac{a(s2)}{a(m2)} = \exp\left(-\frac{F}{RT} \, [E - \Delta\varphi]\right), \tag{1B}$$

where $\Delta\varphi$ is the potential difference across the membrane interior (Eq. 2C), and E and β are defined in Eqs. 1 and 2, respectively (see also footnote 4 in Schwartz, 1971a). Correction may then be made for phase-boundary effects, to yield Eqs. 1. In accord with the usual practice, the equilibria at the boundaries are assumed undisturbed by current, so that β is a function of neither I nor E (Finkelstein and Mauro, 1963, p. 226).

APPENDIX C: THE CASE OF CONSTANT FIELD, HOMOGENEOUS MEMBRANE, AND EQUAL PHASE-BOUNDARY POTENTIALS

When the field is constant and the membrane homogeneous

$$\frac{d\varphi}{dx} = \frac{\Delta\varphi}{\delta} \tag{1C}$$

where

$$\Delta\varphi = \varphi\,(m2) - \varphi\,(m1), \tag{2C}$$

and Eqs. 1 yield

$$Q' = \frac{\gamma}{\omega} \left(\frac{1}{\beta}\right) \frac{\delta}{\Delta\varphi} \ \exp\left[-\frac{F}{RT} \ \varphi(m1)\right] \int_{\varphi(ml)}^{\varphi(m2)} \exp\left(\frac{F}{RT}\varphi\right) d\varphi .$$

(3C)

Integration across the membrane produces

$$Q' = \frac{\gamma}{\omega} \ \frac{RT}{F} \ \frac{1}{\beta} \ \frac{\delta}{\Delta\varphi} \ \left[\exp\left(\frac{F}{RT}\Delta\varphi\right) - 1\right] .$$

(4C)

But

$$\Delta\varphi = E - \eta$$

(5C)

where η is the sum of the two phase-boundary potentials. It follows that

$$I = AFP \left[\frac{\frac{F}{RT}(E - \eta)}{\exp\left\{\frac{F}{RT}(E - \eta)\right\} - 1}\right] \left[a(s2) \exp\left(\frac{F}{RT} E\right) - a(s1)\right] ,$$

(6C)

where

$$P \equiv RT \ \frac{\omega}{\gamma} \ \frac{\beta}{\delta} .$$

(7C)

If the phase-boundary potentials are equal but opposite in sign, $\eta = 0$ and

$$I' = \frac{AF^2 \ E}{RT} P \left[\frac{a(s2) \exp\left(\frac{F}{RT} E\right) - a(s1)}{\exp\left(\frac{F}{RT} E\right) - 1}\right] .$$

(8C)

Goldman, Hodgkin, and Katz worked with concentrations instead of activities, and the mobility used in this paper, ω, is related to theirs, u, by

$$u = F\omega ,$$

(9C)

so that Eq. 8C is identical to that derived by them, and P is the Goldman coefficient.

APPENDIX D

The Nernst-Planck equation for current in the channel due to a single cation

$$I = AF \left(\frac{\omega}{\gamma}\right) \left[RT \ \frac{da}{dx} + Fa \ \frac{d\varphi}{dx}\right] ,$$

(1D)

may be integrated to yield

$$I = AF\left(\frac{\overline{\omega}}{\gamma}\right)\frac{RT}{\delta}\left[a(m2) - a(m1) + \frac{F}{RT}(\Delta\varphi)\ \overline{a(m)}\right], \tag{2D}$$

where $\overline{a(m)}$ is an average defined by

$$\overline{a(m)} = \frac{1}{\Delta\varphi}\int_0^{\delta} a\frac{d\varphi}{dx}\ dx \quad, \tag{3D}$$

and

$$\left(\frac{\overline{\omega}}{\gamma}\right) = \delta/[\int_0^{\delta}(\gamma/\omega)dx] \tag{4D}$$

These averages result from the use of the mean value theorem of integral calculus. To be valid, all functions associated with these integrals must be continuous within the membrane, and $d\varphi/dx$ must not change sign although it does not have to be a smooth function. The only test we can make of this procedure is a pragmatic one: It seems to work and to yield physically reasonable results consistent with those obtained by other approaches.

Using Eqs. 2, 6, 2A, and 2D we obtain

$$I = AF\left(\frac{\overline{\omega}}{\gamma}\right)\frac{RT}{\delta}\ \beta\, a(s1)\left[\exp\left\{\frac{F}{RT}(\eta - E_0)\right\} - 1 + \frac{\overline{a(m)}}{a(m1)}\ \frac{F}{RT}(E - \eta)\right] \cdot \tag{5D}$$

Since

$$E_0 = \frac{RT}{F}\ln\frac{a(s1)}{a(s2)} \tag{6D}$$

we can use Eq. 1 to give

$$\frac{1}{Q'} = \left(\frac{\overline{\omega}}{\gamma}\right)\frac{\beta}{\delta}\left[\frac{\exp\left\{\frac{F}{RT}(\eta - E_0)\right\} - 1 \quad + \quad \frac{\overline{a(m)}}{a(m1)}\ \frac{F}{RT}(E - \eta)}{\exp\left\{\frac{F}{RT}(E - E_0)\right\} - 1}\right] \cdot \tag{7D}$$

This can be rewritten in the form

$$\frac{A}{Q'} = A\left(\frac{\overline{\omega}}{\gamma}\right)\frac{\beta}{\delta}\left[1 - f\right] \tag{8D}$$

where

$$f = \frac{\exp\left[\frac{F}{RT}(E - E_0)\right] - \exp\left[\frac{F}{RT}(\eta - E_0)\right] - \frac{\overline{a(m)}}{a(m1)}\frac{F}{RT}(E - \eta)}{\exp\left[\frac{F}{RT}(E - E_0)\right] - 1} \cdot \tag{9D}$$

Note that $E = \eta$, $\Delta\varphi = 0$ (Eq. 5C). Since $d\varphi/dx$ must not change sign, it follows that a constant field exists at this membrane potential.

APPENDIX E

According to Eqs. 5, and provided $A\,(\overline{\omega/\delta}\,)\,(\beta/\delta)$ is not a function of membrane potential, the normalized A/Q' data can be fitted with an equation of the form

$$\left(\frac{A}{Q'}\right)_N = K(1-f), \tag{1E}$$

where the subscript N denotes normalization, K is a constant given by

$$K = \left[A\left(\frac{\overline{\omega}}{\gamma}\right)\frac{\beta}{\delta}\right]_{N, E = \eta} \tag{2E}$$

and f is a function of $E - \eta$ that is zero when $E = \eta$. The advantage in choosing an equation of this form is that its different parts can then, on theoretical grounds, be assigned physical meaning.

At the start, however, η is unknown so that $(A/Q')_N$ must be determined as a function of E, and not of $E - \eta$. An expression of the form

$$\left(\frac{A}{Q'}\right)_N = K'(1-f'), \tag{3E}$$

where f' vanishes when $E = 0$, was chosen for this purpose. Then

$$K' = \left(\frac{A}{Q'}\right)_{N, E = 0} \tag{4E}$$

A choice of

$$f' = \alpha\left[\tanh\left\{\frac{F}{bRT}\,(E-\theta)\right\} - k\right], \tag{5E}$$

where k, α, b, and θ are parameters to be chosen to shape the curve, was found to do nicely.

Since we want f' to vanish when $E = 0$,

$$k = -\tanh\left(\frac{F}{bRT}\,\theta\right). \tag{6E}$$

We require, also, that $(A/Q')_N$ vanish for large, positive E so that

$$\alpha(1-k) = 1, \tag{7E}$$

and

$$\left(\frac{A}{Q'}\right)_N = \alpha K'\left[1 - \tanh\left\{\frac{F}{bRT}\,(E-\theta)\right\}\right] \tag{8E}$$

results, with three parameters to be determined.

It was noted, on empirical grounds, that fit was best if f'/E was chosen to have a maximum at E_0. Three relationships follow from this requirement (Schwartz, unpublished notes). They are that

$$K' = \left(\frac{A}{Q'}\right)_{N, E_0} - m_0 E_0 \tag{9E}$$

where m_0 is the slope of the graph of $(A/Q')_N$ against E, at $E = E_0$; that

$$\frac{F}{bRT} E_0 = \frac{1}{2} \frac{K'}{\left(\dfrac{A}{Q'}\right)_{N, E_0}} \left[1 - \exp\left(-\frac{2F}{bRT} E_0\right)\right] ; \tag{10E}$$

and that

$$\tanh\left(\frac{F}{bRT} \theta\right) = \coth \frac{F}{bRT} E_0 - \frac{\dfrac{F}{bRT} E_0}{\sinh^2\left(\dfrac{F}{bRT} E_0\right)} . \tag{11E}$$

These relationships provide sufficient information for the remaining parameters to be determined. The procedure is as follows.

1. From the known value of E_0, graphically estimate both $(A/Q')_N$ at E_0, and m_0.

2. Calculate K' from Eq. 9E.

3. Solve Eq. 10E numerically for FE_0/bRT.

4. Calculate F/bRT.

5. Determine tanh ($F\theta/bRT$) from Eq. 11E, and calculate θ.

6. Calculate α using Eqs. 6E and 7E.

7. Calculate $(A/Q')_N$ as a function of E using Eq. 8E.

After η is determined from the graphs of $(A/Q')_N$, f can be calculated from the relationship

$$f = \frac{\alpha\left[\tanh\left\{\dfrac{F}{bRT} (E - \theta)\right\} - \tanh\left\{\dfrac{F}{bRT} (\eta - \theta)\right\}\right]}{1 - \alpha\left[\tanh\left\{\dfrac{F}{bRT} \theta\right\} + \tanh\left\{\dfrac{F}{bRT} (\eta - \theta)\right\}\right]} \tag{12E}$$

derived from Eqs. 1E, 3E, and 5E.

The successul fits achieved by this procedure constitute additional, though rather indirect, evidence for A being constant with membrane potential.

Calculations were performed on a digital computer.

REFERENCES

Ascher, P., and Kehoe, J. S. (1975). Amino and amino acid receptors in gastropod neurones. In "Handbook of Psychopharmacology" (Iversen, L. L., Iversen, S., and Snyder, S., eds.). New York: Plenum.

Ascher, P., Kunze, D., and Neild, T. O. (1976). Chloride distributionin Aplysia neurones. J. Physiol. 256:441–464.

Baker, P. F., Hodgkin, A. L., and Shaw, T. I. (1962). Replacement of the axoplasm of giant nerve fibres with artificial solutions. J. Physiol. 164:330–354.

Brismar, T. (1973). Effects of ionic concentration on permeability properties of nodal membrane in myelinated nerve fibres of Xenopus laevis. Potential clamp experiments. Acta Physiol. Scand. 87:474–484.

Chandler, W. K., Hodgkin, A. L., and Meves, H. (1965). The effect of changing the internal solution on sodium inactivation and related phenomena in giant axons. J. Physiol. 180:821–836.

Dionne, V. E., and Stevens, C. F. (1974). Voltage dependence of agonist effectiveness at the frog neuromuscular junction: resolution of a paradox. J. Physiol. 251:245–270.

Dodge, F. A., and Frankenhaeuser, B. (1959). Sodium currents in the myelinated nerve fibre of Xenopus laevis investigated with the voltage clamp technique. J. Physiol. 148:188–200.

Drouin, H., and Neumcke, B. (1974). Specific and unspecific charges at the sodium channels of the nerve membrane. Pflügers Arch. 351:207–229.

Finkelstein, A., and Mauro, A. (1963). Equivalent circuits as related to ionic systems. Biophys. J. 3:215–237.

Gilbert, D. I., and Ehrenstein, G. (1969). Effect of divalent cations on potassium conductance of squid axons: determination of surface charge. Biophys. J. 9:447–463.

Ginsborg, B. L., and Kado, R. T. (1975). Voltage-current relationship of a carbachol-induced potassium ion pathway in Aplysia neurones. J. Physiol. 245:713–725.

Goldman, D. E. (1943). Potential, impedance, and rectification in membranes. J. Gen. Physiol. 27:37–60.

Hille, B. (1975). Ionic selectivity, saturation, and block in sodium channels. A four-barrier model. J. Gen. Physiol. 66:535–560.

Hille, B., Woodhull, A. M., and Shapiro, B. I. (1975). Negative surface charge near sodium channels of nerve: divalent ions, monovalent ions, and pH. Phil. Trans. R. Soc. Lond. B. 270:301–318.

Hodgkin, A. L., and Katz, B. (1949). The effect of sodium ions on the electrical activity of the giant axon of the squid. J. Physiol. 108:37–77.

Jaffe, L. E. (1974). The interpretation of voltage-concentration relations. J. Theoret. Biol. 48:11–18.

Kado, R. T. (1971). Voltage clamp studies of regional specificity on a single neuron. Dissertation. Dept. of Physiol., University of California at Los Angeles.

Kehoe, J. S. (1972a). Ionic mechanisms of a two-component cholinergic inhibition in Aplysia neurones. J. Physiol. 225:85–114.

Kehoe, J. S. (1972b). Three acetylcholine receptors in Aplysia neurones. J. Physiol. 225:115–146.

Kimizuka, H., and Koketsu, K. (1964). Ion transport through cell membrane. J. Theoret. Biol. 6:290–305.

Kirkwood, J. G. (1954). Transport of ions through biological membranes from the standpoint of irreversible thermodynamics. In "Ion Transport Across Membranes" (Clarke, H. T., ed.). New York: Academic Press, pp. 119–127.

Magleby, K. L., and Stevens, C. F. (1972). A quantitative description of end-plate currents. J. Physiol. 223:173–197.

Mozhayeva, G. N., and Naumov, A. P. (1970). effect of surface charge on the steady-state potassium conductance of nodal membrane. Nature. 228:164–165.

Russell, J. M., and Brown, A. M. (1972). Active transport of potassium by the giant neuron of the Aplysia abdominal ganglion. J. Gen. Physiol. 60:519–533.

Schwartz, T. L. (1971a). Direct effects on the membrane potential due to "pumps" that transfer no net charge. Biophys. J. 11:944–960.

Schwartz, T. L. (1971b). The thermodynamic foundations of membrane physiology. In "Biophysics and Physiology of Excitable Membranes" (Adelman, W. J. Jr., ed.). New York: Van Nostrand Reinhold Company, Chap. II, pp. 47–95.

Schwartz, T. L., and Kado, R. T. (1976). Voltage dependence of both conductance and absolute permeability in the absence of constant field in a cholinergic K^+ channel. Biophys. J. 16:24a.

Schwartz, T. L., and Kado, R. T. (1977). Permeability, phase-boundary potential and conductance in a cholinergic channel without constant field. Biophys. J. 18:323–349.

Teorell, T. (1949). Membrane electrophoresis in relation to bioelectrical polarization effects. Arch. Sci. Physiol. 3:205–219.

Ussing, H. H. (1949). The distinction by means of tracers between active transport and diffusion. Acta Physiol. Scand. 19:43–56.

Author Index

317

Subject Index